Fundamentals of

OTOLARYNGOLOGY

A Textbook of Ear, Nose and Throat Diseases

LAWRENCE R. BOIES, M.D.

Clinical Professor of Otolaryngology
Director of Division of Otolaryngology,
University of Minnesota Medical School

And Associates:

CHARLES E. CONNOR, M.D.   CONRAD J. HOLMBERG, M.D.
ANDERSON C. HILDING, M.D.   KENNETH A. PHELPS, M.D.
JEROME A. HILGER, M.D.   ROBERT E. PRIEST, M.D.
JOHN J. HOCHFILZER, M.D.   GEORGE M. TANGEN, M.D.

W. B. SAUNDERS COMPANY
Philadelphia ☆ London ☆ 1950

PREFACE

This book is the outgrowth of a plan for teaching the undergraduate medical student the fundamentals of otolaryngology. As a textbook it is not only designed to offer this basic instruction to the student but also to provide fundamental information to the physician who is not a specialist. It is not intended as a complete reference textbook. Historical data have been omitted. We believe it represents the opinion of today that has a factual basis. The references that appear at the end of the clinical chapters are offered as a guide to the reader whose interest moves him to further inquiry, but no attempt has been made to make these references complete. For the most part, the references cover literature of only recent years except for the occasional reference to some contribution that has been outstanding and the beginning of some new concept or practice.

Our thanks are due to Jean E. Hirsch, Louise Marshall Follett and Virginia Moore of the Medical Art Department of the University for their painstaking efforts in faithfully reproducing our ideas, and to the W. B. Saunders Company for their aid and their many courtesies.

Minneapolis, Minnesota   LAWRENCE R. BOIES

CONTENTS

PART I. THE EAR

PART II. THE NOSE

CONTENTS

Part I

The Ear

CHAPTER I

APPLIED ANATOMY AND PHYSIOLOGY OF THE EAR

The ear, the organ of hearing and equilibrium, is divided into the external, middle and inner ear. The external ear is outside the head, while the middle and inner components are enclosed in the temporal bone inside the head.

THE EXTERNAL EAR

The external ear is composed of the auricle and the external auditory canal. The *auricle* (Fig. 1) is of interest to the physician chiefly because of skin lesions which may involve its surface, injuries which lacerate it or cause hematoma, and abnormal shapes. The abnormal shapes may consist of unusual protrusions of the ear from the side of the head (Fig. 40, p. 59), an abnormal largeness (macrotia), or abnormally small ears (microtia). Occasionally, newborn children are seen with rudimentary ears, conspicuous by the absence of any well-formed auricle.

EXTERNAL AUDITORY CANAL

The external auditory canal (Fig. 2), when its growth is complete, measures about 2.5 to 3.5 cm. (1¼ inches) in length. The outer one-third of the length of the canal is membranocartilaginous. The outer orifice of the external canal is somewhat elliptical, with its greater diameter from above downward. The outer membranocartilaginous one-third runs slightly upward and backward. The direction of the bony canal is downward and forward so that an angle is formed at the junction of this bony canal with the cartilaginous portion. When the canal is examined, it is necessary to pull the auricle slightly upward and backward in order to get a clear view of the length of the canal.

Nerve Supply. The sensory nerve supply to the external auditory canal is derived from two sources: the auricular branch of the vagus (Arnold's nerve) and the auriculotemporal branch of the trigeminal nerve (the mandibular division). The distribution of the sensory branches overlaps to some extent. Lesions involving other portions of the vagus and trigeminal nerve may cause referred pain to the external auditory canal.

The Epidermal Lining. The epidermal lining is a continuation of the epidermis of the auricle. In the outer one-third of the canal (mem-

branocartilaginous portion) are hair follicles and sebaceous and cerumin-
ous glands. The skin is tightly adherent to the perichondrium and, in
the bony portion, to the periosteum. It is because of this fact that small
furuncles developing in the external canal cannot expand in loose connective tissue, which explains the severe discomfort that may be experienced from a furuncle in the external meatus or within the canal.

THE MIDDLE EAR

Tympanic Membrane (Ear Drum). The tympanic membrane (ear
drum), which closes the inner end of the external auditory canal, forms

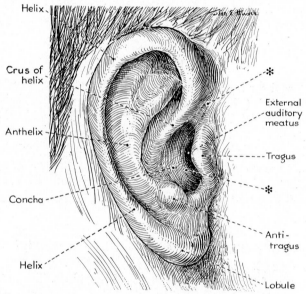

Fig. 1. *The auricle and external auditory meatus.* The names of the external markings
of the auricle are useful to locate lesions accurately when descriptions are made.
The asterisks (*) indicate the sites for the endaural incisions used to expose the
temporal bone for surgical procedures. The upper asterisk indicates the site of a
triangular wedge between the anterior border of the helix and the tragus, which is
relatively free of blood vessels. The lower asterisk indicates the site through which
incision is made through the membranous portion of the posterior wall of the canal
(see Fig. 34).

the *lateral wall* of the middle ear. It is composed of three layers: an outer
layer of epidermis, a middle layer which is fibrous and an inner mucous
layer.

As one views the normal ear drum through the ear speculum, the most
striking mark on it is a nubbin-like projection which is the *short process*
of the *malleus* (Fig. 3). That portion of the ear drum below the level of
this short process is the *tense portion* of the ear drum (pars tensa, membrana tensa, membrana propria) and that part above is the *flaccid portion*

(pars flaccida, membrana flaccida, Shrapnell's membrane). In a slightly oblique direction in a line from the short process is the *handle* of the *malleus*, which is in the middle layer of the ear drum.

The other landmarks on the ear drum are as follows: extending anteriorly and posteriorly at the level of the short process are ligaments which form the *anterior* and *posterior* folds. At the lower tip of the malleus is a slightly prominent rounded area known as the *umbo*. Extending from the umbo and running forward and downward is a triangular segment of shiny ear drum produced by a concentration of light which is reflected

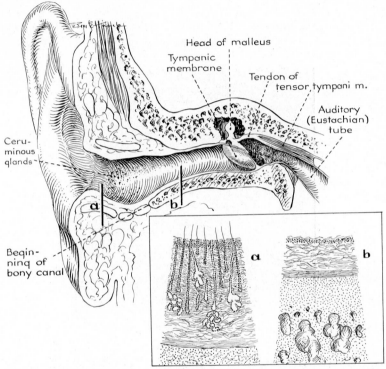

Fig. 2. *The external auditory canal.* The shape, direction and relative dimensions of the external canal are shown.

from the concave surface of the membrane at this point. It is often referred to as the *cone of light*.

The average dimensions of the tympanic membrane, which is almost round, are about 8 mm. in width and 9 mm. in height. It is about 0.1 mm. in thickness.

The pars flaccida (membrana flaccida, Shrapnell's membrane) retracts readily if there is any absorption of air from the middle ear space when the eustachian tube becomes blocked; and it bulges readily when there is any pressure from fluid or inflammatory swelling in the middle ear space. When the ear drum is retracted, the short process of the malleus is prominent; when the ear drum bulges, this landmark becomes obscure.

BOUNDARIES AND CONTENTS

The middle ear space has been described as a wedge-shaped space with six sides. Its measurements from above downward and from behind forward approximate 15 mm. The space is very narrow from side to side, is wider above in the apex and is deeper behind than in front (Fig. 4).

Superior and Inferior Walls. The superior wall, which is part of the floor of the middle cranial fossa, varies a great deal in thickness and may be the site of extension of middle ear infection to the middle cranial fossa above. The inferior wall lies just over the jugular bulb and may

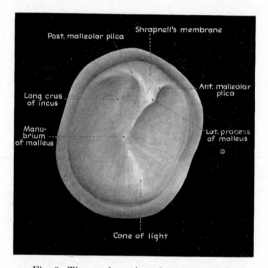

Fig. 3. *The ear drum (membrana tympani).*

be the site of extension of inflammation into the bulb, particularly in infants.

Medial Wall. The medial wall contains the horizontal semicircular canal, the facial canal, the oval and round windows, and the promontory. These structures have been named in order from above downward. The horizontal canal is sometimes eroded in chronic suppurative processes, especially when a cholesteatoma is present. This is also true of the facial canal. The footplate of the stapes fits into the oval window, in which position it is fixed by the annular ligament. The oval window communicates with the perilymphatic space (scala vestibuli) of the vestibule. The round window is a deeper depression, set almost behind a bony prominence in a niche. It faces somewhat posteriorly. This opening is covered with a membrane and connects the middle ear with the scala tympani of the cochlea. The membrane covering the round window is called the *secondary drum membrane*. The medial wall forms the outer, or lateral, wall of the inner ear. The promontory, as the name implies, is a bulge into the middle ear cavity; this bulge is produced by the first turn, or the basilar portion, of the cochlea.

Posterior Wall. The posterior wall is the direct continuation of the posterior wall of the external canal. It contains the facial canal through

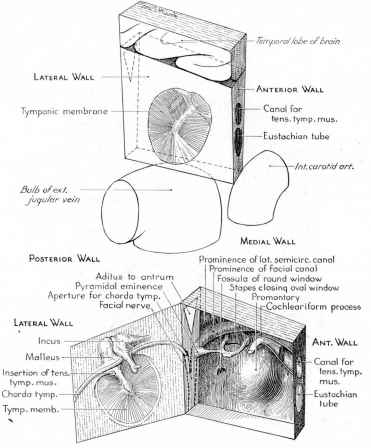

Fig. 4. A diagrammatic scheme of the shape and relationships of the middle ear structures.

which run the facial nerve and artery. This canal contains the descending portion of the facial nerve. The nerve reaches the posterior wall of the tympanic cavity as it passes just above the oval window. Here it turns sharply downward to emerge at the stylomastoid foramen. In this descending portion of the facial nerve are two branches. One is a branch to the stapedius muscle and the other is the chorda tympani nerve. The latter leaves the trunk of the facial nerve a short distance above the stylomastoid foramen and follows a recurrent course upward and through a minute canal in the posterior wall of the tympanic cavity. It crosses the middle ear space (Fig. 5) passing medially to the manubrium of the malleus and exits at the medial end of the petrotympanic (glaserian) fissure and joins the lingual nerve.

Anterior Wall. The anterior wall contains the opening of the *eustachian tube,* a bony canal through which runs the internal carotid artery, and a semicanal containing the tensor tympani muscle. The opening of the eustachian tube connects the tympanic cavity with the pharynx.

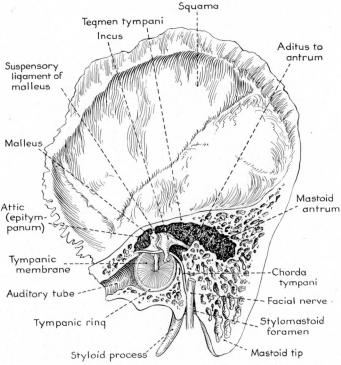

Fig. 5. A drawing (after Fowler) from a section through the mastoid, antrum and middle ear looking from within outward from behind the ear drum.

The total length of the eustachian tube approximates 37 mm. ($1\frac{1}{2}$ inches). Its opening into the middle ear space is in the upper half of the anterior wall.

Muscles. The *tensor tympani* muscle is of considerable size. It arises from the upper surface of the cartilaginous portion of the eustachian tube, the adjacent part of the great wing of the sphenoid and the walls of the semicanal. It ends by a rounded tendon which bends almost at a right angle over a bony, spoonlike projection, the *cochleariform process,* to pass laterally across the tympanic cavity, covered by a mucous membrane, to attach to the handle of the malleus near its neck. The action of this muscle is to draw the handle of the malleus inward, thereby placing the drum membrane under tension. It is innervated by a branch from the motor root of the trigeminal nerve.

The other muscle in the middle ear space, which has already been referred to, is the *stapedius muscle*. This muscle is in the posterior part of the middle ear space just below the *aditus*, which is the opening into the antrum of the mastoid and connects this antrum with the middle ear space. The stapedius muscle arises in a small projection and is attached to the head of the stapes. Its contraction draws the head of the stapes

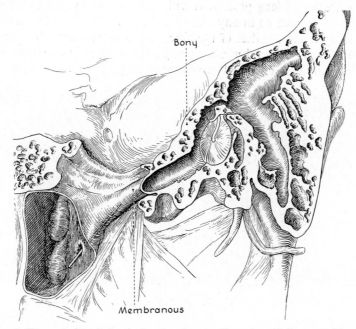

Fig. 6. *The eustachian tube*. A drawing from a dissection of the eustachian tube showing its relationship to the middle ear space on one end and the nasopharynx on the other end.

outward and downward. It is innervated by a branch from the facial nerve.

Eustachian Tube. The portion of the eustachian tube connecting with the middle ear is the osseous portion. From the tympanum, this directs downward, inward and a little forward (Fig. 6). The bony portion forms about one-third of the entire length. The other two-thirds is the cartilaginous portion. The osseous portion is always open, but the cartilaginous portion is closed at its pharyngeal end except during the act of swallowing or yawning, when its lumen is temporarily opened or widened by contraction of the *levator* and the *tensor veli palatini* muscles. The tube is lined in its length by ciliated epithelium which is con-

tinuous with the mucous membrane of the nasopharynx and the middle
ear.

Ossicles. The three ossicles are in a sense suspended in the tympanic
cavity. They form a chain for the conduction of vibrations from the ear
drum to the oval window.

The *malleus* (Fig. 7) has been likened to a hammer because of its shape.
It consists of a head and a neck, the *manubrium* (the hammer handle),
and long and short processes. The manubrium is visible through the
outer layer of the ear drum in a normal ear. The *incus* consists of a body
and a short and long process. It articulates with the malleus laterally,
and has a capsule as in any real articulation. The *stapes* is the medial
ossicle. It is the smallest of the three, but the most important one because it closes the oval window and its vibrations cause movements in
the labyrinthine fluid which are essential to good hearing. It articulates

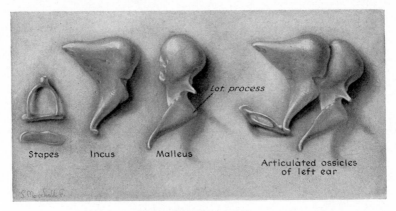

Fig. 7. *The three ossicles.*

with the long process of the incus with a movable joint. Several ligaments support the ossicles in their position within the tympanic cavity.

The ossicular chain acts as a system of levers gaining an advantage in
the force of the impulse transmitted by the stapes to the labyrinthine
fluid of the inner ear.

BLOOD AND NERVE SUPPLY

The blood supply to the middle ear is largely derived from the deeper
auricular branches of the internal maxillary artery. The nerve supply
is through the auriculotemporal branch of the trigeminus, the auricular
branch of the vagus (Arnold's nerve) and the tympanic branch of the
glossopharyngeal (Jacobsen's nerve). The *tympanic plexus* of nerves
passes through grooves over the promonotory. Pain from sources outside of the ear may be referred to the middle ear through the trigeminus,
the glossopharyngeal and the vagus nerves.

DEVELOPMENT OF THE TEMPORAL BONE

At birth, the temporal bone may be separated into three parts: the squamosal, petrosal and tympanic bones (Fig. 8). The petrosal bone encloses the internal ear. It is surmounted by the squamous portion, which forms the covering for the antrum and the attic of the middle ear. A suture line between the petrous and the squamous portions (petro-

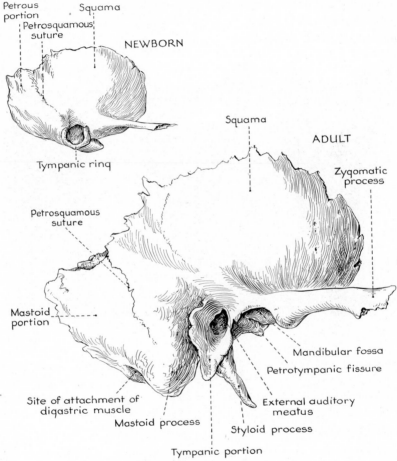

Fig. 8. The temporal bone at birth and in the adult.

squamous suture) passes through the tegmen (roof) and outer wall of the antrum. This line remains open through early infancy and childhood, which accounts in some instances for the early development of postaural swelling and abscess in infancy as a complication of otitis media.

Pneumatization. The temporal bone is pneumatized by the extension of an epithelial sac from the middle ear into the bone marrow in the region of the mastoid process. Pneumatization begins in infancy and is said to be due to an expansion of this sac by air pressure produced through the eustachian tube and middle ear cavity. Any interference with this developnent will cause a cessation of the pneumatizing process and thus cause an interference with pneumatization. The *diploic* type of bone is one that is only partly developed. The *sclerotic* bone is one in which no pneumatization has taken place at all.

The *tympanic portion* of the temporal bone is a small bone shaped like a horseshoe, which attaches to the inferior margin of the squamosal portion. It serves for the attachment of the ear drums.

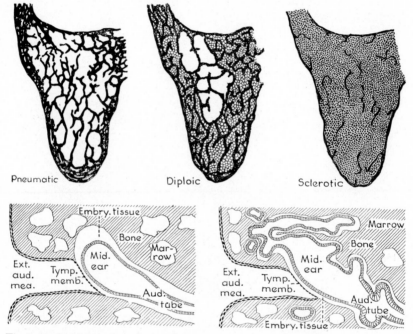

Fig. 9. A schematic representation of the role of the epithelium in pneumatization and the types of mastoid development. (In part, after Fowler.)

Mastoid Process. The mastoid portion is formed by the union of processes of the squamous and petrous portions of the temporal bone. It does not exist at birth but begins its development shortly thereafter. The antrum is at birth formed by the squamosal and petrous portions and later, as the mastoid develops, is considered part of the mastoid process. The entrance into this antrum from the middle ear is through the *aditus* (aditus ad antrum).

The mastoid process is pneumatized by an extension into it of the mucous membrane of the antrum (Fig. 9).

Pneumatization begins in the first year of life and at the end of four to six years the entire mastoid is normally pneumatized. The mastoid tip becomes prominent as the attachment of the sternocleidomastoid muscle increases its pull when the infant begins to hold up his head.

Pneumatization may extend into the petrous portion of the temporal bone even to the tip, and inflammation of these deep cells may complicate middle ear and mastoid infection. Pneumatization may be extensive or slight, or there may be no pneumatic cells at all in the mastoid process. In the latter state, we refer to the mastoid as a sclerotic one.

Sclerosis of Mastoid. A sclerotic mastoid bone occurs under two conditions. The more common condition is due to a lack of development or pneumatization of the mastoid process. The other cause of sclerosis is from inflammatory changes resulting from suppuration of the middle ear and mastoid.

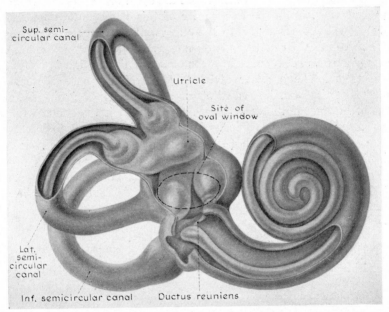

Fig. 10. The osseous and membranous labyrinths. (Redrawn from McHugh.)

Sigmoid Sinus. An important structure coursing through the mastoid structure is the sigmoid sinus. This may become involved in a thrombophlebitic process during the course of a middle ear or mastoid inflammation.

THE INNER EAR

The inner ear is called the labyrinth because of the complexity of its shape. It is completely formed at birth and, in fact, changes little in size as the temporal bone enlarges around it. It consists of two parts (Fig. 10): (1) the osseous labyrinth, a series of cavities within the petrous portion of the temporal bone, and (2) the membraneous labyrinth, which is a series of communicating sacs and ducts within the bony labyrinth.

OSSEOUS LABYRINTH

The osseous labyrinth has three main parts: the vestibule, the bony semicircular canals and the cochlea. The vestibule is the central part of the osseous labyrinth. It is situated just medial to the tympanic cavity of the middle ear. The oval window, into which fits the footplate of the stapes, is in the lateral wall of this vestibule. The three semicircular canals open into the vestibule.

Cochlea. The bony cochlea lies horizontally in front of the vestibule. Its shape resembles a snail shell of two and a half turns. The central conical axis of the cochlea is called the modiolus. The outer wall of the central axis in its spiral two and a half turns forms the inner wall of a canal. A thin shelf of bone called the osseous spiral lamina projects from the modiolus and partially subdivides the canal into two parts throughout its length. From the free border of this lamina, a tough basilar membrane stretches across to the outer wall of the bony cochlea and thus separates the canal into two passages except for a small communicating opening between them at the apex. This opening is called the helicotrema. The cochlear division of the eighth nerve enters the modiolus at its base. This canal of the cochlea at its beginning is about 3 mm. in diameter. It has three openings. One is the round window, or fenestra cochlea, which looks into the cavity of the middle ear but is closed by a membrane (secondary tympanic membrane). Another opening leads into the vestibule. A third, much smaller than the others, opens into a tiny canal leading from the lowest turn of the cochlea through the temporal bone to the subarachnoid cavity at the base of the brain. This canal is called the cochlear aqueduct.

MEMBRANOUS LABYRINTH

This labyrinth lies within the bony labyrinth and has its same general form, but it is considerably smaller than the bony labyrinth and is separated from the walls by the perilymph (Fig. 10). The membranous labyrinth is filled with endolymph, a fluid of higher specific gravity than the perilymph. Within the vestibule, the membranous labyrinth does not form a single chamber but consists of two sacs, the utricle and the saccule. These contain sensory epithelium and are supplied by nerve fibers from the vestibular portion of the eighth cranial nerve.

Ductus Cochlearis

The sensory cells concerned with hearing are contained in the ductus cochlearis, which is a portion of the membranous labyrinth. It is formed as a spiral tube in the bony cochlea and lies along its outer wall on the basilar membrane. This basilar membrane forms the floor of the ductus cochlearis. A second and much more delicate membrane, Reisner's membrane (Fig. 11), forms the roof. It extends diagonally from the osseous spiral lamina to the outer wall of the cochlea some distance above the outer edge of the basilar membrane. The ductus cochlearis is also termed the *scala media*. It ends as a blind sac (*caecum cupulare*) at the helico-

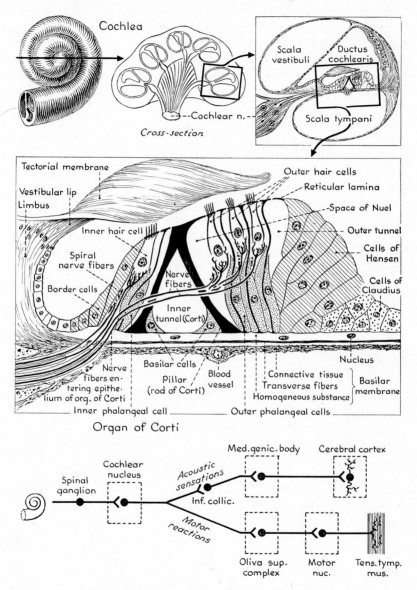

Fig. 11. Structural arrangements within the cochlea, the organ of Corti, and central connections of auditory nerve. (In part, after Rasmussen.)

trema. The portion of the canal of the cochlea above the scala media is the *scala vestibuli;* the portion below the basilar membrane is the *scala tympani.* The basilar membrane is attached to the outer wall of the ductus cochlearis by the spiral ligament, which is formed by greatly thickened periosteum. The under surface of the basilar membrane is covered by a vascular connective tissue. The vas spirale, an artery, runs lengthwise with the basilar membrane.

Blood Supply. The blood supply of the cochlea is from the internal auditory artery, which is a branch of the basilar artery or anterior inferior cerebellar artery, which enters through the internal auditory meatus.

The Organ of Corti. The organ of Corti is an epithelial structure (Fig. 11) which extends the entire length of the ductus cochlearis resting on the basilar membrane. It is divided into an inner and an outer portion by a tunnel which is composed of two rows of rods. These rods, called the inner and outer pillars, or rods of Corti, form a triangle with the basilar membrane between them. The inner rods of Corti are at the site of the attachment of the basilar membrane to the spiral lamina. There is a single row of hair cells on the inner side of these inner rods. These are referred to as the inner hair cells. Their name is derived from the cilia or tiny hairs which project from their upper ends into the endolymph of the ductus cochlearis. They are the most important sensory cells of the organ of hearing. The outer hair cells on the outer side of the outer rods are more numerous. They form three or four rows of small external hair cells. The hair cells are accompanied by supporting cells. The terminal fibers of the auditory nerve end in contact with these hair cells.

A semisolid structure called the *tectorial membrane* is situated above the organ of Corti. It consists of fine, colorless fibers embedded in a transparent matrix. It is attached at its inner end to the superior lip of the osseous lamina near the attachment of Reissner's membrane.

The cross section of the canal of the cochlea becomes smaller as it approaches the apex of the cochlea. However, the change is somewhat irregular. On the other hand, the basilar membrane is narrowest at the end near the round window, attains its maximum width at a point about one-half a turn before the apical end, and then narrows rapidly once more. The tunnel of the organ of Corti also becomes progressively larger. The inner and outer rods and the span of the arch increase. The spiral ligament decreases in size from the base to the apex while the tectorial membrane increases in size. These progressive systematic changes in dimensions form an essential part of the anatomic basis of the theories of hearing.

Innervation. The spiral ganglion of Corti within the modiolus contains an average of 31,000 ganglion cells. Each inner hair cell receives innervation from two nerve fibers; each nerve fiber makes connection with one or two hair cells. The external hair cells have a richer innervation in that a nerve fiber may connect with many hair cells extending over a range of as much as half of a turn, and each hair cell may be connected with several nerve fibers.

The Physiology of Hearing

The phenomenon of hearing is still explained in a large measure on the basis of theoretical considerations which continue to be the subject of research inquiry. Our present knowledge of the physiology of hearing may be summed up as follows:

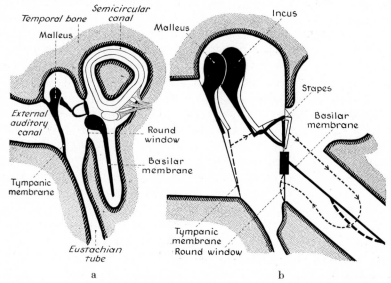

a   b

Fig. 12. a, A schematic diagram of the middle ear and also the vestibule semi-circular canals, and cochlea. The cochlea is here represented as straight although actually it is coiled in the form of a snail-shell of two and one-half turns. (After Bekesy.)

b, "Schematic diagram of the tympanic membrane, the ossicles and the basilar membrane. The solid figures of the ossicles and the solid lines for the tympanic, basilar and the round window membranes show the position of these structures at rest. The open outlines of the ossicles and the broken lines for the membranes show their positions following inward displacement of the tympanic membrane by a sound wave." (From Stevens, S., and Davis, H.: Hearing: Its Psychology and Physiology, New York, John Wiley & Sons.)

1. Sound waves reach the inner ear by three routes. The most important route is by way of the ossicular chain across the middle ear from the tympanic membrane to the oval window. The other routes are (1) directly across the middle ear by means of air waves (instead of by movements of the ossicles) with resultant vibrations of the round window membrane, and (2) by bone transmission when sound energy is taken up by the walls of the external canal and transmitted by bone conduction to the inner ear by way of the bony structure around the middle ear.

The function of the intra-aural muscles is apparently a protective one. By reflex contraction, these muscles diminish the sensitivity of the ear to low tones.

2. Vibrations of the footplate of the stapes produces waves which are transmitted through the fluid of the scala vestibuli to the basilar membrane (Fig. 12), in which corresponding vibrations are set up. There is experimental evidence to show that there is a selective frequency reception on the basilar membrane. Low tones cause vibrations at the apex and high tones near the round window. This forms the basis of discrimination of pitch.

3. The mechanical vibrations of the basilar membrane and the organ of Corti generate electric potentials ("cochlear microphonics"). These correspond in form and frequency to this mechanical activity in the inner ear. It is believed that the hair cells of the organ of Corti generate the cochlear microphonics.

4. Nerve impulses which are set up in the auditory nerve as a result of cochlear microphonics occur in a one-to-one relationship to the incident sound waves, so far as the refractory period of the nerve fibers permits. The maximal frequency in a single nerve fiber is 1000 per second. For higher frequencies, the fibers respond to alternate or to every third or fourth sound wave. Above 4000 per second, the impulses are not synchronized with sound waves.

The particular nerve fibers stimulated apparently determine the pitch, and the number of active nerve fibers determines primarily the loudness. The central connections of the auditory nerve are well established.

The Vestibular Apparatus

The vestibular mechanism serves for the maintenance of equilibrium and the production of vertigo. The end-organs for this function consist of three semicircular canals, a common cistern into which these canals enter—the *utricle*—and the *saccule*. The vestibular apparatus is discussed in detail in Chapter IX.

The semicircular canals are concerned with the movements of the head and represent the *kinetic* (movement) function of the labyrinth. The utricle and saccule interpret changes from the normal and thus constitute the *static* part of the labyrinth (see Chapter IX).

It seems probable that vertigo would result from a stimulation of either the kinetic or static structures of the internal ear.

The nerve fibers from the cristae acusticae of the semicircular canals and the maculae of the utricle and the saccule unite after coming in contact with Scarpa's ganglion in the vestibular nerve, which enters the medulla by way of the internal auditory meatus (Fig. 13). These fibers terminate in one of four ganglionic masses to mark the end of the first neuron: (1) the lateral nucleus (Deiters), (2) the principal, or medial, nucleus (triangularis), (3) the superior nucleus (Bechterew), and (4) the spinal, or descending, nucleus.

The second neuron is more complicated in its course. It involves the following: (1) superior vestibular nuclei send fibers in the medial lon-

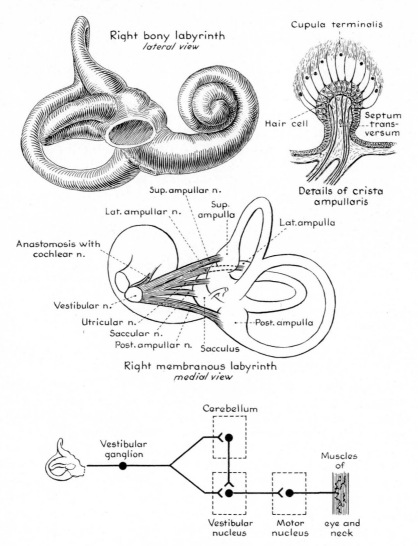

Right bony labyrinth
lateral view

Cupula terminalis

Hair cell

Septum
-trans-
versum

Details of crista
ampullaris

Sup. ampullar n.

Lat. ampullar n.

Sup.
ampulla

Lat. ampulla

Anastomosis with
cochlear n.

Vestibular n.

Utricular n.

Saccular n.

Post. ampullar n.

Post. ampulla

Sacculus

Right membranous labyrinth
medial view

Cerebellum

Vestibular
ganglion

Muscles
of

Vestibular
nucleus

Motor
nucleus

eye and
neck

Central connections of vestibular nerve

Fig. 13. Nerve relationships of the vestibular portion of the labyrinth. (In part, after Rasmussen.)

gitudinal fasciculus of the same side; (2) fibers from the principal, or medial, nucleus and the lateral nucleus extend to the posterior longitudinal bundle (medial longitudinal fasciculus) on the same and, chiefly, on the opposite side, some descending to the motor cells of the cord, some ascending to the level of the oculomotor nuclei and some terminating in the end-nuclei of the posterior longitudinal bundle at the level of the midbrain; (3) fibers from the lateral nucleus to the cerebellum; (4) from the lateral nucleus by way of the uncrossed lateral vestibulospinal tract to the anterior motor-horn cells of the spinal cord; and (5) from the vestibular nuclei of the substantia reticulosa to reach the oculomotor nuclei and the vegetative centers.

The end-organs are mounds of ciliated or hair cells projecting into endolymph channels. This is a bilateral mechanism. No motion of the head, however slight, is possible without causing some fluid disturbance which in turn affects the ciliated cells. Thus the kinetic equilibrium is affected. A forward movement of the body in a linear direction will disturb the cilia and otoliths of the macula in the utricle (static equilibrium); a linear motion of the body sideways produces a disturbance of the cilia and otoliths of the macula in the saccule. A rotary movement of the body or head disturbs the endolymph in one or more of the semicircular canals and the cilia or hairs in the corresponding cristae.

In addition to these effects, the semicircular canals and otolithic structures are in a state of constant tonic activity which exerts an influence upon various portions of the body musculature.

REFERENCES

Batson, O.: Surgical Anatomy of the Temporal Bone. In Kopetzky, S. J.: Surgery of the Ear. New York, Thomas Nelson & Sons, 1947.

Fowler, E. P., Jr.: Medicine of the Ear. New York, Thomas Nelson & Sons, 1947.

Lindsay, J. R.: Petrous Pyramid of Temporal Bone: Pneumatization and Roentgenologic Appearance. Arch. Otolaryng., *31*:231, 1940.

Mellaway, P.: Cochlear Microphonics. *Ibid.*, *39*:203. 1944.

Rasmussen, A. T.: The Principal Nervous Pathways. 3d ed. New York, The Macmillan Co., 1945.

Singleton, J. D.: Pneumatization of the Adult Temporal Bone and the Mastoid Portion. An Anatomic and Clinical Study. Laryngoscope, *54*:324, 1944.

Stevens, S. S., and Davis, H.: Hearing: Its Psychology and Physiology. New York, John Wiley & Sons, 1938.

CHAPTER II

EXAMINATION OF THE EAR

Examination Form. The undergraduate medical student who is to receive his first instruction in otology or the physician in general practice who wishes a guide for the routine examination of his patients who have ear complaints will find the following history and examination form for diseases of the ear a practical one.

This form suggests one or more of the complaints which a majority of patients have when they seek medical aid for symptoms of an ear disease. They represent the important complaints.

In the examination form, the directions offer a guide for a systematic examination of the ear beginning with the external ear, going on to the middle ear, the function of the eustachian tube, the hearing ability of the patient and the status of the vestibular mechanism.

This history and examination form has been in use for the past ten years in the teaching of senior medical students. As the permanent clinical record of the patient, it has proved practical, and, if followed completely, offers a guide to the steps in making an examination of the patient's history in relation to his ear trouble and of the objective part of the actual clinical examination.

HISTORY FORM FOR DISEASES OF THE EAR

Name...................... Sex...... Age.... Date.......... No........

(Circle where indicated. Fill in all blank spaces.)

CHIEF COMPLAINT: 1. Discharge. 2. Hearing impairment. 3. "Head noises" (Tinnitus). 4. Earache. 5. "Dizziness" (Vertigo). 6. ....

1. DISCHARGE

R. or L. ear?........ *Character:* pulsating, serous, mucoid, bloody, purulent, fetid. *Amount:* slight, moderate, profuse. *Duration:*......wks. ....mos. ......yrs. *Nature of onset:* preceded by head cold?.... earache?.... hearing impairment?.... other disease?...... History of previous discharge?........................

....

2. HEARING IMPAIRMENT

R. or L. ear?........ *Duration:* ....wks. ....mos. ....yrs. ......(Age at onset?) Is the impairment a handicap?.... Is the hearing better or worse in the presence of noise?.... Is the onset of hearing impairment associated in the patient's mind with "head colds"?........ "abscess" in the ear?........ injury?..........

21

Indicate whether the patient has had any of the following diseases. Record the date. If there is any known relationship of the defect in hearing to any of these diseases, specify. . . . .

| Measles | Scarlet Fever | Influenza | Arthritis |
| Mumps | Pneumonia | Poliomyelitis | Other diseases: |

Is there any indication that any of the following might be related to the hearing impairment: operations on the ears, nose, or throat?. . . . . .Occupation?. . . . . Medication of mother before or during delivery?. . . . . .Forceps delivery?. . . . . Use of any drugs? . . . . Have any members of the family defective hearing?. . . . .

Indicate to the best of the patient's knowledge the present age (if living), the age of onset, and the cause of hearing defect in the:

Father:. . . . . .Mother:. . . . . .Brothers:. . . . . Sisters:. . . . . .Aunts:. . . . . .Uncles:. . . . . Grandparents:. . . . .

3. "HEAD NOISES" (Tinnitus)

Referred to R. or L. ear?. . . . . . . What is the nature of the noise (a ringing, sound of escaping steam, low hum, etc.)?. . . . . What makes these sensations worse?. . . . . . . Are the sounds continuous?. . . . . . . intermittent?. . . . . . . worse at any time of day?. . . . .

4. EARACHE

Which ear?. . . . . . Duration?. . . . . . Continuous or intermittent?. . . . . Is the patient subject to earaches?. . . . . . In the patient's mind, with what is the onset associated?. . . . .

5. "DIZZINESS" (Vertigo)

Duration of present attack. . . . . . Characteristics of this attack: position of the patient at the onset. . . . . direction of seeming rotation. . . . . direction of fall or tendency to fall. . . . . Did the patient become nauseated?. . . . . vomit?. . . . . perspire?. . . . . If there have been previous attacks, how long has the patient been subject to these experiences. . . . . with what frequency?. . . . .

6. . . . .

Summary of past treatment for any of the symptoms mentioned:. . . . .

THE EXTERNAL EAR

Describe any abnormalities: (evidence of local inflammation, hematoma, "cauliflower" changes, the presence of interstitial deposits, macrotia, microtia, "flop ears," etc.). . . . .

Describe any changes in the zygomatic or postaural areas (evidence of an inflammatory process, cyst formation, glands, scars, etc.)..........................
....

External auditory canal: cerumen..

    furunculosis (describe)..

    generalized external otitis (describe)..

    fungus infection......... exostoses......... congenital malformation.........

THE MIDDLE EAR

Drum membrane (Membrana tympani): dull, thickened, retracted, relaxed, perforation, discharge, fluid level, calcareous deposits. *Perforation:* central, marginal, complete absence. Describe size and present state of perforation (recent, healed, etc.)
............................Is there a promontory "flush" present?........
Discharge: thin, serous, mucoid, mucopurulent, frankly purulent, bloody, pulsating.
Odor: of fresh pus, fetid, characteristic of bone necrosis; evidence of cholesteotoma
............................Mobility of drum membrane..............

THE EUSTACHIAN TUBE

Describe the condition of the eustachian tube as determined by inflation with catheter or Politzer method: open?........ evidence of stenosis? .... congestion?....................:

THE VESTIBULAR MECHANISM

(*Note:* When a detailed study of the vestibular mechanism is indicated, this should be preceded by a complete neurologic examination. A special record is used for this objective study. Record, however, the results of a preliminary study of any case in which the history findings indicate a vestibular dysfunction.)

Nystagmus: horizontal, rotary, oblique; quick component to the right or left?........
    Is it spontaneous or induced?...... Is there a tendency to fall in any definite direction?............ *Romberg Test:*.......... *Fistula Test:*..............

INSTRUMENTS FOR MAKING AN EAR EXAMINATION

Speculum. The first instrument which the otologist employs when he starts to examine an ear is the simple aural speculum which requires reflected light and the use of a head mirror. In modern practice, the head mirror (Fig. 14) is not utilized as much as it seems to have been in the past, particularly by the general physician. For that reason, many physicians find that it is not too satisfactory when it is only occasionally used. Medical students and general practitioners are urged to use it constantly because by this practice they become much more confident in their ability to utilize its reflected light easily and successfully.

The aural speculum (Fig. 15) is supplied in several sizes. It is important to use the largest size which can be employed. When the speculum is inserted, it is often found that the canal has to be cleaned of cerumen, desquamated epithelium and any secretions or accumulations which may obstruct the clear view of the ear drum. In order to insert the speculum adequately and gently, it is usually necessary to grasp the auricle between the thumb and forefinger of the free hand (Fig. 16) and pull it slightly upward and then backward.

External Canal Instruments. The instruments necessary for cleaning the external auditory canal are applicators (Fig. 15), cerumen spoons (Fig. 15) and often an ear syringe (Fig. 17).

Applicators. An applicator for cleaning the external auditory canal should be small and malleable. In many cases, the ordinary wooden

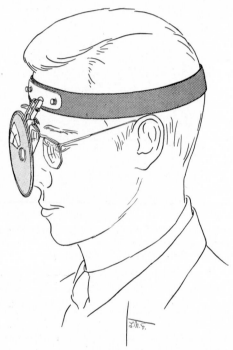

Fig. 14. *Use of the head mirror.* The head mirror becomes useful to the student only after its use is practiced. It may be worn over either eye. Both eyes should be kept open and binocular vision utilized by looking through the central hole with the eye behind the mirror. The mirror most commonly used is one of a focal length of 14 inches.

applicator is too thick. A proper preparation of the applicator is very important. A wisp of cotton should be thinned or flattened out and the applicator twisted in this so as to leave a thin layer of cotton at the tip of the applicator with a protective tuft beyond the point (Fig. 18).

Many patients exhibit a certain amount of apprehension and discomfort when the external canal is wiped with an applicator. The gentle use of the instrument, therefore, is extremely important. The applicator should be used through the aural speculum under direct vision.

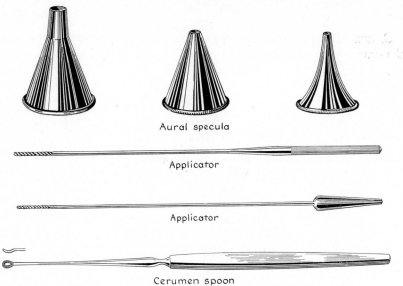

Aural specula

Applicator

Applicator

Cerumen spoon

Fig. 15.

The largest aural speculum which will fit into the external meatus should be employed. Applicators should be thin and malleable. Some physicians prefer to bend the shaft of an applicator at an angle so that the fingers that grasp and manipulate the applicator will be out of the line of vision. The cerumen spoons in several sizes may be obtained with a fenestrated tip in the form of a loop. This tip should be thin, serrated, without sharp edges and bent at a 30 to 45 degree angle.

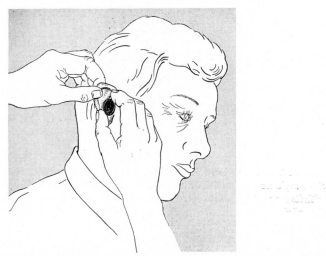

Fig. 16. *Technic of examining the external auditory canal and the ear drum.* The technic of examining the external auditory canal and the ear drum through a speculum is as follows: Grasp the auricle with the thumb and index finger of the free hand and gently pull it backward and slightly upward. The speculum held between the thumb and index finger of the other hand is then inserted gently into the external meatus. As the light from the head mirror is reflected through the speculum, the direction in which the speculum points needs to be altered slightly so as to visualize the margins of the canal and whole of the ear drum.

Cerumen Spoon. Cerumen spoons should not be sharp or pointed and the proper size is necessary for their skilful use.

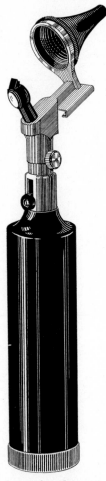

Fig. 17. As a supplement to inspecting the external canal and the ear drum with the simple aural speculum and reflected light, inspection with an electric otoscope with its magnifying lens is often desirable. Also, it is usually preferable in the examination of children, especially under circumstances in which accurate reflection of light might be difficult because of difficulties in maintaining the small patient's auricle in the proper position. When a cleaning of the external canal is necessary, the simple aural speculum is superior for exposure and manipulation. Therefore, it is wise to have both types available.

There are several different models available.

Ear Syringe. The syringe should have a capacity of several ounces and should have tips of several sizes. Usually the small tip is the one to employ. The patient should be properly protected with a towel around his neck and a light, waterproof apron fastened over the towel. A basin is placed below the ear and held snugly against the side of the neck. The physician then grasps the auricle with his free hand and pulls it

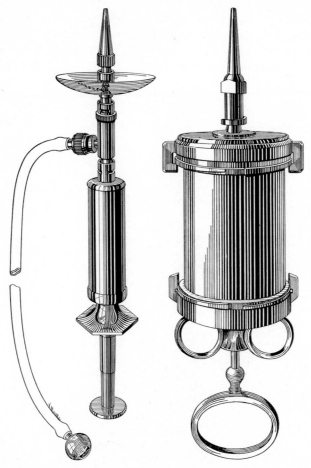

Fig. 18. *Syringes for irrigating the external canal.* A good ear syringe is not an ordinary metal syringe. It should have a mechanically perfect plunger which fits smoothly into a barrel which is solidly constructed so that it will not become easily bent if dropped or bumped. It is well to have a capacity of 6 ounces or more. Most syringes when purchased have tips in several sizes. A small conical tip with a blunt point is most commonly used. It should be of a size which will not fill more than half of the diameter of the canal when it is in the working position. This allows for the ready escape of the fluid and bits of cerumen.

For use with children and in small adult canals, I prefer a special type of syringe made by the Becton-Dickinson Company. This is small and has an "automatic" flow. The fluid is drawn up into the barrel through a tube connecting the barrel with a dish containing the irrigating fluid.

This special syringe is perfectly satisfactory in all adult cases.

slightly upward and backward, and the tip of the syringe is introduced either just within the external meatus along the floor of the canal or superiorly along the roof of the canal (Fig. 19). Gentle use of the stream of water from the syringe will often evacuate the wax very promptly. Occasionally, repeated syringing is necessary. When the cerumen or foreign material has been removed from the canal, it is well to place a cotton wick in the canal for a few moments to absorb the excess moisture.

Otoscope. As a supplement to the ordinary aural speculum through which the external ear and the ear drum are viewed from reflected light

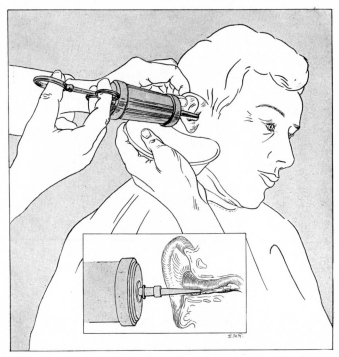

Fig. 19. *The use of the irrigating syringe.* When the external canal is irrigated, it is important to protect the patient with a light waterproof apron which can be snugly fastened over a folded towel around his neck. A basin curved so that it can be easily pressed against the side of the neck just below the auricle receives the irrigating fluid and the material washed out. The irrigating tip is placed just within the meatus and pointed along the floor of the canal.

from the head mirror, the electric otoscope finds a useful place (Fig. 17). I prefer, as a rule, to inspect an ear through the simple speculum and then to supplement this inspection with the electric otoscope, which has a magnifying glass. Certain practitioners, such as the pediatrician, rely on the electric otoscope entirely and rarely use the head mirror either in their office practice or in the home. This is because much of their examining is on small children on whom it might be difficult to adjust lights.

A useful accessory instrument for the examination of the ear drum is provided in an otoscope in which the speculum is closed externally by a magnifying lens. A small rubber bulb and a length of tube are attached to a vent on the side of the speculum. This allows positive and negative pressures within the speculum so that the movements of the drum can be observed. When the speculum is inserted snugly in the external

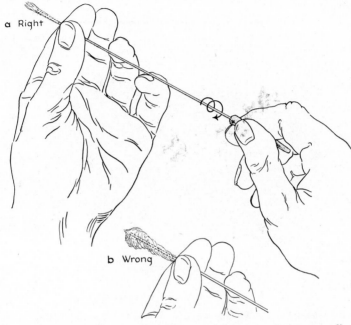

Fig. 20. *Winding a cotton applicator.* The properly wound cotton applicator is important to the efficiency with which one works and the patient's comfort in cleaning out an external auditory canal. It should be madc as follows: A wisp of cotton, small in size and flattened out, is held between the thumb and index finger of the free hand. The tip of the applicator with the point well back of the edge of the cotton is then laid against the wisp. The applicator is then rotated clockwise until the cotton is tightly wonnd on the tip, leaving a "feather duster" end which will scarcely be felt when it is inserted and which is loose enough to take up moister easily (a).

When the piece of cotton used is too large and the end of the applicator is too near the edge of the cotton, a club-shaped mass is obtained which is too large for the canal. Also, it absorbs moister less freely than the "feather duster" tip (b).

auditory canal and light is reflected through its magnifying glass, pressure on the bulb will cause the ear drum to move inward, and release of of this pressure will allow it to return to its previous position. Mobility of the ear drum, the increased mobility of certain portions of the ear drum which have been previously the site of infection, and so on, can be determined with the use of this instrument.

THE TESTING OF HEARING

A large variety of tests have been employed to determine the ability of the patient to hear. A number of these, such as the watch test, the coin click, testing with the acoumeter, and so on, which were once used by the otologists are now considered more or less obsolete. A monochord and calibrated whistles were once used for testing high notes. These are now rarely employed by the average clinical otologist. A description of all of the tests, together with a discussion of their relative values, is

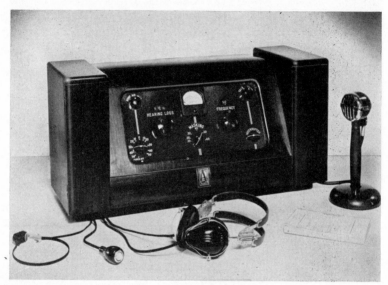

Fig. 21. *The audiometer.* Audiometers are equipped with a push button with a connecting cord for flashing a red light on the panel of the audiometer. This signals the patient's responses. Many otologists prefer to have the patient signal with a raised finger that he hears the sound. It is thought that push button arrangement adds chances of distraction and that the raised finger is the more natural way to signal a response.

not within the purpose of this book. For that reason, only the tests that are commonly employed in the daily practice of the modern otologist will be considered.

These tests utilize the modern electrically operated audiometer and certain tuning forks to test air and bone conduction.

Audiometer. The audiometer has three essential parts: (1) a frequency oscillator, (2) a device for regulating the volume of sound and (3) a receiver (Figs. 21 and 22). Acoustically, it generates approximately pure tones which can be varied in pitch and intensity. The vacuum tube audiometers are widely used and produce a range of the octave and semioctaves from 128 to 11,584 double vibrations, ten tones in all. The same method of testing is used for measuring both air conduction and bone conduction. The instrument has a special bone conduction receiver.

The advantage of the audiometer is that it provides a uniform standard of measurement of hearing loss with tones of greater intensity than those of forks. In addition, a graphic record of hearing is made for future reference. Considerable time is saved by this method of testing. The instrument is, however, both expensive and cumbersome.

The record which is made is known as an audiogram (Fig. 23). The loss is expressed on this audiogram as a loss of sensation units, or *decibels*.

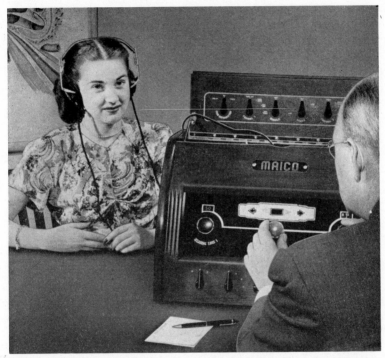

Fig. 22. The audiometer is also equipped with a switch button by which the examiner can interrupt the sound without the patient being aware of this fact.

For obvious reasons, the patient is seated so that he does not observe the panel of the audiometer.

For accuracy, the examiner must be thoroughly familiar with the working of the instrument, procedures which most accurately determine thresholds of hearing for the various frequencies, and so on.

Two well known makes of audiometers are shown.

A simple definition of decibel states that a decibel, or sensation unit, is the smallest difference in intensity of sound appreciated by the normal ear.

Spoken or Whispered Words. Spoken or whispered words provide an important and a useful means for determining hearing acuity. An ideal setup for these tests requires, however, relatively soundproof surroundings and a space large enough so that the examiner can approach the patient slowly from a distance of at least twenty feet. Consideration must, of course, be given to the fact that there is a considerable variation in the ability with which certain words are heard. For instance, the sibilants are of a higher pitch and are more easily heard than some consonants; the word "sixty-six" is more easily heard than the word "twenty-three." Also, there is a variation in the ease with which different voices are heard. In relatively soundproof surroundings, the patient with perfectly normal hearing may hear many spoken words at a distance as great as forty feet and whispered words at thirty feet. However, for practical purposes, ability to hear conversational voice well at twenty feet and whispered voice at fifteen feet is considered to be roughly

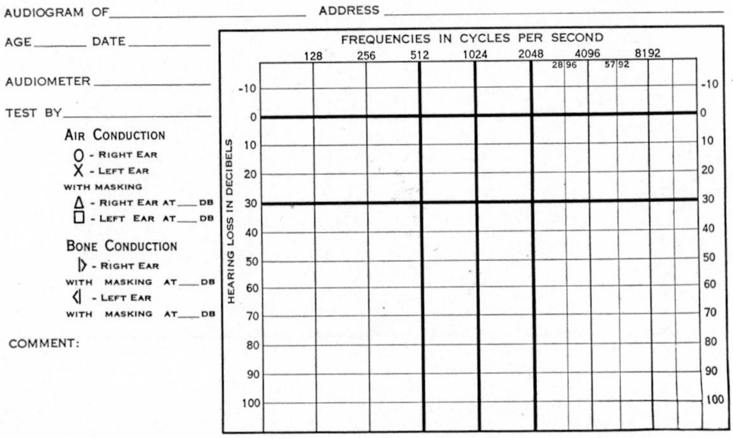
AUDIOGRAM OF
ADDRESS
AGE
DATE
AUDIOMETER
TEST BY
AIR CONDUCTION
O - RIGHT EAR
X - LEFT EAR
WITH MASKING
Δ - RIGHT EAR AT ___ DB
□ - LEFT EAR AT ___ DB
BONE CONDUCTION
|> - RIGHT EAR
WITH MASKING AT ___ DB
<| - LEFT EAR
WITH MASKING AT ___ DB
COMMENT:
FREQUENCIES IN CYCLES PER SECOND
128
256
512
1024
2048
2896
4096
5792
8192
HEARING LOSS IN DECIBELS
-10
0
10
20
30
40
50
60
70
80
90
100

Fig. 23. *The audiogram.* The heavy black vertical lines indicate the most important frequencies for ordinary speech. The most important frequency of these three is the 2048; the 1024 is second in importance.

The heavy black horizontal line at the 30 decibel level indicates the "critical" level relative to speech. When the patient's air conduction curve is above this level through the speech frequencies, he usually has adequate hearing for ordinary social and economic contacts.

normal hearing. It has been customary, therefore, to express the ability to hear normally when the patient is tested by spoken words as 20/20, and whispered words as 15/15.

The patient should be seated so that the ear being tested is faced by the examiner, who starts at a point twenty feet away and slowly approaches the patient. The ear which is not being tested should be occluded by having the patient insert the tip of his index finger into the external canal.

Recently, speech tests using phonetically balanced words and dissyllabic words of the spondee stress pattern have been developed. These tests combined with pure tone audiometric tests are proving valuable for more exact diagnoses of the suitability of a particular case for fenestration surgery, and in the fitting of hearing aids.

Tuning Forks. Tests with tuning forks are used to determine rapidly the lower and upper tone limit within the speech range, A set of five forks of 128 to 2048 double vibrations are a commonly used set (Fig. 24).

Forks are the standard method for differentiating between the two types of impairment, the conduction and perception type. The tests

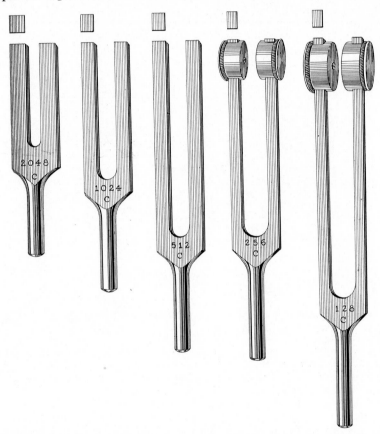

Fig. 24. *Set of tuning forks.* A commonly used set of five forks known as the Hartman set is suitable for ordinary purposes. These are available in a magnesium alloy, are light and are relatively inexpensive.

which are commonly employed are: the Weber test, the Rinne test and the Schwabach test.

Weber Test. The Weber test is used to determine whether monaural impairment is of obstructive or nervous origin by comparing the bone conduction of both ears. A tuning fork of 256 double vibrations is struck a moderate blow and the stem of the fork is placed against the patient's forehead or on top of the head (vertex) (Fig. 25). The patient is asked in which ear he perceives the sound. If he hears the sound in the diseased ear, the bone conduction must be greater in this ear than in the opposite ear, and the impairment is of the conduction type. If he hears the vibrating fork better in the normal ear, the hearing loss in the diseased ear is of the perception type.

Rinne Test. The Rinne test is used to compare the duration of bone conduction with that of air conduction for the ear tested. For this test, a fork of 512 double vibrations, is struck a moderate blow and held

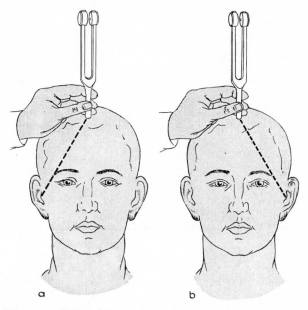

Fig. 25. *Weber test.* This test determines whether monaural impairment is of obstructive or nervous origin by comparing the bone conduction of both ears. A tuning fork of 256 double vibrations is struck a moderate blow and the stem of the fork is placed on the top of the head (vertex). In (a), the right ear is the diseased one. The sound of the vibrating fork is heard in this ear, indicating that the bone conduction must be greater in this than in the opposite ear. Therefore, the impairment must be of the conduction type. In (b), the right ear is also the diseased one but the vibrating fork is heard in the left (normal) ear. Therefore, the impairment in the diseased ear is of the perception type.

by its shank firmly against the mastoid bone of the ear being tested (Fig. 26). When the patient signals that he no longer hears the vibrating fork, note the duration of his bone conduction and immediately move the fork so that the prongs are about one inch away and broadside to the external auditory meatus. When the patient signals that he no longer hears by air the sound of the vibrating fork, note the duration of air conduction. In a normal ear, the fork is heard approximately twice as long by air conduction as by bone conduction $\left(\dfrac{\text{air} \quad 2}{\text{bone} \quad 1}\right)$.

Tuning forks in good condition have a known vibrating period, depending, of course, on the force with which they are set in vibration. A steel fork of 512 d.v. set in motion with a brisk blow may have a ratio of about $\frac{40}{20}$ seconds. Magnesium forks vibrate for a longer period. When the air conduction is greater than the bone conduction, we refer to the result as a "positive Rinne." If there is conduction deafness of a degree sufficient to make the air conduction less than the bone conduction, it is spoken of as a "negative Rinne." If the duration of both air and bone

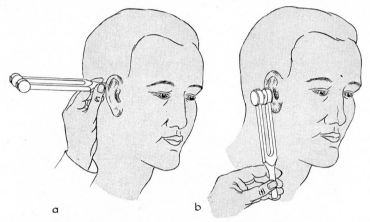

a   b

Fig. 26. *Rinne test.* This test is used to compare the duration of bone conduction with that of air conduction for the ear being tested.

A fork of 512 double vibrations is struck a moderate blow and held by the stem firmly against the mastoid bone (a). When the patient signals that he no longer hears the vibrating fork, the duration of bone conduction is noted and the fork is immediately transferred to position (b) so that the prongs are about one-half inch away from the external auditory meatus. When the patient no longer hears by air the sound of the vibrating fork, note the air conduction.

In a normal ear, the fork is heard approximately twice as long by air conduction as by bone.

A "positive Rinne" = air conduction greater than bone.

A "negative Rinne" = bone conduction greater than air.

conduction are approximately equal, it will usually be found that both have been shortened, but that air conduction has suffered most and that a perception or mixed type of deafness is present.

For a complete evaluation by forks of the patient's air and bone conduction, the Rinne test should be performed with the 512, 1024, and 2048 forks (the speech frequencies).

Schwabach Test. The Schwabach test is used to compare the bone conduction of the person being tested with normal hearing. For this test, forks of 512, 1024, and 2048 double vibrations are struck a moderate blow and the shank of the fork is placed on the mastoid of the patient.

When he no longer hears the tone, the fork is transferred to the examiner's mastoid. If the tone is still heard (assuming the examiner's hearing to be normal), the patient may have a perception deafness. The result is expressed in the plus or minus seconds above or below normal.

TESTS FOR PATENCY OF THE EUSTACHIAN TUBE

In a complete ear examination, it is often necessary to determine the patency of the eustachian tubes. Inflation of the tubes is also frequently important as a matter of therapy.

Patients often learn auto-inflation of their own tubes by what is known as the *Valsalva* procedure. The nostrils are compressed between the thumb and forefinger so as to occlude the nasal passageways. With lips compressed, the patient swallows and can usually sense the passage of air up through his tubes to his middle ear on each side. This act gives him a "fluttering" sensation referred to each ear. Failure of the air to

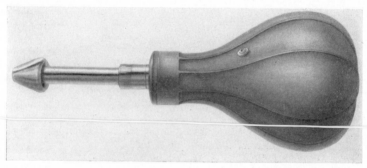

Fig. 27. *Politzer bag.* A specially constructed rubber bag designed by Politzer, an Austrian otologist, is useful for inflating the eustachian tube without catheter by a special procedure (see Fig. 28) and for performing the fistula test (see Fig. 46).

pass up the tube is readily sensed. More positive pressure may be obtained by blowing up the cheeks with air and then swallowing.

Use of Air. The physician uses two methods to test or treat the eustachian tubes: by compressed air or eustachian catheter. The simplest way is to force air through a nostril as the patient swallows water. A Politzer bag equipped with a nasal tip (Fig. 27) is gently inserted in one nostril and the other nostril is occluded by pressure from the physician's finger. As the patient swallows a sip of water, pressure on the Politzer bag forces air into the nasopharynx and eustachian tubes. The physician listening through a rubber tube connecting his ear with one of the patient's can hear the air coming into the middle ear (Fig. 28). Then he examines the ear drums and may detect a bulging in cases of flaccid drums, especially those with old healed-over perforations or bubbles or levels of fluid in cases of serous exudate in the middle ear. This method inflates both tubes at the same time from compression of air through either nostril.

However, the examiner can only listen through his tube to one ear at a time.

Eustachian Catheter. A more exact means of testing or therapy is by the eustachian catheter (Fig. 29). The surface of the nasal mucosa and the area adjacent to the tubal orifice in the nasopharynx is treated lightly with a weak solution of cocaine (1 per cent). The catheter is gently passed with tip down into the nasopharynx and against the posterior pharyngeal wall. When it touches the posterior wall, it is

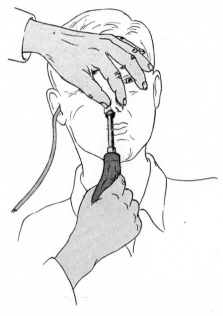

Fig. 28. *The Politzer procedure.* This method of inflating the eustachian tubes is a simple one. The patient is directed to take a tiny sip of water and to retain it in his mouth until he is told to swallow. The tip of the tube connected with the bag is placed in one nostril and the other nostril is occluded by pressure from the side. When the patient swallows, the bag is forcibly compressed and air is forced through the nasal fossa and out through both eustachian tubes. The physician listens through the tube connecting his ear with one of the patient's and hears the passage of air into the patient's middle ear.

gently turned so that the tip is outward and then it is gently drawn forward. The experienced examiner can usually tell as the tip passes over the posterior lip of the eustachian orifice and slips into the mouth of the tube. A Politzer bag attached to a short piece of tubing, the opposite end of which is equipped with an adapter to fit into the outside end of the catheter supplies the air, which is forced through the catheter. The passage is heard through a rubber tube fitted with ear pieces, one of which is inserted into the examiner's ears and one into the patient's ear which is being tested.

Difficulties. There are, of course, some difficulties in a successful performance of this procedure. It is not always easy to get the catheter into the nasopharyngeal orifice of the tube. Trauma should be avoided.

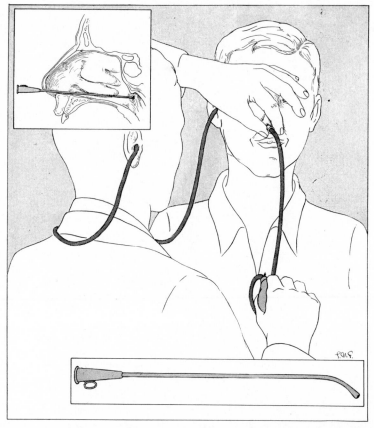

Fig. 29. *The use of the eustachian catheter.* The nasal fossa is usually treated with a 1 per cent solution of cocaine prior to the passage of the catheter. This produces light surface anesthesia and vasoconstriction.

The catheter is then passed gently along the floor of the side being examined or treated until it reaches the posterior wall of the nasopharynx. It is then rotated gently laterally until it is approximately horizontal. Then the catheter is withdrawn slightly and the tip is felt to pass over the posterior margin of the eustachian orifice and slip into the mouth of the tube. It is then rotated slightly upward.

The passage of air is then tested by listening through a rubber tube connecting the physician's ear with the patient's ear being tested.

Catheters are available in several sizes. The curve of the tip needs alteration in curvature for different cases.

Instances are recorded where air has been forced into the soft tissues of the pharyngeal wall with subsequent infection. Anatomical irregularities in the nose or the relationships of the eustachian orifice may prohibit success. Also, in the event a passage of air through the tube cannot be heard, it is not always certain that this is due to tubal stenosis, as there may be some other cause of failure, particularly that of the position of the tip of the catheter.

TESTS FOR VESTIBULAR FUNCTION

In certain patients with the symptom of *vertigo*, it is important to test the reaction of the vestibular function so far as this can be examined through tests on the end-organ. Chapter IX describes these tests in detail. The testing of hearing is, of course, one of the tests which gives information as to the function of the cochlear portion of the end-organ or inner ear. The other test would be to determine the function of the vestibular portion of the end-organ as it functions through the semicircular canal.

Bárany Chair. A special chair was once quite widely used for this. This was known as the Bárány chair. It was constructed so the patient's head could be placed in one of several positions and the chair could be turned rapidly for a certain number of turns in either the right or the left direction. In a normal person, this turning produced vertigo and the effect of the stimulation on the end-organ could be observed in the matter of the patient's nystagmus, his tendency to fall in a definite direction and his past pointing when, with his eyes closed, he attempts to approximate a certain point with his arm outstretched in front of him. These turning tests have limited value in the matter of providing accurate information as to the function of the vestibular system of a particular side, so are not widely used in solving ordinary clinical problems in otology. The tests are useful in determining whether or not there is any vestibular function in a patient who is completely deaf.

CALORIC TESTS

Cold Water. A test which can be easily performed with very simple equipment to determine the functioning of the vestibular system as regards end-organ function is to stimulate the end-organ by the use of cold water. If water at a temperature of 68° F. (20° C.) is allowed to flow against the ear drum, the cold effect of this causes a movement of the fluid within the semicircular canals and produces nystagmus, falling and past pointing in the normal person. An irrigating can which will hold a quart or two of water tested by a thermometer, a few feet of rubber tubing, and a small nozzle, such as may be made from the glass tip of an ordinary medicine dropper for the end of the tube are all the instruments needed for this test. The irrigating can is placed about a foot above the level of the head and the water is allowed to run slowly into the external auditory canal and against the ear drum. It is important, of course, to have an external canal free of cerumen, and such tests are not performed in the presence of infections of the middle ear, either

acute or chronic, or perforations of the ear drum. The patient's head is
in the upright position. The time is noted when the water is first allowed
to flow into the canal. As soon as the patient expresses a sense of
dizziness, or nystagmus is noted, the cold water is discontinued. The
time interval elapsing between the onset and the production of symptoms is noted. The patient's tendency to fall when he is allowed to stand
with his eyes closed is also noted, and his ability to point correctly is
determined. The stimulation in this instance involves the vertical semi-

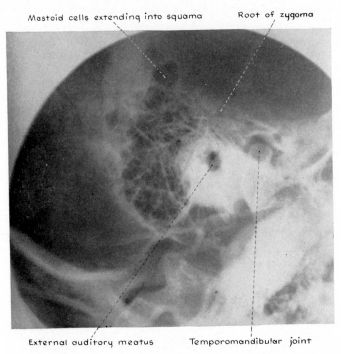

Fig. 30. *Roentgenogram of a normally pneumatized mastoid taken in the Law position.*
This is the most commonly used position for an x-ray study of the temporal bone.
When properly made, the external and internal auditory meatuses superimpose. The
information obtained from this view concerns the degree of pneumatization, the extent
of cell structure in the squama and zygoma, the matter of decalcification, destruction,
sclerosis, etc. Other positions supplement this one to show the degree of pneumatization of the petrosa and define the outlines of the mastoid antrum.

circular canal. If the head is tipped backward, the horizontal canal
assumes a vertical position and is stimulated. Because of its position in
relation to the middle ear space, it is the one which can be most easily
stimulated.

Ice Water and Minimal Stimulation. Another method of performing the caloric test is to use ice water and minimal stimulation. It requires
the injection of a few cubic centimeters of ice water into the external
auditory canal against the ear drum. The test is begun with 5 cc. of ice

water; if no reaction is observed, the amount is increased to 10 cc., then 15 cc., and finally 20 cc. To perform this test with minimal discomfort to the patient, a pair of special glasses with magnifying lenses is worn by the patient so that the very smallest movements of the eyeball in nystagmus can be noted.

Value. The value of these caloric tests for testing vestibular function lies chiefly in the fact that one can determine whether the end-organ functions normally or does not function at all. This information is used to supplement a neurologic examination as well as tests for cochlear function, and will give the otologist a more complete idea as to the

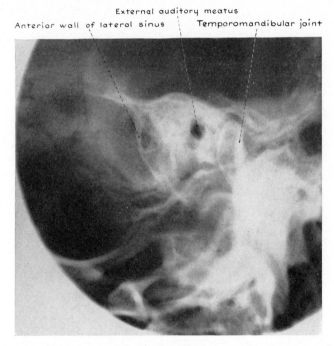

Fig. 31. *An undeveloped mastoid.* This view in the Law position shows an undeveloped mastoid with one small cellular area.

status of the end-organ. Information may also be obtained as to hyper- or hypo-activity of the end-organ, although there are certain variations which are within normal limits; these must be taken into consideration in interpreting the results.

X-RAY STUDIES OF THE TEMPORAL BONE

In those cases in which the otologist is dealing with inflammation within the middle ear space, x-ray studies form an important item of examination. The information to be obtained from these studies may be listed as follows: (1) the type of mastoid development, (2) the extent of pneumatic cell structure and (3) the evidence of decalcification or abscess formations in the acute cases, and sclerotic change and the presence of cholesteatoma in the chronic cases.

The simplest x-ray study which gives a considerable amount of information is taken in the Law position (Figs. 30 and 31). When properly performed, the external and internal auditory meatuses are superimposed. Other positions supplement the information obtained from the Law position and usually are required by the otologist who wants special information about the petrous portion of the temporal bone, the enlargement of the mastoid antrum by cholesteatoma and so on.

CHAPTER III

HEARING LOSS

It has been customary to refer to all persons who have an impairment of the function of hearing as deafened. However, for psychological reasons, there is now a tendency to employ the term "deaf" only in cases of extreme loss, while the term "hearing defect" or "impairment of hearing" is applied to the milder form.

Types of Hearing Loss. Hearing loss is of two general types: a *conduction* type and a *perception* type. There may be an element of both types in a patient and then it is called *mixed*.

Any impairment of the conduction of sound impulses through the external canal, the drum membrane, the middle ear space, and in the transmission of the stimulus through a normal movement of the stapes causes a hearing loss of the conductive type.

Any interference with the perceiving of the impulse (after it has been transmitted into the inner ear) because of injury to the organ of Corti, the cochlear nerve, or the acoustic nerve in its course in the temporal bone or centrally, causes a perception type of hearing loss. This is also known as *nerve* deafness.

Two other types of deafness, not usually classified under the conduction or perception type, are: (1) simulated deafness and (2) congenital deafness.

The simulated type occurs in two forms: (1) hysterical and psychic and (2) malingering.

Congenital deafness of a profound degree is essentially a perception type and may be due to abnormal development of the cochlea or as a result of congenital syphilis, birth injury, or the effect of quinine (taken by the mother) on the unborn child.

CONDUCTION DEAFNESS

A conduction type of hearing impairment may be caused by the following:

1. Obstruction to passage of the sound waves through the external auditory canal. Impacted cerumen, otomycosis, swelling of the canal walls if marked and foreign bodies in the canal are common causes. The impairment is usually not marked in these cases, but it is a definite one.

2. Abnormalities of the tympanic membrane, such as marked thickening, retraction, scarring, or perforation. Usually when there has been a

43

marked change in the tympanic membrane, there is also an abnormal middle ear condition which also is a factor in the hearing impairment.

3. Pathologic change in the middle ear which interferes with the mobility of the ossicular chain. This may be in the form of a fixation of the ossicular joints, adhesive bands from scarring which tend to interfere with the movements of the ossicles, secretions, granulations and so on (Fig. 32).

4. Pathologic change in the capsule of the labyrinth causing a fixation of the stapes in the oval window, a condition known as *clinical otosclerosis*.

The mechanism of the impairment in these first three groups is obvious. The causes of these conditions are understood. The condition mentioned

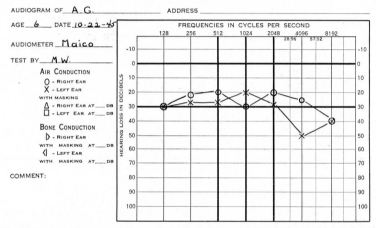

Fig. 32. An audiogram in a case of hearing loss caused by the presence of secretion in the middle ear. The loss had been present for approximately one month. Examination of the ear drums revealed a yellowish tint with moderate retraction of the drum. Inflations of the eustachian tube had produced temporary hearing improvement. Myringotomy was performed and stringy mucoid secretion was aspirated. The hearing promptly improved and was sustained at a low normal level.

in the fourth group and known as *otosclerosis* is of a very different character. It will be discussed later.

PERCEPTION DEAFNESS

Perception (nerve) type of hearing impairment may be caused by:

1. Toxic neuritis of the acoustic branch of the auditory nerve. This may occur in mumps, influenza, diphtheria, diabetes, and so on. Mumps is a common cause of unilateral deafness.

2. Trauma. Blows or falls which produce concussion of the labyrinth, fractures of the base of the skull which, if transverse, may injure the bony and membranous labyrinth, and gunfire, industrial noises and other loud noises are common causes of traumatic deafness (Fig. 33).

3. Certain drugs and poisons. It is now believed that quinine and the salicylates may cause degeneration of the nerve cells of the spiral ganglion. Alcohol is said to cause a degeneration of the hair cells. Tobacco is also toxic to some people. Arsenic, lead and mercury are known to cause hearing impairment.

4. Meningitis. The meningitis of the meningococci type, or that which may complicate influenza, scarlet fever, or measles may cause a loss of function of one or both parts of the internal ear (cochlea and semicircular canal function) by destruction of the nerves, nerve ganglia, or structures of the labyrinth.

5. Senility. There is a physiologic loss of hearing for the high-pitched tones as age advances. This is known as *presbycusis*. It is due to arteriosclerotic and degenerative changes, and consists of an atrophy of the

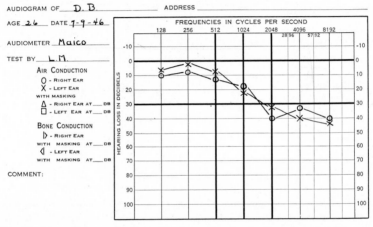

Fig. 33. An audiogram showing the air conduction in the case of a thirty-seven year old foundry worker who had been subjected to the acoustic trauma attendant to the prolonged use of a pneumatic hammer. At first he noted that he suffered some hearing loss while at work but that it would improve after a night or weekend of rest.

ganglion cells, changes in the hair cells and in the blood supply to the acoustic nerve and its connections.

6. Endolymphatic hydrops. An advanced stage of this disorder produces nerve deafness.

7. Miscellaneous causes. A tumor of the eighth nerve or in the cerebellopontile angle may cause progressive unilateral hearing loss; it may be associated with vertigo and tinnitus and disturbances of branches of the trigeminal and facial nerves. Degenerative lesions such as atypical otosclerosis, multiple sclerosis, and so on must also be considered.

THE TREATMENT OF HEARING LOSS

At the present time, there is no known effective therapy for hearing loss due to nerve injury. Our hope lies in prevention. Progress is being made in the prevention and control of the diseases which cause this type of loss (measles, scarlet fever, diphtheria, meningitis and so on) and in understanding the effect of certain drugs and poisons on the function of the acoustic nerve. Hearing loss due to trauma can be prevented.

In the matter of actual therapy, it is only for certain conductive types of loss that active treatment is effective. For the simple types of external canal causes, the remedy is obvious. There will be progress in the prevention of the disorders which affect the middle ear and leave impairment in their wake (such as measles, scarlet fever and respiratory infections) in the form of perforations, scars, adhesions and so on.

Today, the most effective remedial measures are concerned with: (1) nasopharyngeal disorders causing eustachian tube congestion and hearing loss, and (2) the surgical therapy of otosclerosis.

NASOPHARYNGEAL DISORDERS

In recent years, there has been considerable emphasis on the role of lymphoid tissue in the nasopharynx as a cause of eustachian tube congestion and hearing loss. It is definitely established that congestion in the eustachian tube is a common cause of minor losses of hearing in childhood. This is the age in which congestive changes in the nasopharynx are common. Some children apparently have a disposition toward hypertrophy and infection of lymphoid tissue. This disposition seems to exist through the age of adolescence. Regressive changes then set in.

Some children experience a considerable hearing loss due to the effect of hypertrophied or infected nodules of lymphoid tissue adjacent to or within the orifice or lumen of the pharyngeal end of the eustachian tube.

The deleterious effect of this lymphoid tissue on eustachian tube function seems to be controlled by *irradiation* of this lymphoid tissue. This irradiation is relatively simple to accomplish. The effect is largely biologic. Twelve minutes of irradiation with 50 mg. of radium, screened to allow the effects of the more caustic beta rays, disturbs the life cycle of the lymphocytes and prevents their reproduction. The clinical effect is adequate. (Fig. 42.)

OTOSCLEROSIS

Otosclerosis is a common cause of hearing impairment. It is a disease or disorder of the bony wall (capsule) of the labyrinth (Fig. 34). It is a localized osteodystrophy which has some similarity to osteitis fibrosa cystica (Recklinghausen's disease) and osteitis deformans (Paget's disease). It usually becomes manifest (clinical otosclerosis) when the bony disorder has involved the oval window and interfered with the normal movement of the stapes. This produces a conduction deafness (Fig. 35). The hearing impairment usually becomes noticeable at some time between puberty and thirty years of age. Hereditary and familial occurrence are quite common.

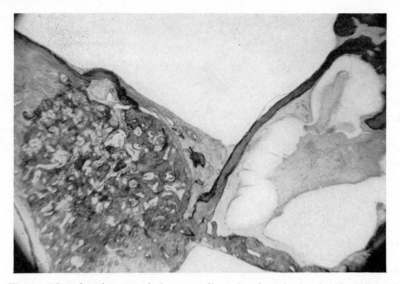

Fig. 34. "Otosclerosis as seen in hematoxylin and eosin stain showing the differentiation between normal and pathological bone. Note ankylosis of the foot plate of the stapes and the flecks of calcium deposited in the scar tissue lying between the crus and the cochlear wall." (Eggston and Wolff: Histopathology of the Ear, Nose, and Throat. Baltimore, Williams and Wilkins Co.)

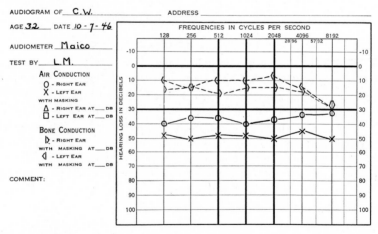

Fig. 35. Audiogram for air and bone of a thirty-year-old woman with a history of familial hearing loss, tinnitus and paracusis. The loss had first been noted eight years previously in one ear and a year later in the second one. It seemed to have become definitely worse after a pregnancy three years ago. The ear drums appeared to be normal. A diagnosis of otosclerosis was made.

Usually both ears are affected, though not to the same degree. The onset is often insidious. Most people with otosclerosis suffer from tinnitus. In mild cases of clinical otosclerosis, it may be the tinnitus which troubles the patient most.

3

The disorder is more common in women than in men. In some women, pregnancy may be a precipitating factor.

Usually the ear drum is normal or may appear to be somewhat thin. In some cases, a redness may be seen through the drum. It is thought to represent the vascularization of an otosclerotic focus on the inner wall of the middle ear. This is known as Schwartze's sign, and has also been referred to as a "promontory flush."

Knowledge regarding the presence of otosclerotic lesions without clinical manifestations in humans has been increased through the work of Guild, who has examined the temporal bones from 1161 routine autopsies. Some aspects of his findings have been summarized as follows:

The incidence in children under five years of age was less than 0.6 per cent.

In persons over five years of age, it was approximately 4 per cent.

Only one-half of those with otosclerosis showed active lesions, with the incidence of activity greatest under twenty and least over sixty years of age.

The approximate rate of incidence in white males was one in fifteen; in Negro males, one in eighty-seven; in white females, one in eight; in Negro females, one in 135. (The 4 per cent incidence in persons over five years of age would be higher if the sex and racial proportions of those coming to autopsy had been similar to the proportions in the general population.)

The cause of otosclerosis is not known, although a great deal of time and thought has been spent in a study of the disease.

Treatment

Medical. No medical therapy has ever proved effective in staying the progress of this disorder, although reports have appeared from time to time supporting the use of some particular medication.

Surgical. Surgical therapy for otosclerosis is not new. Several European otologists (Passow, Bárány, Jenkins, Holmgren, Sourdille) have tried to open and maintain an opening in the bony capsule of the labyrinth which would allow sound waves to by-pass the stapes fixed in the oval window and reach the membranous labyrinth directly. Some success was achieved in a temporary improvement in hearing, but the great obstacle to the success of the fenestration operation was the tendency of the fistula to close because of the formation of new bone. The most successful of these procedures was done in more than one stage.

Lempert's Technic. In 1938, Lempert reported a technic which involved an exposure and exenteration of the mastoid through endaural incisions. The fenestra was made through the most accessible portion of the horizontal canal. Later, he discovered that there is less tendency to bony closure if this fistula is made farther forward through the ampullated end of the horizontal canal. A flap of thin canal wall continuous with the thin membrana flaccida (Shrapnell's membrane) is stretched up over the fenestra to form its covering. The removal of the incus and the excision of the head of the malleus was found to provide better exposure of the site for the fenestra and to allow a better placement of the membrane over the fenestra.

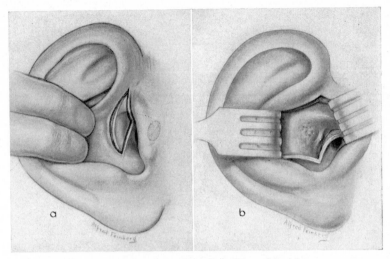

Fig. 36. Surgery of otosclerosis. a, Lines of endaural incision.

b, Exposure of the cortex through the endaural approach. (Courtesy of Dr. Julius Lempert. From: Jackson and Jackson: Diseases of the Nose, Throat and Ear.)

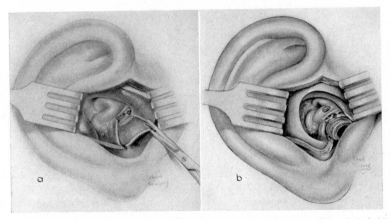

Fig. 37. *Surgery of otosclerosis*. a, The exenteration of the mastoid and definition of the lateral horizontal semicircular canal, removal of the incus, amputation of the head of the malleus, and construction of the plastic flap.

b, Completion of the fenestra. (Courtesy of Dr. Julius Lempert. From: Jackson and Jackson: Diseases of the Nose, Throat and Ear.)

Lempert's technic involves the use of a motor-driven dental polishing burr to make the fenestra. The exenteration of the mastoid and the skeletonization of the semicircular canals is accomplished with curettes and burrs (Figs. 36, 37, 38).

Much of the success of the operation depends upon painstaking technic, a clean, thin, intact flap, a well-made fistula, no bone dust or blood in the perilymphatic space, a minimum amount of reaction in the flap from trauma and so on. As experience has accumulated, some new refinements in technic have been added by otologists who had their original training with Lempert.

Evaluation of Treatment. In the present state of our knowledge, it can be said that:

1. A patient with clinical otosclerosis with good bone conduction through the speech frequencies has a good chance of obtaining a recovery of permanent practical hearing.

2. There is a slight risk that a further impairment of the hearing may occur in the operated ear, owing to the immediate effect of trauma to

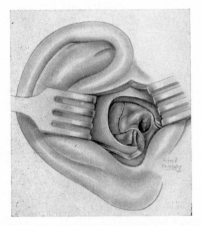

Fig. 38. Surgery of otosclerosis: the plastic flap in position over the fenestra. (Courtesy of Dr. Julius Lempert. From: Jackson and Jackson: Diseases of the Nose, Throat and Ear.)

the membranous labyrinth at the time of surgery or as a result of a condition of serous labyrinthitis developing in the immediate postoperative period.

3. A certain percentage of fenestra tend to close postoperatively. (The percentage has been variously estimated by several workers in this field; it probably approximates 15 to 20 per cent.) With improvements in technic, this percentage is being reduced. If there has been a good improvement in hearing which is gradually lost again within six months or a year and in some cases within the second postoperative year, this invariably means a bony closure. A relatively simple procedure consisting of an elevation of the flap and a removal of the lid of new bone will restore the hearing to its previous level in some cases.

REFERENCES

Boies, L. R.: Irradiation of Nasopharyngeal Lymphoid Tissue. An Evaluation. Arch. Otolaryng., *44*:129, 1946.

Cantor, J. J.: Rupture of Tympanic Membrane Due to Blast. Ann. Otol., Rhin. & Laryng., *54*:554, 1945.

Craig, D.: Blast Injuries of the Ear. J. Laryng. & Otol., *59*:443, 1944.

Crowe, S. J., Guild, S. R., Langer, E., Loch, W. E., and Robbins, M. H.: Impaired Hearing in School Children. Laryngoscope, *52*:790, 1942.

Crowe, S. J., and Baylor, J. W.: The Prevention of Deafness. J.A.M.A., *112*:585, 1939.

Davis, H., et al.: Temporary Deafness Following Exposure to Loud Tones and Noise. Laryngoscope, *56*:9, 1946.

Day, K.: Appraisal of Fenestration Operation: Report of 100 Cases. Arch. Otolaryng., *44*:547, 1946.

Decker, R. M.: Relation of Eustachian Tube to Chronic Progressive Deafness. *Ibid.*, *36*:926, 1942.

Emerson, E. B., Jr., Dowdy, A. H., and Heatly, C. A.: Use of Radium in Treatment of Deafness by Irradiation. *Ibid.*, *35*:845, 1942.

Farrior, J. B., and Richardson, G. A.: Nasopharyngeal Applicator. *Ibid.*, *35*:811, 1942.

Fisher, G. E.: Recognition and Radium Treatment of Infected and Hypertrophied Lymphoid Tissue in the Nasopharynx. *Ibid.*, *37*:434, 1943.

Fowler, E. P., Jr.: Causes of Deafness in Flyers. *Ibid.*, *42*:21, 1945.

Fowler, E. P., Jr.: Non-Surgical Treatment of Deafness. Laryngoscope, *52*:204, 1942.

Fricke, R. E., and Pastore, P. N.: The Radium Treatment of Granular or Hypert ophied Lateral Pharyngeal Bands. Proc. Staff Meet., Mayo Clin., *18*:307, 1943.

Guild, S. R., Polvogt, L. M., Sanstead, H. R., Lock, W. E., Langer, E., Robbins, M. H., and Parr, W. A.: Impaired Hearing in School Children. Laryngoscope, *50*:731, 1940.

Hall, I. S.: Fenestration Operation for Otosclerosis. Brit. M. J., *2*:647, 1946.

Hill, F. T.: Problems of Diagnosis in the Obstruction of the Eustachian Tube. Ann. Otol., Rhin. & Laryng., *57*:324, 1948.

House, H.: Fenestration Operation: Survey of 500 Cases. *Ibid.*, *57*:41, 1948.

Jones, E. H.: Irradiation of the Nasopharynx in Office Practice. Arch. Otolaryng., *37*:436, 1943.

Juers, A. L., and Shambaugh, G. E., Jr.: Indications for and End Results of Fenestration Surgery. Ann. Otol., Rhin. & Laryng., *57*:397, 1948.

Lempert, J.: Lempert Fenestra Nov-ovalis Operation for Restoration of Serviceable Unaided Hearing in Patients with Clinical Otosclerosis. Present Evolutionary Status. Arch. Otolaryng., *46*:478, 1947.

Lindsay, J. R.: Fenestration Operation: Observations on Evaluation of Hearing Tests. Laryngoscope, *57*:367, 1947.

Loch, W. E.: The Effect on Hearing of Experimental Occlusion of the Eustachian Tube in Man. Ann. Otol., Rhin. & Laryng., *51*:396, 1942.

Lurie, M., Davis, H., and Hawkins, J.: Acoustic Trauma of Organ of Corti in Guinea Pig. Laryngoscope, *54*:375, 1944.

MacLaren, W. R., and Chaney, A. L.: Evaluation of Some Factors in Development of Occupational Deafness. Indust. Med., *16*:109, 1947.

Martin, N.: Psychogenic Deafness. Ann. Otol., Rhin. & Laryng., *55*:81, 1946.

McCoy, D.: Industrial Noise Hazard. Arch. Otolaryng., *39*:327, 1944.

Moorhead, R. L.: Fenestration for Otosclerosis: Report of 123 Cases. *Ibid.*, *45*:49, 1947.

Polvogt, L. M., and Babb, D. C.: Histologic Studies of the Eustachian Tube of Individuals with Good Hearing. Laryngoscope, *50*:671, 1940.

Popper, O.: Fenestration of the Labyrinth: Transtympanic Route. J. Laryng. & Otol., *61*:24, 1946.

Ruedi, L., and Furrer, W.: Acoustic Trauma: Origin and Prevention. Schweiz med. Wchnschr., *76*:843, 1946.

Semenov, H.: Some Observations on the Histopathology of Inflammation in the Eustachian Tube and Middle Ear. Tr. Am. Laryng., Rhin. & Otol. Soc., *42*:563, 1936.

Shambaugh, G. E., Jr., and Juers, A. L.: Surgical Treatment of Otosclerosis: Preliminary Report on Improved Fenestration Technic. Arch. Otolaryng., *43*:549, 1946.

Shilling, C. W., Haines, H. L., Harris, J. D., and Kelley, W. J.: Prevention and Treatment of Aerotitis Media. U. S. Nav. M. Bull., *46*:1529, 1946.

Stewart, J. V., and Barrow, D. W.: Concussion Deafness. Arch. Otolaryng., *44*:274, 1946.

Sullivan, J.: Indication for and End Results of Fenestration Operation. Canad. M.A.J., *53*:543, 1945.

Taylor, H. M.: Deafness from Drugs and Chemical Poisons. In: Fowler, E. P., Jr.: Medicine of the Ear. New York, Thomas Nelson & Sons, 1947.

Wolff, D.: Microscopic Observations of the Eustachian Tube. Ann. Otol., Rhin. & Laryng., *40*:1055, 1931.

CHAPTER IV

DISEASES OF THE EXTERNAL EAR AND EXTERNAL AUDITORY CANAL

A majority of the diseases of the external ear and auditory canal are within the special province of the dermatologist as much as of the otologist. However, because of their association with a special part with more or less relationship to the function of that part, these conditions are often encountered first hand by the practicing otologist. If he is equipped with a basic knowledge of the pathology involved and some experience in the management of the disease, his familiarity with the diagnosis of possibly associated diseases, such as might be present in the middle ear in some conditions involving the deeper parts of the external canal, places him in a position of advantage to care for certain of these conditions.

A practically complete list of the diseases of external ear and auditory canal encountered by the otologist would include the following in an approximate order of their frequency:

1. Excessive accumulation of cerumen in the external auditory canal.
2. Furuncle in the external canal.
3. Fungous infections in the canal.
4. Eczematous dermatitis.
5. Diffuse dermatitis of the canal.
6. Intertrigo and fissures related to the auricle.
7. Perichondritis.
8. Hematoma of the auricle.
9. Eruptions such as impetigo, erysipelas, herpes zoster oticus and so on, more commonly observed involving the auricle, and hemorrhagic eruptions involving the tympanic membrane and adjacent meatal wall.
10. Malformations, usually congenital, of the auricle. Imperforate external canal. Stenosis.
11. New growths in the external canal.

EXCESSIVE CERUMEN

This is not a disease. Some people produce an unusual amount of it, just as some persons perspire profusely. In some, the cerumen tends to cake and form a solid plug; in others, a large amount of a buttery consistency blocks the canal. The disorder is one of a sense of blockage, sometimes pressure and in some people, a conduction impairment of

53

hearing. When the solid form of plug becomes moistened, as from bath-
ing, the distress may become acute. Excessive cerumen is, in most cases,
best removed by syringing with the proper equipment (Figs. 17–18).
The opposite extreme, which is rather common, is an absence of cerumen.
This is unfortunate in some cases, since it predisposes to a dryness often
accompanied by a sense of scaling and itching, for which the victim
scratches with his fingernail or with sharp objects and inflicts a surface
abrasion.

FURUNCULOSIS (OTITIS EXTERNA CIRCUMSCRIPTA)

This is a common condition which is confined to the fibrocartilaginous
portion of the external auditory meatus. It begins in a pilosebaceous
follicle and is usually caused by *Micrococcus pyogenes* (*Staphylococcus
aureus* or *albus*) (Fig. 39).

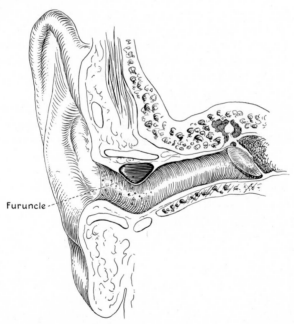

Fig. 39. A furuncle in the external auditory canal may be extremely painful because
it develops in a membranocartilaginous area where there is little room for expansion.
Invariably this cause of pain in the area of the ear is suspected when passive movements of the auricle cause discomfort.

Symptoms. The first symptom is one of acute tenderness localized
within the meatus. Passive movements of the auricle cause pain. Discomfort may be felt on movements of the temporomandibular joint in
chewing, or in the jaw movements while talking. The factor of tension
accounts for the extreme discomfort often experienced by victims of this
type of infection. There is little expansile tissue in the area involved. The
amount of discomfort suffered by the victim of this small infection may

be extreme. Often the infection slowly localizes and then extends so that more than one furuncle may be present. In some cases, the canal wall may become almost completely occluded, owing to swelling. Postaural swelling may simulate a postaural abscess from acute mastoiditis, making differential diagnosis somewhat difficult.

Treatment. Treatment depends upon the stage of the disease in which it is instituted. When the treatment is started early, the infection may be aborted. This can be accomplished in some cases with therapeutic doses of *penicillin*. When swelling is marked, some abscess formation has usually taken place, which usually must localize and be drained. Relief is needed from the extreme sensitiveness of the canal and the pain. In some cases, *incision* under gas anesthesia is indicated. In others, the local application of *meta-cresylacetate* (cresatin) on a wick inserted into the canal brings relief. (See page 413.)

FUNGOUS INFECTIONS (OTOMYCOSIS, OTITIS EXTERNA MYCOTICA)

Several fungi are found as a cause of inflammatory reaction in the external auditory canal or sometimes without meatal reaction and only blocking the canal. The two common fungi are the pityrosporum and several varieties of the aspergillus (niger, flavus and so on).

The pityrosporum organism may only cause a superficial scaling similar to dandruff of the scalp, it may be associated with an inflammatory seborrheic dermatitis, or it may form a basis in which more uncomfortable infections develop, such as furuncles or eczematous changes. The same is true of the aspergillus organism. It is sometimes found in the canal in the absence of any symptoms except a sense of blockage of the canal, or an inflammatory process invading the epithelium of the canal or drum membrane may cause acute symptoms.

Treatment. Treatment consists in gently *cleansing the canal* by wiping and by irrigation when necessary. A 2 per cent solution of *salicylic acid in alcohol* is practically specific for the average case. The fluid should be warmed to body temperature, and one-half a dropperful is then instilled into the canal, allowed to remain in place for about five minutes and then allowed to run out. This process should be performed twice daily for several days.

If eczematous changes have developed, treatment appropriate to this is indicated and likewise in the case of furunculosis.

During World War II, American physicians developed a considerable experience with these disorders, through the higher incidence of fungous infections in the tropics. New medications have had a trial and are now appearing in our literature.

ECZEMATOUS DERMATITIS

Apparently the dermatologists have differed in what should be considered a correct usage of the term "eczema," and in the past have included many dermatoses under this term. With increasing knowledge, a number of entities have been removed from this group. There is even a tendency to drop the term "eczema" and substitute the word "dermatitis."

The practicing otologist not infrequently encounters a lesion in the external canal and adjacent portions of the meatus and concha which is characterized by redness, itching, swelling and a stage of watery exudation followed by crusting. On removal of the epithelium, exudate, or crusts, a raw, bleeding surface is exposed. Perhaps it is correct to regard these lesions as bacterial in origin and the skin reaction as an eczematous type of change brought on through sensitization of the skin tissue cells to the causative microorganism or its antigen.

The diagnosis of this eczematous dermatitis is rather easy because of the characteristic appearance of the lesion.

Chronic Stage. If the acute stage is not controlled, chronic changes characterized by thickening of the skin and even stenosis of the external canal may develop. This chronic stage may be troublesome because of periods of uncomfortable itching with a tendency on the part of the victim to resort to scratching and further irritation.

Treatment. *General. Sulfathiazole* or *sulfadiazine cream* in 5 or 10 per cent strength, and *penicillin ointment*, 1000 units per gram, may be used effectively. Three types of *wet dressings* are as follows:

1. Penicillin, 1000 units per cubic centimeter in sterile isotonic saline solution

	Gm. or cc.
2. Aluminum subacetate	60
Distilled water	120
3. Boric acid	2
Distilled water	90
Alcohol, 70 per cent	90

Acute Stage. In the acute stage, washing of the involved area, particularly with soap, should be avoided. If crusts or secretions need removal, an applicator dipped in *olive* or *mineral oil* should be used. In the average case, protection with a *bland ointment* is adequate to effect a cure. The following ointments meet this requirement:

1.	Gm.	2.	Gm.
Naftalan	10	Crude coal tar	2
Zinc oxide	5	Zinc oxide	2
Starch	5	Starch	16
		Petrolatum	16

Chronic Stage. In the chronic stage, the lesion usually involves a portion of the auricle and may even have extended beyond the auricle. Scales or crusts are often present and need removal after softening with an *emollient ointment.* The surface of the lesion, particularly in the canal, may need cleansing with *warm boric acid irrigations,* after which it is well to dry the surface with *95 per cent alcohol.* Then a protective ointment with the ingredients mentioned previously is applied. In some cases, a more stimulating ointment is needed. The addition of *2 per cent salicylic acid* to the ingredients of the ointments mentioned previously is often adequate.

X-ray therapy has been successfully used on limited areas of chronic eczematous dermatitis.

DIFFUSE DERMATITIS OF THE EXTERNAL CANAL

A diffuse inflammatory process—a cellulitis—occasionally is seen in which the signs and symptoms resemble furunculosis but in which there is no limited localization as with a furuncle. The causative organism is usually a streptococcus or *Pseudomonas aeruginosa (Bacillus pyocyaneus)* and, rarely, other organisms.

Treatment. Treatment consists of the *control of pain* and the *local application of heat.* A solution of *penicillin,* 1000 units per cubic centimeter in isotonic saline applied topically, may be beneficial. Occasionally *incision through the canal wall* for drainage is indicated.

meta-Cresylacetate (cresatin) promptly relieves pain. A wick should be saturated with the medication and inserted into the canal. The patient should be supplied with about a dram of the medication and instructed to instill 4 or 5 drops of the medication against the wick every four to eight hours. The wick is left in place for forty-eight hours.

INTERTRIGO AND FISSURES

Intertrigo is an erythematous inflammation which results from two adjacent skin parts rubbing together. Fissures occur in the depth between two adjacent surfaces where the skin changes are usually superficial at first and then increase from irritation. Intertrigo is most common in the postauricular fold; fissures are also found there, beneath the lobe of the ear and in angles in the meatal orifices.

Treatment. Simple treatment is usually effective. A satisfactory *bland ointment* is made as follows:

	Gm.
Tincture benzoin compound	1.25
Zinc oxide	1.75
Petrolatum	8.00

In extreme cases, it may be necessary to keep contacting parts separated by a dressing.

PERICHONDRITIS

This condition develops from trauma or inflammation causing an effusion of serum or pus between the layer of perichondrium and the cartilage of the external ear. In most cases of trauma, the injury is in the form of a laceration or is surgical trauma incident to some operation on the ear. Occasionally, it follows simple bruising without hematoma. An inadequately treated furuncle provides a ready source for a potent causative agent. Usually the organism is a virulent type of micrococcus (staphylococcus), streptococcus, or *Pseudomonas aerugenosa* (*Bacillus pyocyaneus*). The diagnosis is simple; the involved part of the auricle swells, is reddened and warm and tender upon palpation.

Treatment. In early cases, *hot packs* may be all that is necessary to effect a cure. In more advanced cases, the parenteral use of *penicillin* is indicated. If the condition seems to be spreading and there is evidence of fluid under the perichondrium, *incision* for the evacuation of fluid is indicated. Cartilage stands infection poorly. Necrotic cartilage, therefore, should be *incised* and *drainage maintained.* Gross permanent deformity of an auricle has resulted from perichondritis.

HEMATOMA OF THE AURICLE

This condition usually develops from trauma, such as bruising or blows in athletic contact. Small hematomas may be disregarded. If large, they should be *aspirated* under aseptic conditions. The lesion often tends to refill, and repeated aspiration on separate days may be indicated.

ERUPTIONS

Impetigo. When impetigo occurs on the auricle, it is often associated with an inflammation of the external canal. It is often a mixed infection, micrococcal (staphylococcal) and streptococcal. The primary lesion begins as a red spot which becomes papular, vesicular and then a pustule of thin clear pus. When it drains, the exudate dries into a small, yellow crust which when removed reveals an exudative surface. The spread is by auto-inoculation.

Treatment. Response to treatment is usually rapid, especially in the limited lesions usually encountered by the otologist. If crusts are present, they should be removed with *warm water.* Then the lesion should be protected with an ointment containing from 2 to 5 per cent of *ammoniated mercury* in equal parts of *zinc oxide* and *petrolatum.*

Herpes Zoster Oticus. Herpetic eruptions on the auricle and in the canal are of virus origin and are considered to be part of a geniculate ganglion involvement (Hunt's disease) in which there may occur facial palsy, tinnitus and even vertigo.

Treatment. The eruption is self limiting and as a rule needs no therapy. Occasionally the vesicles break down or become infected. The application of the usual local *antiseptics* is then indicated.

Erysipelas. When erysipelas begins on the auricle, it is usually a complication of an otitic inflammation. It is suspected when a spreading superficial cellulitis extends to adjacent skin and onto the face. The edges are sharply demarcated. More often when this disease is encountered on the auricle, it has spread there from a facial erysipelas.

Treatment. The modern treatment seems to be *chemotherapeutic* with *sulfonamides.*

Hemorrhagic Eruptions (Otitis Externa Hemorrhagica). These occur as a complication of influenza. Purple blebs or blood-filled blisters are found on the tympanic membrane or the adjacent meatal wall. The chief symptom is earache, more or less severe. The blebs rupture spontaneously or become absorbed. No treatment is usually necessary.

MALFORMATIONS

A variety of conditions which are considered to be defects in shape and position are encountered. The more common of these are abnormal prominence of the auricle (protruding ears) (Fig. 40), abnormal size of the pinna and defects through partial or complete loss of substance.

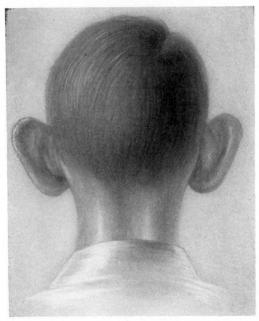

Fig. 40. An unusual protrusion of the auricle from the side of the head is the most common deformity of the external ear. Skillful plastic surgery will provide a marked improvement in appearance.

Congenital defects such as rudimentary ear appendages and total abscess of the ear are occasionally encountered. In some of the more severe forms of congenital abnormality, an imperforate canal may be found. Stenosis of the external canal may follow chronic inflammatory changes and trauma.

Many of these conditions can be remedied by plastic surgery performed by the surgeon experienced in this work.

NEW GROWTHS

ˊCarcinoma of the external auditory canal is amenable to cure if diagnosed early and properly treated in the early stages. Chronic discharge, often serosanguineous, or free bleeding, pain and swelling within the canal are manifestations which single or in combination should arouse in the examiner's mind the possibility of a new growth. Benign polyps from the middle ear sometimes fill the external canal. All polyps when removed should be sectioned. Granulomas sometimes develop in the external canal outside of intact middle ears.

Exostoses of the external canal are rather common. If these cause no significant morbidity, they should be let alone.

REFERENCES

Brown, L. G.: Inflammation of the External Ear and External Auditory Meatus. In: Fowler, E. P., Jr.: Medicine of the Ear. New York, Thomas Nelson & Sons, 1947.

Morey, G.: Herpes Zoster Oticus. J. Laryng. & Otol., 61:131, 1946.

O'Neill, H.: Herpes Zoster Auris ("Geniculate" Ganglionitis). Arch. Otolaryng., 42:309, 1945.

Senturia, B.: Etiology of External Otitis. Laryngoscope, 55:277, 1945.

Senturia, B., and Wolff, F.: Treatment of External Otitis: Action of Sulfonamides on Fungi Isolated from Cases of Otomycosis. Arch. Otolaryng., 41:56, 1945.

Tschiassny, K.: Site of Facial Nerve Lesion in Cases of Ramsay Hunt's Syndrome. Ann. Otol., Rhin. & Laryng., 55:152, 1946.

CHAPTER V

ACUTE OTITIS MEDIA

Acute otitis media occurs in two forms. In one, the fluid content of the middle ear is serous; in the other, it is purulent. An accumulation of serum in the middle ear may occur from closure or congestion of the eustachian tube from a cause that is not inflammatory, or it may represent an early change in a sequence of pathologic events leading to an acute suppuration in the middle ear.

The serous form which remains as such has been described under a number of titles, such as catarrhal otitis media, acute exudative catarrh and acute otitis media with effusion. The manifestations in all serous otitis media are the same. When a transient stage of serous otitis media develops in an otitic infection destined to become a suppurative process within a matter of hours, the limited serous stage is usually observed, if seen at all, during a phase in which the ear drum is undergoing increasing injection and thickening, with landmarks rapidly becoming obscure. This depends, of course, on a virulent organism. Cases are frequently seen, however, in which a mild inflammation in the middle ear does not progress beyond the serous stage and in which the first symptoms, moderately acute, begin to subside rapidly. This sequence of events is apparently seen more frequently now, when early therapy is instituted with adequate doses of a sulfonamide or penicillin. From a clinical standpoint, this type of case usually offers no particular problem in therapy. The process usually subsides gradually but rather promptly as the host's resistance to the causative organism limits the infection.

Serous otitis media which is not part of an acute middle ear infection has become a problem. It is of common incidence and, its importance from the standpoint of morbidity is too often overlooked by the family doctor and the pediatrician.

ACUTE SEROUS OTITIS MEDIA

Etiology and Pathogenesis. Acute serous otitis media characterized by an exudate into the middle ear is caused by the following:

1. A mild inflammatory process beginning in the nasopharynx or extending to the nasopharynx from adjacent infection (in the nasal space or the oropharynx) with subsequent extension through the eustachian tube and which limits itself on reaching the middle ear, so that the end result of the inflammatory changes in the middle ear does not

61

progress beyond the serous stage. This is common in children, particularly in the age group in which lymphoid hyperplasia around and in the mouth of the tube is common. Irradiation of this lymphoid tissue may be an effective method of controlling this type of disease.

2. Allergenic phenomena cause eustachian tube blockage extending from nasal congestive changes. The blockage of the tube creates negative middle ear pressures which persist long enough to create edema of the middle ear mucosa and subsequent collection of serum in the middle ear. This is also most common in children, but occurs in all ages.

3. Changes in atmospheric pressure, as occur in air travel, may produce blockage of the tube because of factors predisposing to this blockage; that is, edema in the nasopharynx incident to nasopharyngitis, anatomical irregularities in the nose and possibly within the tube, limited pneumatization of the mastoid process and so on.

SYMPTOMS AND SIGNS

Most patients with serous otitis media have some impairment of hearing as their principal symptoms. A few experience tinnitus. In the early stages, especially if the onset is abrupt, some pain may be experienced. The ear drum is usually retracted. In some cases, it appears injected. In others, it has a grayish color or a yellowish cast. At times one may see bubbles of fluid through the drum or a definite meniscus of fluid (Fig. 41). The ear drum may have a diffuse grayish color and a shiny cast. If air is blown through the tube to the middle ear by catheter or the Politzer bag (Figs. 28 and 29), the ear drum tends to bulge outward. The patient usually senses an improvement in hearing, often temporary.

DIAGNOSIS

Most of the diagnostic points have already been mentioned. Sometimes actual decision as to whether or not there is fluid in the ear rests on the effect of blowing air through the tube. Occasionally, when the ear drum seems scarred and thickened and retracted, as from previously active processes, a ballooning of a thin portion of the ear drum will follow inflation and a straw-colored serum is observed through the bulging portion of the ear drum.

The hearing loss in serous otitis media is from the disease alone, and is never very marked. In early stages, particularly in children, the first loss is for the very high notes, above 2048 frequencies. In more advanced cases, all notes may be down, approximating the 30 to 40 decibel line through the speech frequencies (512, 1024, 2048). The hearing loss is of the conductive type (Fig. 32).

TREATMENT

Many cases of acute serous otitis media are self limiting. If an inflammation in the nasopharynx is the cause, as this resolves, the primary factor in the tubal disease is removed, and healing with return to function follows. However, there is a common occurrence in children in which the process remains subacute, a considerable mucoid content is part of the middle ear exudate, hyperplastic lymphoid nodules in and around

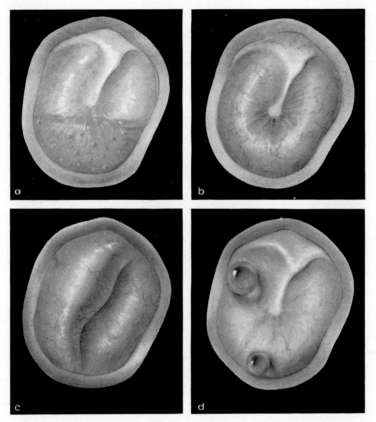

Fig. 41. a, A serous exudate into the middle ear may occur in an initial stage of an acute inflammatory middle ear infection or as secretion which is non-inflammatory in origin such as occurs from an allergic change or from the effect of physical factors, such as a rapid change of altitude in flying (otitic barotrauma, aero-otitis media).

b, The inflamed ear drum characterized by injection and thickening is the direct result of bacterial infection of the middle ear.

c, The swollen bulging ear drum results from inflammatory exudate under pressure in the middle ear.

d, Myringitis bullosa occurs in virulent middle ear inflammation such as occurs in the infections caused by virulent streptococcal or influenzal organisms.

the tubal orifice in the nasopharynx are present and the tubal function is not a normal one. This is the type of case in which *irradiation of these lymphoid nodules* is now being widely used as a means of controlling the important causative factor in the development of the tubal congestion and occlusion (Fig. 42). In very mild cases, the only objective finding of significance may be a high-tone loss above the 4096 frequency. In the more severe cases, the hearing loss is prominent. The parents or teacher suspect some impairment and when the child is examined, a moderate loss through all frequencies of the audiometric scale is found.

It has been the practice in these cases to force air through the eustachian tubes either by the Politzer method or, when possible, by catheter inflations. The actual benefits from this are only temporary, although in adult patients, a sense of relief is often expressed as a result of an improvement in the hearing.

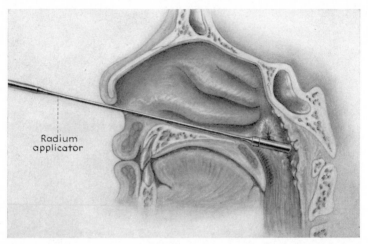

Radium applicator

Fig. 42. Irradiation of the nasopharynx with an application containing 50 mg. of radium screened so as to employ chiefly the more caustic beta rays is now a common procedure. The twelve minute dosage to each side of the nasopharynx is calculated to be sufficient to disturb the life cycle of the lymphoid cell and thus exert a "biologic" effect. This therapy is thought to be valuable in controlling the disorders in which nasopharyngeal lymphoid tissue infection plays an important role, i.e., congestive changes in the middle ear causing hearing loss, asthma in children in which nasopharyngeal infection is an important factor, nasal obstruction from infection in the nasopharynx, and so on.

In patients in whom improvement is not obtained within a few days from the onset, or in patients seen after the condition has been present for three or four weeks, simple *myringotomy* is indicated. The fluid is then forced out by Politzer inflation or, if it is largely mucoid, it may be aspirated by inserting a thin suction tip into the canal and placing it against the opening in the ear drum. A "string" of mucus can thus be aspirated. The hearing is promptly recovered and the incision in the ear drum heals promptly, usually without scarring (Fig. 43).

In adult patients, the ear drums in these cases may be incised without anesthesia, since they are not very sensitive. In children, a few seconds of gas or vinyl ether anesthesia is used.

The causative factor may need attention. In adults, the fluid tends to reform in the presence of chronic nasal conditions and in debilitated persons. Attention to these factors is sometimes necessary before the middle ear is relieved.

ACUTE PURULENT OTITIS MEDIA

Etiology. In most cases, the infection extends up the eustachian tube from an acute inflammation in the nasopharynx. On rare occasions, the pathway of infection to the middle ear is by vascular routes through blood vessels or lymphatics, or by way of the external or internal auditory meatus. The streptococci are responsible for over half of the pyo-

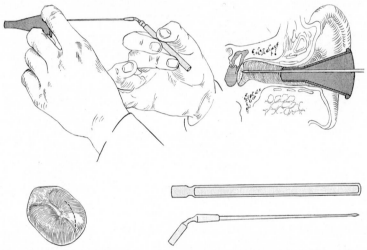

Fig. 43. The most important essentials to a skilfully performed myringotomy are (1) accurate visualization of the ear drum, and (2) perfect immobilization of the patient as obtained under the relaxation of general anesthesia when children are concerned. The myringotomy knife should incise only the ear drum and should not penetrate the mucosa over the promontory.

genic infections of the middle ear. Pneumococcic organisms and micrococci (staphylococci) account for about one-third. Uncommonly, organisms such as *Streptococcus viridans*, *Hemophilus influenzae* and *Proteus vulgaris* are found.

PATHOLOGY

A stage of acute serous otitis media undoubtedly precedes a purulent change in the middle ear in a majority of cases. In a virulent process, it is often only a matter of a few hours from the time a fulness or some slight twinges of pain are felt until the advanced changes have taken place. The pathogenesis of these changes are those of any inflammatory process, plus the fact that the blockage of the eustachian tube causes a negative middle ear pressure with its resultant effect on the membrane of the middle ear. Cellular elements from the blood vessels and bacteria are found in the fluid in the middle ear. Gas forms, which adds to the discomfort. A particularly virulent process produces the more visible changes of a cellulitis in the ear drum—as pressure continues from the gas and accumulating fluid, the ear drum bulges outward and the stage is set for a rupture of the drum. Or, if the process is less virulent, the fluid content of the middle ear becomes frankly purulent and the ear drum in time may actually appear yellow in color.

SYMPTOMS AND SIGNS

The local symptoms include a sense of fulness or pressure, often a mild tinnitus and pain. In severe cases, the pain is deep and boring and difficult to control except by strong analgesics. In other cases, there may be severe twinges of spasmodic pain. Infants tend to tug at their ears or roll their heads in lieu of an ability to complain of the pain.

The general symptoms are fever, malaise, sometimes headache in addition to the earache and, in children particularly, anorexia and sometimes nausea and vomiting. The fever may be rather high in small children.

TREATMENT

Prior to 1937, when chemotherapy in the form of sulfanilamide came into usage in acute ear inflammations, the ear drum was incised (myringotomy, paracentesis) for drainage of the middle ear to prevent extension of the inflammatory process to the mastoid cells and toward other complications.

Sulfonamide Therapy. After sulfonamide therapy came into general usage, fewer ear drums were incised. There were reports that most cases of acute middle ear suppuration could be controlled by the administration of adequate doses of the sulfonamides; other reports indicated that sulfonamide therapy tended to quiet down the infection in some cases but failed to heal it and that a subsequent sudden occurrence of such complications as meningitis, lateral sinus thrombophlebitis, petrositis and so on could be expected. This was referred to as the "masking" effect of sulfonamide therapy. However, we hear little about that today. Most of the diseases of which acute suppurative otitis media is a common complication (acute tonsillitis, pharyngitis, rhinitis and sinusitis with suppuration, lower respiratory tract inflammations such as pneumonia) are now receiving penicillin or a sulfonamide or the combination, and acutely discharging ears are now a relatively uncommon experience in the practice of most otolaryngologists.

Ear Drops. It was and still is a common practice to prescribe ear drops for the pain accompanying otitis media. Formerly, phenol incorporated in glycerin (phenol, 10 grains; glycerin, 1 ounce) was widely used. From 5 to 10 drops were warmed and instilled every 2 hours. The phenol produced surface anesthesia of the ear drum and rendered the condition less painful. A disadvantage of this medication was the surface desquamation of the ear drum caused by the phenol. Today, a more widely used preparation, *auralgan*, contains antipyrine and benzipyrine in glycerin. The dose is from 5 to 10 drops warmed and instilled every 2 hours. Its use in the milder type of cases seems to be beneficial. Its effect is less marked in the more virulent or fulminating infections.

Penicillin Therapy. Before penicillin was available, the administration of a sulfonamide early in a severe form of otitis media combined with drainage of the middle ear was an effective method of a prompt cure in a majority of cases. Today, a considerable percentage of cases of acute suppurative otitis media respond to penicillin therapy without the need of drainage of the middle ear. The medication must be administered in adequate doses. At the present time, an adequate dosage means the blood levels equivalent to that maintained by administering approximately 30,000 units or more parenterally every three hours. A substitute method of parenteral administration is being clinically evaluated at this time. Intramuscular administrations of 300,000 units in beeswax or an oil in single doses once daily, apparently can maintain an adequate blood level. The disadvantage to this method is local discomfort at the site of injection; actual necrosis has been reported. Oral administration is also being used. With this method, the drug has to be taken every three hours in approximately five times the dosage given parenterally, and fluid and food intake are restricted to midway between the three hourly dosage of the oral penicillin.

Myringotomy. Prior to the use of the sulfonamides and penicillin, myringotomy was indicated when the ear drum was found to be swollen and thickened, with obliteration of the landmarks, and earache or fever was present. Usually the color of the drums was that of acute infection. Occasionally one encountered a middle ear abscess which had been present without drainage for several days. Myringotomy was also indicated in various degrees of ear drum swelling, often without complete obliteration of the landmarks when there was continued earache, fever, or evidence of toxicity, particularly in children.

Today, myringotomy is indicated when the infection does not respond promptly to sulfonamide or penicillin therapy. The course of the inflammation will be shortened and the hearing more promptly and safely restored if this is done.

Technic. The first requisite for performing a myringotomy properly is adequate illumination of the ear drum. The otologist usually prefers a head mirror for this. General anesthesia is preferable because a myringotomy on an acutely inflamed ear drum is extremely painful. The duration of the anesthesia need be only for a few minutes. Vinyl ether, a short administration of "drop" ether, or intravenous administration of pentothal sodium in older patients is adequate.

Any special preparation of the ear drum or external canal with skin antiseptic is unnecessary, although it has been a common practice to fill the canal with alcohol prior to incising the ear drum. This probably only adds to local tissue morbidity, particularly of the ear drum.

With proper illumination and visualization, a curvilinear incision is usually made about a millimeter from the posterior margin of the drum, starting below and carrying the incision up to the posterior fold (Fig. 43).

The knife should not be inserted deeply, so that it will not touch the medial wall of the middle ear. This would add unnecessary trauma;

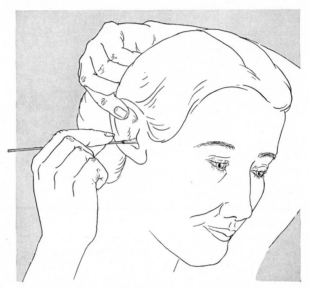

Fig. 44. Dry wiping of the middle ear by the patient must be demonstrated to the patient in order to insure accuracy. The auricle of the ear being treated is grasped between the thumb and forefinger of the side opposite to the one being treated. The auricle is gently retracted upward and backward. A properly wound applicator (Fig. 20) is grasped between the thumb and forefinger of the free hand. It is gently inserted until the cotton tip touches the ear drum and then it is withdrawn. Repeated maneuvers of this type will wipe the external canal free of secretion.

instances have been reported in which the stapes has been dislocated and the facial nerve injured.

As the ear drum is incised, actual gas may escape, or thin, purulent secretion may half fill the external canal. A variable amount of blood is usually mixed with the drainage.

A wick of cotton is fashioned to the approximate size of the canal and inserted so that the end of the wick touches the ear drum. This wick aids early drainage.

After-Care. General supportive care and the continuation of sulfonamide or penicillin therapy are important after the ear is draining.

Locally, the instillation of any medication is probably useless. Dry wipes with sterile cotton should be carried out every two or three hours when drainage is profuse (Fig. 44). In the presence of fever, the patient should be confined to bed, lying on his affected ear most of the time so as to promote drainage by posture. The application of external heat is desirable when pain persists.

REFERENCES

Allman, C.: Pencillin in Otology: Use in 511 Cases of Otitis Media and 74 Cases of Mastoiditis. J.A.M.A., *129*:109, 1945.

Boies, L. R.: Middle Ear Disease in Children. Journal Lancet, *64*:36, 1944.

Eagle, W.: Secretory Otitis Media. Ann. Otol., Rhin. & Laryng., *55*:55, 1946.

Fowler, E. P., Jr.: Diseases of the Middle Ear. In: Medicine of the Ear. New York, Thomas Nelson & Sons, 1947.

Fox, M. D., and Mining, V.: Incidence of Otitis Media and Mastoiditis in Scarlet Fever. Ann. Otol., Rhin. & Laryng., *57*:489, 1948.

Hoople, G., and Blaisdell, I.: Clinical Observations on Acute Catarrhal Otitis Media. Proc. Roy. Soc. Med., *37*:270, 1944.

Wilcox, J. G.: Penicillin Treatment of Acute Middle Ear and Mastoid Infection. Pennsylvania M. J., *50*:574, 1947.

CHAPTER VI

CHRONIC SUPPURATIVE OTITIS MEDIA

The occurrence of chronic middle ear suppuration is based on certain pathologic incidents. An ordinary case of acute suppurative otitis media in a normally pneumatized temporal bone rarely becomes chronic.

ETIOLOGY AND PATHOGENESIS

Chronic suppuration in the middle ear is usually the result of one of three developments.

1. A severe infection causing necrotic changes in some portion of the tympanum. This is not uncommon in severe middle ear infections, such as occur in scarlet fever, measles and diphtheria. The necrotic change may be marked enough so that the ear is destined to chronicity from the time of occurrence of this necrotic change. This change may involve the mucosa, the ossicles and the bony walls, in addition to the invariable destruction in the drum membrane. Granulations and polyps are common. A marginal tympanic perforation involving the annular rim of bone allows a ready pathway for an ingrowth of squamous epithelium. This epithelial ingrowth is an attempt on the part of nature to heal the infection; it may invade the space rapidly, proliferate, desquamate and form a cholesteatoma.

2. An acute inflammation occurring in an ear in which there has been an interference with the normal development of the tympanic mucosa so that it has remained hyperplastic through the effect of otitis media neonatorum or catarrhal otitis media in early infancy. This mucosa is considered to be poorly resistant to infection. Acute otitis media developing in this hyperplastic mucosa is thought to be destined to chronicity because of the limited capacity of this type of mucosa to heal. Granulations and polyps are common to this type of disease, but unless there is a marginal perforation, the formation of cholesteatoma is uncommon.

3. The formation of a cholesteatoma from an ingrowth of epithelium from Shrapnell's membrane without pre-existing perforation or otitis media. This ingrowth of epithelium results from a negative pressure in the attic. Two factors may produce this negative pressure. It may result from the closing off of the attic by persistent hyperplastic subepithelial connective tissue in the epitympanic recess, or it may result from a prolonged occlusion of the eustachian tube, owing to nasopharyngeal disease. When Shrapnell's membrane is drawn in, a blind pouch forms by the invagina-

tion. The neck of this pouch is too constricted to allow escape of the desquamating squamous epithelium. Thus a cholesteatoma forms. Its presence becomes known when it becomes large enough to extend out of the attic or when saprophytic infection of the epithelial debris causes discharge through the small perforation.

There are occasional instances of a type of acute otitis media occurring in a normally pneumatized mastoid which does not produce initial necrosis, and which, because of the patient's inability to limit the infection, acquires the characteristics of chronicity. It may eventually heal, but with some impairment of aural function and with a sclerotic change in the mastoid picture. These cases are uncommon.

Cholesteatoma. In otology, cholesteatoma refers to an accumulation of horny and desquamated epidermis and cholesterin crystals. The cholesterin results from decomposition of organic matter out of contact with oxygen.

In reality, there are but two types of cholesteatoma, true and pseudocholesteatoma. It is the pseudo type which we encounter in chronic middle ear suppuration. There are two types of pseudocholesteatoma; primary and secondary. The primary type develops from an epithelial invagination in Shrapnell's membrane, a result of the production of a negative pressure in the attic from absorption of air from this space.

The secondary type is commonly encountered in chronic suppurative otitis media subsequent to an ingrowth of squamous epithelium through a marginal tympanic perforation.

Definition. From these considerations, it is evident that a definition of chronic suppurative otitis media cannot be simply constructed because of the varied pathologic possibilities. The following definition is made on the basis of the modern concept of the disease.

Chronic suppurative otitis media is a continued suppuration from the middle ear, following an acute necrotic otitis media or a primary suppuration in a middle ear with hyperplastic mucosa; uncommonly it occurs following an invagination of epithelium from Shrapnell's membrane to form a cholesteatoma without pre-existing perforation, or ordinary otitis media in a previously normal middle ear.

CLASSIFICATION

The use of a classification of the several types of chronic suppurative otitis media is helpful in visualizing the pathologic process. An empirical, clinical one suggested by Lillie is useful. It is based on the location of the most important pathologic process.

In this classification are four types:

Type I. A thin mucoid discharge with little or no odor characterizes this type. The discharge comes from a perforation in the anterior quadrant of the drum membrane, and is chiefly from the eustachian tube. Evidence of destructive disease in the middle ear is lacking. The discharge is increased and more purulent during head colds. Contributing factors in the continuation of the discharge are pathologic conditions of the nose and the nasopharynx (Fig. 45).

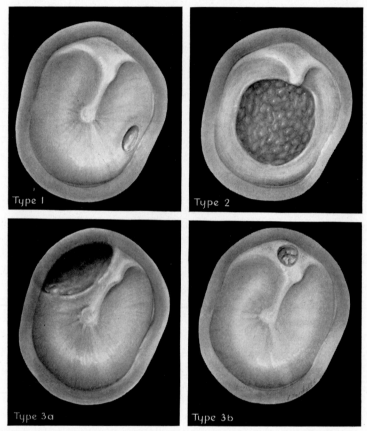

Fig. 45. In Type I chronic suppurative otitis media, the perforation is anteriorly near the tympanic mouth of the eustachian tube. It may be difficult to visualize. The disease is essentially an involvement of the mucosa of the eustachian tube and middle ear. In Type II, the perforation is large and central and one sees the products of chronic middle ear suppuration which is practically confined to the mucosa although there may be bony necrosis involving the ossicles. Granulations and polyps are common. In Type III, the perforation is marginal (a) or through Shrapnell's membrane (b). The disease is often confined to the attic. Cholesteatoma is invariably present. The discharge may be scanty. For clinical convenience, the classification includes a Type IV in which there may be combined elements of Types II or III but in which there are positive signs for surgical intervention, such as a positive fistula test indicating a circumscribed labyrinthitis, or a facial paralysis, or symptoms of impending meningitis.

Type II. There are pathologic changes confined to the middle ear. The perforation is central, usually large, and the middle ear is filled with mucopurulent or purulent secretion. The odor is fetid, but saprophytic changes may suggest caries or cholesteatoma. Granulation tissue or polyps may be present over the promontory. No definite caries is evident, although the ossicles may have been destroyed. There may be evidence that the tube is open and discharging. There is no evidence of disease in the attic (Fig. 45).

Type III. The most striking pathologic change is in the attic, although the conditions described in Types I and II may be associated. The discharge has a foul odor and may be scanty. The perforation is in Shrapnell's membrane or along the posterior margin of the tympanic membrane. Cholesteatoma is usually present (Fig. 45).

Type IV. All cases in which there are signs of extension of the disease to the labyrinth, meninges, brain, or facial nerve are designated as this type. Cholesteatoma is invariably present. Surgical intervention is positively indicated.

IMPORTANT SYMPTOMS AND SIGNS

Discharge. The character of the discharge in chronic suppuration of the middle ear may indicate at first examination the nature of the pathologic process. For example, the very foul-smelling discharge of a dirty grayish-yellow color suggests cholesteatoma and its degenerating epithelial and osseous association. Small, white, shiny, greasy flakes may be seen in the discharge, which definitely indicate cholesteatoma.

Bacteriologic examination of the discharge from chronic middle ear suppuration offers little of practical value. Secondary invaders such as the micrococci (staphylococci), *Proteus vulgaris* and *Pseudomonas aeruginosa* (*Bacillus pyocyaneus*) are invariably found in aural discharge which has acquired the characteristics of chronicity.

In cases of primary pseudocholesteatoma, the discharge from the small perforation in Shrapnell's membrane may be very scanty, almost dry and consist chiefly of flakes of cholesteatoma.

Aural discharge in cases of chronic middle ear suppuration which is not characterized by any of the aspects just mentioned has little diagnostic importance. It should be emphasized, however, that a thin, fetid discharge, occasionally or frequently bloodstained, suggests the possibility of malignancy.

Objective Signs. Exclusive of the discharge, objective signs in the middle ear are of considerable diagnostic value. Marginal and attic perforations invariably are associated with cholesteatoma in cases of longstanding suppuration. Granulation tissue is indicative of an attempt at repair. A firm bed of granulations in the middle ear as seen through a large central perforation may indicate a disease confined to the mucosa. When the granulations are large and loose, bare bone can usually be palpated with a probe.

The presence of a polyp is not in itself an indication of the extent of the pathologic process. The polyp may be simply a part of a mucous membrane change or it may be attached to a site of bone necrosis. Usually removal of the polyp is necessary to study the condition of the middle ear. Removal should be performed by snare or punch and not by pulling the growth free from its attachment, since this latter method carries the risk of opening pathways for infection.

Hearing. Hearing loss in chronic middle ear suppuration varies in degree according to the site and type of the disease. In primary pseudo-cholesteatoma, hearing may be practically normal as long as the disease is confined to the attic.

The average case of chronic middle ear suppuration has a definite loss of useful hearing, which is dependent upon the degree of involvement of the medial wall of the tympanic cavity. Any interference with the mobility of the stapes in the oval window may be a greater factor in hearing loss than the perforation in the drum or necrosis of the ossicular chain.

Very marked hearing loss indicates that there has been a deeper involvement than that of the conducting mechanism alone. Absolute deafness associated with chronic suppuration suggests that labyrinthitis has been the cause for this loss. A toxic neuritis not related to a labyrinthitis would be the only other cause to consider.

Pain. This is an uncommon symptom in the ordinary case of chronic middle ear suppuration, and may be a serious sign. It may mean that:

1. Tension has developed, owing to a stoppage of secretion (pus or cholesteatoma), or

2. The dura or sinus wall has been exposed by the disease and a localized pachymeningitis is present, or a perisinus abscess, or

3. A brain abscess is present.

Vertigo. Vertigo occurring in the presence of a chronic middle ear suppuration is a serious symptom. Transient attacks with positive fistula test may mean an erosion of the bony labyrinth, usually of the horizontal semicircular canal. Persistent vertigo with nystagmus denotes an actual labyrinthitis in which the membranous labyrinth has been invaded by the inflammatory process.

Fistula Test. The fistula test should be performed in every case of chronic middle ear suppuration of Types III and IV. It may be performed by compressing air in the external canal. This can easily be accomplished by use of a Politzer bag fitted with a tip which fits snugly into the orifice of the external canal (Fig. 46).

The onset of vertigo and nystagmus by compression and rarefaction of air in the external canal indicates that there is a fistula through the bony labyrinth with the membranous labyrinth intact. When a fistula is present, it is usually in the external semicircular canal.

When the fistula test is negative, it usually means that the labyrinth is intact, although it can mean that there has been a total destruction of labyrinthine function. This latter possibility should be considered when there is an absolute hearing loss; it can be substantiated by the turning tests in a Bárány chair.

A positive fistula test is indication for surgical intervention in the form of a tympanomastoidectomy (radical mastoidectomy).

Facial Paralysis. Facial paralysis occurring during the course of chronic suppurative otitis media is an indication for surgical intervention. Usually it means that an expanding cholesteatomatous mass has eroded the wall of the fallopian canal. The most common site for such

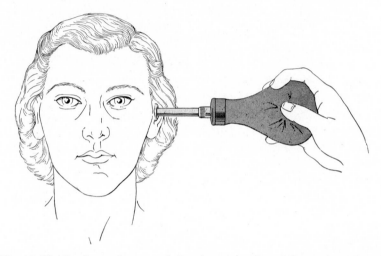

Fig. 46. The fistula test in cases of chronic suppuration of the ear is used to determine the presence of an erosion through the horizontal semicircular canal. The Politzer bag fitted with an atomizer tip supplies a convenient means of compressing the air in the external canal. If a fistula is present, the compression of the air will cause vertigo and usually nystagmus. If the test is negative, there is no fistula or the labyrinth is dead. In the event of the latter, one would expect to find a total deafness in the involved ear.

A positive fistula test may often be obtained in cases in which there is erosion through the bony semicircular canal simply by probing through the perforation in the ear drum with a cotton-tipped applicator.

an erosion is close to the mastoid antrum or within the tympanic cavity. Surgery for the relief of this complication requires complete tympanomastoidectomy (radical mastoidectomy). Occasionally, an actual decompression of the facial canal might be indicated.

X-ray studies of the temporal bone are necessary in chronic middle ear suppuration before an evaluation of the clinical problem is made. For this, we routinely use the Law, Stenvers and Towne positions. The latter will reveal any definite enlargement of the tympanic antrum owing to an enlarging cholesteatoma.

TREATMENT

Conservative therapy is indicated in Types I and II of chronic middle ear suppuration. This therapy includes one or more of the following procedures:

1. The local use of certain antiseptic solutions or powders.

2. Minor surgical procedures designed principally to remove diseased tissue, proliferative change, and to improve the drainage.

3. Removal of any pathologic processes of the upper respiratory tract which might contribute to inflammation of the middle ear.

ANTISEPTIC SOLUTIONS AND POWDERS

The well-known alcoholic solution of boric acid owes its usefulness to the alcohol rather than to the boric acid content. In addition to its antiseptic properties, the alcohol inhibits to some extent the development of granulations. In an instance of a secreting membrane such as lines the middle ear space, alcohol may stimulate this membrane to continue to secrete as long as the medication is in use. Ear drops of the following prescriptions are effective.

	Gm. or cc.
1. Boric acid	0.6
Alcohol, 95 per cent	30.0
2. Urea	3.0
Sulfathiazole	2.12
Ethyl aminobenzoate	0.2
Glycerol	20.0
3. "Glycerite of Hydrogen Peroxide"	
Hydrogen peroxide	1.446 per cent
Urea (carbamide)	2.554 per cent
8–Hydroxyquinoline	0.1 per cent
Anhydrous glycerin	q.s.

Evolves active oxygen

Several powders have been popular in the treatment of chronic middle ear suppuration. The usefulness of any ear drop or powder depends upon whether the chronic suppurative process is limited and whether the medication will reach the diseased area. Powdered boric acid, boric acid and potassium iodide in combination, Sulzberger's iodine powder in two strengths, and more recently, powdered sulfonamides have all seemed to have merit. The following are three commonly used formulas:

	Gm.
1. Boric acid, finely powdered	15
Sulfanilamide, finely powdered	15
2. Sulfanilamide, finely powdered	
Zinc peroxide, finely powdered āā	7.5
3. Iodine	0.3
Ethyl oxide (solvent ether)	4.0
Boric acid, finely powdered	30.0

(Dissolve the iodine in the ether and mix thoroughly in a mortar with boric acid until dry again.)

Powders for use in chronically discharging ears are usually blown in by a special powder blower or dropped in by the patient. A simple, inexpensive powder blower is shown in Fig. 172. One end of a detachable tip may be dipped in the supply of powder, the blower assembled and the soft rubber end of the tip inserted in the external meatus and canal. The powder is then insufflated when the soft rubber bulb is compressed. It is my belief that diagnosis as to the type of disease and the care with which the medication is used are essential to an evaluation of the end result.

Zinc ionization once had a transient popularity. It was probable that the careful cleansing preparations prior to the application of the zinc sulfate solution were an important factor in the good result.

MINOR SURGERY

It is important to remove any proliferative tissue changes which may impede drainage and the process of repair. With large perforations, compact granulations can often be reduced with topical applications of silver nitrate in strength ranging from 10 to 50 per cent, or with use of the silver nitrate stick. Large granulations should be removed with small biting forceps. Polyps are removed with a small snare threaded over the polyp. The growth should not be pulled from its attachment, since there may be attachment of the polyp to an ossicle, particularly the stapes, the dislodgment of which would open a pathway for infection. After cutting through the polyp as close to its base as feasible, the base is treated with applications of silver nitrate.

In selected cases, surgical tympanic and attic drainage should be considered. This consists of enlargement of the perforation by surgical incision or biting forceps, then breaking down attic adhesions, cureting away granulations which block drainage and removal of necrotic ossicles.

Chronic rhinitis, sinusitis, nasopharyngeal lymphoid tissue and chronic tonsillitis all play important roles in stimulating certain types of chronic suppurative otitis media to continued activity. This is particularly true in Types I and II, in which there is evidence that the infection elsewhere in the respiratory tract seems to be responsible for an occasional exacerbation of the inflammation. This relationship is more commonly encountered in the chronic aural infections in children than in adults. The most common offender in the former group is the lymphoid tissue of the nasopharynx, either in the form of the whole adenoid mass, a recurrent growth of adenoids, or the lymphoid tissue in Rosenmüller's fossa.

Conservative treatment is indicated in Type I and most of Type II. When the cholesteatoma is limited to the attic in Type III, some cases may be successfully treated with attic irrigations, although the perforation may have to be enlarged to accomplish this.

MAJOR SURGERY

The proper choice of a specific major surgical procedure for chronic middle ear suppuration and mastoiditis depends upon the site and type of the disease process. The objective in the radical management of any case of chronic suppurative otitis media and mastoiditis is first to remove the disease and thus the danger to life, and second, to preserve as much hearing as possible. The preservation of hearing will in a degree be dependent upon the healing of the internal wall in relation to the amount of scar tissue involving the stapes and, to a lesser extent, the round window.

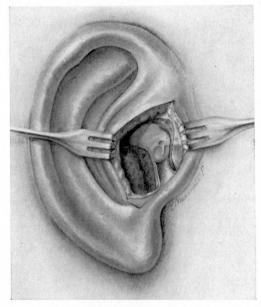

Fig. 47. The purpose of the modified radical mastoidectomy is to preserve hearing although all of the disease must be eradicated. With proper indications and skilful surgery, this procedure has excellent results.

Modified Radical Mastoidectomy. A modified radical mastoidectomy is indicated in certain cases when there is an adequate opportunity to eliminate the disease without disturbing the ossicular chain or the pars tensa. This means that the disease is limited to the attic, antrum and mastoid. This type of operation is usually suited to the cure of cases of primary pseudocholesteatoma of the attic.

Complete Radical Mastoidectomy. The complete radical mastoidectomy is indicated in all cases of chronic suppurative otitis media and mastoiditis with extensive secondary cholesteatoma and in any case in which there are signs of extension of the disease to the labyrinth, facial nerve, lateral sinus, meninges, or brain.

An operation of this extent is required to eliminate the disease from

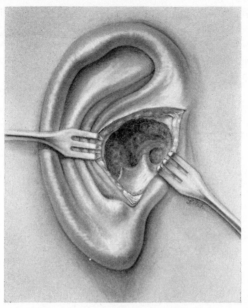

Fig. 48. The purpose of the complete radical mastoidectomy is to remove all of the disease even though the hearing may suffer further impairment.

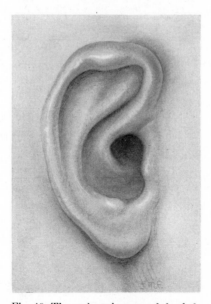

Fig. 49. The endaural approach healed.

the middle ear, the antrum and mastoid space. When this has been accomplished, these areas are converted into one smooth-walled cavity. A lining of squamous epithelium usually follows.

4

Endaural Approach. The endaural approach (Fig. 36), a modern improvement to surgery of the middle ear and mastoid in cases of chronic suppuration, has some definite advantages over the postaural route. These advantages are:

1. There is less soft tissue disturbance.

2. The operative maneuvers are directly over the middle ear and mastoid antrum, where the most important work is centered.

3. The construction of the plastic flap is simplified.

4. Postoperative discomfort and care are lessened.

The exposure through this approach, the modified radical mastoidectomy, complete radical mastoidectomy and the healed external ear are illustrated in Figs. 47, 48, 49.

REFERENCES

Babbitt, J. A.: Surgery in Chronic Middle Ear Infection. Ann. Surg., *101:*407, 1935.

Boies, L. R.: Chronic Suppurative Otitis Media. Ann. Otol., Rhin. & Laryng., *54:*265, 1945.

Brown, E. A., and Owen, W. E.: Treatment of Chronic Purulent Otitis Media with Glycerite of Hydrogen Peroxide. Arch. Otolaryng., *43:*605, 1946.

Hochfilzer, J.: Myringitis Granulosa. Laryngoscope, *55:*509, 1945.

Kopetsky, S. J.: Chronic Mastoiditis and its Therapy. J. Iowa M. Soc., *26:*665, 936.

Lempert, J.: Endaural, Antauricular Surgical Approach to the Temporal Bone. Arch. Otolaryng., *27:*555, 1938.

Lillie, H. I.: Indications for the Bondy Type of Modified Radical Mastoid Operations. Ann. Otol., Rhin. & Laryng., *44:*307, 1935.

Lillie, H. I.: An Empirical Clinical Classification of Chronic Suppurative Otitis Media. Atlantic M. J., *31:*559, 1928.

Smith, J. M.: Surgical Technic for the Conservation in Hearing in Chronic Mastoiditis. Laryngoscope, *48:*499, 1938.

Trommelfell und Gerhorknochelchen: Totalaufmeisselung mit Erhalting. Monatschr. f. Ohrenh., *44:*15, 1910.

Wittmaack, K.: Wie entsteht ein genuines Cholesteatom? Arch. f. Ohren-, Nasen- u. Kehlkopfh, *137:*306, 1933.

Woodruff, G. H., and Henner, Robert: Endaural Mastoidectomy: Experience in a Series of 76 Cases. Arch. Otolaryng., *35:*777, 1942.

CHAPTER VII

COMPLICATIONS OF SUPPURATIVE OTITIS MEDIA

Prior to the advent of sulfonamide therapy and, more recently, the use of penicillin, complications of acute suppurative otitis media were rather common. In order of their relative frequency of incidence, these complications were:

1. Acute surgical mastoiditis and petrositis.
2. Lateral sinus thrombophlebitis.
3. Meningitis.
4. Brain abscess.

At the present time, most of the infections in which there is involvement of the nasal space and pharynx are treated with a sulfonamide or penicillin. Consequently, acute otitis media as a complication of these conditions is less common than it once was, because the infections of which otitis media is a complication are controlled earlier in their course. Likewise, acute otitis media occurring seemingly as a primary infection is usually treated with a sulfonamide or penicillin and in most instances is controlled often without surgical drainage and usually without any of the previously mentioned complications. Figure 50 indicates the change in the incidence of acute surgical mastoiditis in my experience over the past sixteen years.

ACUTE SURGICAL MASTOIDITIS

Pathogenesis. In an acute suppuration in the middle ear, a certain amount of inflammatory reaction is bound to develop promptly in the mucosa of the mastoid process adjacent to the mucosa of the middle ear. The virulence of the infecting organism, the ability of the host to limit the infection (resistance) and the type of middle ear mucosa (normal or hyperplastic) and mastoid structure (sclerotic, diploic, or pneumatic) will determine to a degree the extent of the involvement.

The type of organism and its virulence may vary from season to season. *Streptococcus haemolyticus* is most commonly found, with some reports indicating an incidence as high as 60 per cent. The various types of pneumococcus are next in frequency, sometimes as high as 30 per cent. Less common are *Micrococcus pyogenes* (*Staphylococcus aureus* and *albus*), then *Streptococcus viridans*, *Hemophilus influenzae* and several other organisms.

81

The early microscopic changes in the mucosa of the pneumatized mastoid are those characteristic of any mucosal inflammatory reaction. Edema of the mucosa develops; in some areas there may be actual ulceration. Inflammatory exudate and pus fill the cells, resulting in pressure on the blood supply of the bony intercellular framework. As a consequence, necrosis appears, then coalescence, granulations develop, an abscess cavity forms and the only route for drainage out through the aditus from the middle ear is blocked. In the well-pneumatized mastoid, there is considerable variability in the extent of the cell structure. An

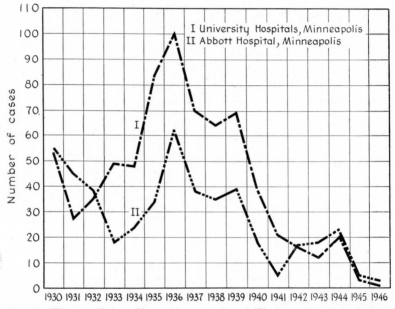

Fig. 50. The use of the sulfonamides and of penicillin has reduced the incidence of acute surgical mastoiditis to a point where surgery for this condition is a rarity. This chart depicts the incidence of surgery for acute mastoiditis over a period of sixteen years, both on a public ward service (University Hospital) and a private pediatric service (Abbott Hospital). The first sulfonamide (sulfanilamide) was used in 1937; penicillin came into general usage in 1945.

anatomic factor, therefore, may influence to some extent the course of the infection. If the mastoid process is well pneumatized, there is often a degree of pneumatization of the petrous pyramid and undoubtedly a certain degree of inflammation of the petrous cells develops in all cases of acute mastoiditis in which a partially or extensively pneumatized petrosa exists. When this gives clinical symptoms, we refer to it as *petrositis.* Just as the effect of pus and granulations accumulating without drainage may result in destruction of the bony cell partitions, the inner table of bone over the dura of the middle fossa or lateral sinus may undergo necrosis. This usually causes granulations to form over the dura and in some instances causes an actual extradural or perisinus abscess formation.

This necrosis of some portion of the bony confines of the mastoid may likewise lead to an extension of the inflammatory process to the soft tissue overlying the mastoid cortex to form a postauricular or zygomatic swelling, or an inflammation medial to the tip to cause a swelling in the neck ("Bezold's abscess").

Types of Mastoiditis. Two types of acute mastoiditis have been described, each of which has been considered by some otologists to represent clinical entities. The one just described represents a common type, the so-called "acute coalescent mastoiditis." The other type has been known as an acute "hemorrhagic mastoiditis." Some otologists have contended that this latter represents only an early stage of an infection which in time would progress to a stage of coalescence.

In this so-called "hemorrhagic mastoiditis," the findings when the mastoid has been opened are in contrast to those in the acute coalescent state. The intercellular walls are intact, the mucous membrane is thickened and swollen, but it is injected and bleeds readily when touched. A bloody serum fills the spaces; there is no pus. Microscopically the vascular channels present the picture of engorgement and thrombosis. Complications such as lateral sinus thrombophlebitis are common. Clinically, the patient is septic. Often the fever is high and there is prostration and restlessness. The ear drums may present only the picture of an acute injection.

SYMPTOMS AND SIGNS

Discharge. In acute mastoiditis of the coalescent type, the ear is usually discharging more or less profusely. When the purulent secretion is wiped from the external canal, a new supply can be seen coming through the perforation in the swollen ear drum. Usually the discharge pulsates, owing to a vascular impulse transmitted through the swollen congested mastoid mucosa.

Pain. Pain is significant of tension within the infected mastoid. It is less common in large pneumatic mastoids. In the diploic type, there is more fibrous tissue and a richer blood supply. This accounts for more tension and a greater likelihood of pain in this type of structure.

Postaural Edema. Postaural edema indicates that the inflammatory process has extended through the cortex of the mastoid process to cause inflammation in the soft tissue over the mastoid. This is more common in small children where islets of cartilage may persist in the cortex over the antrum or suture lines may not be tight. In older persons, it is more common in pneumatic mastoids in which large cells are close to the cortex; because of their size, these cells may have very thin walls. Postaural abscess is not uncommon in children; it is uncommon in adults. The pneumatic extent of the cells may be a factor in the development of zygomatic swelling or swelling below the mastoid tip (Fig. 51). When there is an extension of mastoid cells into the zygoma or up into the squama, infection may break through the cortex to produce edema or actual abscess beneath the soft tissue covering these sites. The same situation holds true at the mastoid tip. Abscesses have actually formed in the neck ("Bezold's abscess"), owing to a perforation on the medial surface of the tip inside the attachment of the sternomastoid muscle.

X-ray Findings. X-ray studies may reveal changes indicative of decalcification of cell partitions, such as actual coalescence of cell groups and extensive abscess formation. This information supplements the clinical picture in deciding on surgical therapy.

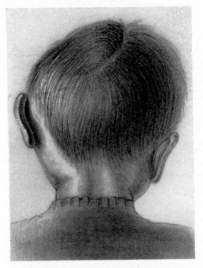

Fig. 51. A common picture in acute mastoiditis in children was the development of postaural edema and often of swelling extending into the zygomatic area. This will probably continue to be seen occasionally as one of the first indications for surgical intervention in cases in which sulfonamide or penicillin therapy or their combination has not been administered in adequate dosage and in cases in which the infecting organism is not susceptible to the effect of one or both of these drugs.

In the so-called "hemorrhagic mastoiditis," the discharge is thin and serosanguineous, pain and tenderness are common manifestations, the fever is high and toxicity is marked. X-ray findings are less reliable than in the coalescent type.

Indications for Surgical Intervention. At the present time, even in the presence of some x-ray evidence of destruction, the use of sulfonamide therapy and penicillin has produced cures. The indications for surgical intervention which were considered as definitely established prior to the advent of sulfonamide therapy or the use of antibiotics hold for the present time. In the presence of acute mastoiditis, the well-defined indications for surgery are:

1. Superiosteal abscess or postauricular edema.

2. The development of persistent mastoid tenderness (at tip, antrum, emissary vein), accompanied by fever, pain, or headache and a profuse discharge. These symptoms may be present in the first week of mastoiditis, but with indication of improvement, and the disease may go on to complete resolution. If the symptoms persist, however, without indication of definite improvement, surgical intervention is indicated.

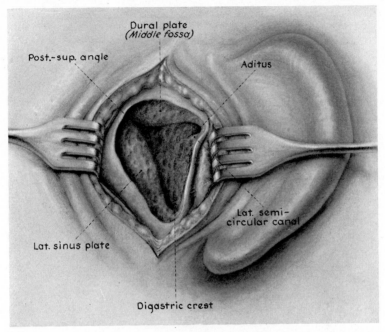

Fig. 52. The surgery for acute mastoiditis entails a systematic exenteration of cell structure so that when the operation has been completed, the dural bony plates of the middle fossa and the lateral sinus have been exposed and are clean, the horizontal semicircular canal is in view, and the tip has been reduced so as to obliterate its cell structure.

3. The development of:
   a. Symptoms of septic absorption (such as chills, septic temperature and sweats)
   b. Symptoms of vestibular irritation (such as vertigo, vestibular nystagmus, nausea and vomiting)
   c. Abducens paralysis
   d. Facial paralysis (except when it occurs early in the disease)

4. Prolonged profuse middle ear suppuration (four weeks or more) in the absence of other significant symptoms and which has resisted all rational nonoperative methods of treatment. The persistence of this profuse purulent discharge indicates that the chief source of this dis-

charge is beyond the limits of the tympanum and antrum. When the external canal is cleaned and the drum membrane exposed, a fresh supply of pus will soon appear and pulsate. There is usually sagging of the posterior superior canal wall or edema of the external canal. An x-ray study usually shows a considerable cell coalescence.

SURGICAL TREATMENT

The postaural incision has been preferred for this because the site of the work is in the mastoid process and drainage postoperatively seems

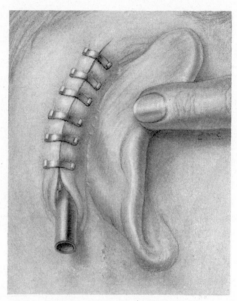

Fig. 53. A majority of otologists still favor the postaural incision for the surgery of acute mastoiditis. When the operation is complete, a simple rubber tube is used for drainage and the wound otherwise closed completely. Usually the wound heals promptly and the drain is removed by the fifth to seventh postoperative day and is not replaced. The middle ear is usually dry and healing of the incision is complete in two weeks from the date of surgery.

better assured by this approach. However, an increased experience with the endural approach for the treatment of acute surgical mastoiditis has demonstrated that the mastoid can be adequately exenterated through this approach. The surgical steps involve:

1. Exposure and removal of mastoid cortex.

2. Systematic exenteration of cell structure. When this has been completed, the bony plate over the middle fossa, dura, and over the lateral sinus are visible, the zygomatic cells have been removed, the horizontal semicircular canal is visible and the tip is reduced so as to obliterate its cell structure (Fig. 52).

3. Closure of the wound with a small rubber drain in the dependent portion of the wound (Fig. 53).

If mastoidectomy has been thoroughly performed and if the tissue infection was well localized, the drain can usually be removed in five to

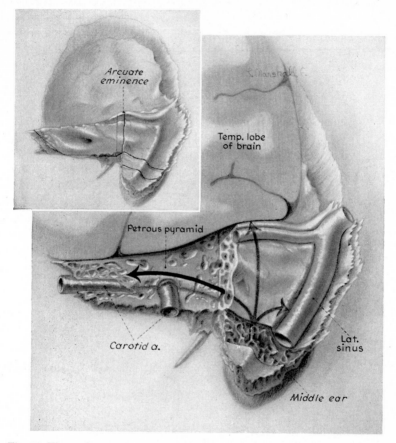

Fig. 54. The pathways of extension of an inflammatory process in the middle ear and mastoid in order of frequency are:

1. To the petrous pyramid by way of a spread through cellular structure.

2. To the lateral sinus by way of coalescence and necrosis involving the lateral sinus plate or by a retrograde thrombophlebitic process involving the vascular channels.

3. To the meninges and brain by the same process as indicated in 2.

seven days, and healing and convalescence are uneventful. As a rule, hearing returns to normal if it was normal prior to the onset of the infection.

The pathways of extension of an inflammatory process in the middle ear and mastoid, in order of frequency, are illustrated in Fig. 54.

PETROSITIS

A few years prior to the advent of the sulfonamides, a condition known as petrositis was introduced as a clinical entity. This involved inflammation of the petrous portion of the temporal bone. Today, with chemotherapy and the antibiotics, relatively little concern is shown regarding petrositis. It is, however, important to recognize it as a possibility and to provide adequate drainage when indicated through complete mastoidectomy with attention to cell tracts entering the pyramid and, in isolated cases, an actual exenteration or evacuation of the pyramid by way of exposure of intracapsular cell routes or actual drainage of isolated abscesses.

LATERAL SINUS THROMBOPHLEBITIS

Pathogenesis. Invasion of the sigmoid sinus as it courses through the mastoid develops in two ways. In the coalescence of a pneumatic mastoid, an abscess formation in contact with the sinus wall produces an inflammatory change in the venous wall. A perisinus abscess forms, the blood stream is slowed, involvement of the inner wall of the vein results in a mural change and in time the lumen may be completely occluded. In the acute fulminating type of mastoiditis without coalescence, the so-called "hemorrhagic" type, no pus is seen in the external auditory canal. The ear drum is thickened and injected; the discharge is thin and bloody. No purulent secretion is noted. Involvement of the lateral sinus is by a retrograde thrombophlebitis which involves the wall of the sinus to become the focus from which the blood stream is involved.

Symptoms and Signs. Fever unexplained by other findings is the first sign of blood stream invasion. It tends to fluctuate considerably and in the fully developed case is of the septic or "picket fence" type. Chills often accompany a rise in temperature. Pain is relatively uncommon, but it may be present if there is a perisinus abscess. Blood cultures may reveal a positive result, particularly if the culture is made at the time of the chill. Manometer tests on the spinal fluid (the Tobey-Ayer test) will record a sinus occlusion by thrombus if the thrombus is complete.

Treatment. Treatment consists in *removing the focus of infection* in infected mastoid cells, a necrotic lateral sinus plate, or an infected and often necrotic lateral sinus wall. If a thrombus has formed, *drainage of the sinus* and *evacuation of the infected plot* may be indicated, and occasionally a *ligation of the internal jugular vein* to prevent escape of infected emboli into the lung and then to other parts of the body.

MENINGITIS

Meningitis as a complication of acute middle ear and mastoid infection may result from an extension through the lateral sinus, from an extradural abscess forming in a coalescent state in the mastoid, from petrositis, or through labyrinthitis. The symptoms of sustained fever, headache, vomiting, a stiff neck and so on, indicate this diagnosis. Prior to the use of the sulfonamides or penicillin, meningitis with organisms in the spinal fluid was seldom cured. Today, the mortality has been greatly reduced, usually through the use of a combination of a sulfonamide and penicillin. Surgery is effective only to remove the focus from which the complication originates.

BRAIN ABSCESS

A brain abscess complicating an acute middle ear infection is most apt to follow lateral sinus thrombophlebitis, petrositis, or meningitis. Continued toxicity, headache, fever, vomiting, or a lethargic state suggests a cerebral involvement. A slow pulse and convulsive seizures are most significant signs. Sulfonamide therapy and penicillin have been thought to cure an acute abscess, but surgical drainage of a localized disease combined with this therapy seems more rational.

REFERENCES

Almour, H.: Surgery of Suppurative Petrositis. In: Kopetsky, S. J.: Surgery of the Ear. New York, Thomas Nelson & Sons, 1947.

Boies, L. R.: Acute Mastoiditis: 1931–1941. Ann. Otol. Rhin. & Laryng., *51:*60, 1942.

Boies, L. R.: Lateral Sinus Thrombosis: Review of One Hundred and Eighty-four Cases. *Ibid., 41:*227, 1932.

Boies, L. R.: Extradural Inflammation; A Study of Its Occurrence in Acute Surgical Mastoiditis. Tr. Am. Acad. Ophth. & Otolaryng., *41:*150, 1936.

Fowler, E. P., Jr., and Swenson, P. A.: Petrositis—A Roentgenologic and Pathologic Correlation. Am. J. Roentgenol., *41:*317, 1939.

Kopetsky, S.: Otogenic Meningitis. In: Fowler, E. P., Jr.: Medicine of the Ear. New York, Thomas Nelson & Sons, 1947.

Lempert, J.: Complete Apicectomy: New Technic for Complete Exenteration of Apical Carotid Portion of Petrous Pyramid. Arch. Otolaryng., *25:144*, 1937.

Lillie, H.: The Surgery of Sepsis of Otitic Origin. In: Kopetsky, S. J.: Surgery of the Ear. New York, Thomas Nelson & Sons, 1947.

Lillie, H. I.: Suppuration of the Temporal Bone Accompanied by Infection of the Blood Stream. Arch. Otolaryng., *18:*630, 1933.

Meltzer, P. E.: Treatment of Thrombosis of the Lateral Sinus. *Ibid., 22:*131, 1935.

Rosenwasser, H.: Thrombophlebitis of the Lateral Sinus. *Ibid., 41:*117, 1945.

CHAPTER VIII

TINNITUS

CHARLES E. CONNOR, M.D.

Definition. Tinnitus is a sound originating in the body of the patient and heard by himself, the observer, or both. Sounds physiologic in origin, such as those attending mastication or swallowing, are not considered tinnitus; those which are the result of pathologic conditions or processes are true tinnitus.

It is a very common symptom found in many conditions.

TYPES OF TINNITUS

Tinnitus may be periotic, arising about the ear, or entotic, arising within the ear; it may be internal, arising within the cochlea, or external, arising without the cochlea. Its origin may be central to the terminal hair cells, in the auditory nerve, spiral ganglion, or cerebral centers, or peripheral in the ductus cochlearis, scala tympani or scala vestibuli. It may be subjective, heard only by the patient, or objective, heard by the observer, or both. It may be vibratory or nonvibratory, caused by irritative or degenerative changes in the hair cells, the auditory nerve, spiral ganglion, or cerebral centers.

CAUSES OF VIBRATORY TINNITUS

Muscular. Tinnitus, being a symptom and not a disease, calls for search for its cause. Vibratory tinnitus depends upon the origin in and transmission through the tissues of the body of vibrations; these vibrations may originate in the muscles of the eustachian tube, the tensor veli palatini and levator veli palatini, and cause faint crackling sounds, or they may be caused by the contraction and relaxation of the intratympanic muscles, the tensor tympani and stapedius. Such action of the tympanic muscles, caused reflexly by sensory stimuli such as sudden variation in the intensity of sound, produces a faint fluttering sound and sensation. Rhythmic contraction of the palatopharyngeal musculature may not only be visible but also heard by the patient (and occasionally by the observer) as a regular clicking sound; the sounds arising from the action of the muscles of chewing and deglutition are always heard by a normal person when he is attentive to them. Patients with cervical arthritis may not only feel but also hear the grating of the cervical vertebrae when the head is turned. These sounds, with the exception of those caused by idiopathic rhythmic contractions of the palatal and pharyngeal musculature, are physiologic and heard by normal persons; they do not constitute tinnitus in the exact definition of the word.

Cardiovascular. The cardiovascular system is frequently responsible for tinnitus. Patients not only feel but hear their pulse in the ear when it becomes accentuated as the result of sudden pressure changes; they describe a faint throbbing sound synchronous with the pulse. This may be either physiologic or pathologic, depending on the cause of the change in pressure.

Temporary changes in blood pressure, such as elevation after violent exercise or depression attendant on syncope, may cause tinnitus, as may permanent changes in pressure, the elevation of hypertension, or the depression of exhaustion and debilitation. Change in pressure is more apt to produce tinnitus than is an evenly sustained level.

Tinnitus originating in the blood stream is apt to be humming, rushing, or roaring in quality; if of arterial origin, it has a rhythmic or pulsating character, while that originating in the venous stream is a regularly sustained sound, the so-called "venous hum."

Various pathologic conditions in this system may be responsible for tinnitus; among these are arteriovenous aneurysm, dilated blood sinuses in the dura, valvular lesions, and blood changes such as anemia resulting in the so-called "hemic murmur."

Anatomic variations may be responsible for tinnitus. The internal carotid artery in its course through the temporal bone may be close enough to the cochlea so that the flow of blood is perceived by the internal ear; the same thing occurs when the jugular bulb bears an unusually close relation to the cochlea.

CAUSES OF NONVIBRATORY TINNITUS

Biochemical Changes. Nonvibratory tinnitus is caused not by vibrations reaching the cochlea from sources elsewhere in the body but by biochemical changes occurring in the nerve mechanism of hearing, usually irritative or degenerative in type, such as the degeneration responsible for the deafness and tinnitus of presbycusis or that caused by absorption of toxins from sources such as acute or chronic infection, metabolic disturbances such as diabetes, or endocrine disturbances such as hyperthyroidism. It may result from the ingestion of drugs and chemicals such as quinine and the salicylates; from the prolonged use of alcohol and tobacco; and from substances such as arsenic, lead, phosphorus, carbon monoxide, carbon bisulfide, morphine, atropine and aniline dyes. Theoretically, any substance to which the nerve tissue of the auditory mechanism is sensitive may cause nonvibratory tinnitus.

Head Trauma. Nonvibratory tinnitus may occur as the result of head trauma. The pathologic changes may consist of swelling, hemorrhage, laceration, or even disintegration of the delicate nerve structures within the cochlea; fracture through the latter structure is often present.

The same changes may be seen in the auditory nerve in severe cases; autopsy studies have revealed edema and hemorrhage in the cerebral auditory centers in cases of concussion and skull fracture. Long-continued noise, especially when of great intensity, acts as trauma and may cause degenerative changes in the organ of Corti where sounds of like pitch, usually in the upper register, are perceived; these changes are responsible for impaired hearing for high tones and for high-pitched ringing tinnitus seen in patients, such as boiler makers, operators of punch machines and air hammers, and aviators, who have been long employed in noisy environments.

Disease in Ear. Diseases within the ear itself, by disturbing the circulation or pressure within the labyrinth, may cause nonvibratory tinnitus. In the external ear, foreign bodies, such as impacted cerumen, or marked inflammatory processes may be a cause; in the middle ear, either acute inflammatory or chronic adhesive processes or metaplastic bone changes, especially in the region of the round or oval windows with fixation of these structures, may be responsible. The latter changes are seen in otosclerosis, which is often accompanied by tinnitus of great intensity and long duration.

Changes within the acoustic labyrinth itself, congestion, anemia, edema and hemorrhage may be responsible; labyrinthine hydrops (Ménière's disease) is often attended by severe intermittent tinnitus which may be the first of the three diagnostic symptoms, deafness, tinnitus and vertigo, to make its appearance. The pathologic change in this condition is an edema, possibly of a physical allergic origin, in the ductus cochlearis.

Nervous System Diseases. Tumors of the acoustic nerve and of the cerebellopontine angle may, by pressure, cause tinnitus, as may various diseases of the central nervous system involving the auditory nerve and cerebral auditory tracts and centers, such as syringomyelia, disseminated sclerosis and multiple sclerosis. Tinnitus may be present in various psychoses and neuroses and increase the gravity of the prognosis, especially when it takes the form of organized phrases, sentences, or musical strains, as in patients who hear voices or music.

TREATMENT

From this brief consideration it becomes evident that tinnitus is but a symptom of a large number of conditions, not only in the ear itself but also elsewhere in the body; tinnitus is frequently the first warning of a beginning hearing impairment. The treatment of tinnitus, therefore, is the treatment or removal of its cause. A review of the various suggested treatments indicates at once that there is no universally satisfactory treatment; each of the long array of suggested therapeutic measures has been reported as effective in some cases but has failed when given broader application. This means that the treatment of tinnitus is more often than not difficult and unsatisfactory, either because we cannot discover its cause or, having discovered the cause, we can do nothing about it. Tinnitus frequently fails to respond to long-continued and intelligent treatment, only to disappear spontaneously and for no known reason or following the correction of some apparently unrelated condition.

Characteristics of Tinnitus. There are several characteristics of tinnitus, explanation of which helps in understanding its clinical behavior. Its intensity is increased by anything which increases the bone conduction of sounds to the ear in which it is heard, such as impacted cerumen, acute otitis media, chronic adhesive otitis media, or otosclerosis; its intensity is diminished by external sounds, especially those near its own pitch. Tinnitus audible at night may not be heard in the noise of daily occupation; it may increase hearing impairment for sounds of its own pitch. Tinnitus may be attended by the illusion that it is of much greater intensity than is really the case; patients frequently complain bitterly of the loudness of the noise in their ears when audiometric measurement shows it to be of relatively low decibel intensity.

The nerve mechanism of hearing is, phylogenetically, one of the youngest tissues in the body and therefore is one of the first to reflect through impaired function deleterious influences, whether local or general; it follows from this that tinnitus, representing functional activity of the nerve mechanism of hearing, is diminished by anything that promotes the general health and well-being, both physical and mental, of the patient, and is increased by anything that has a deleterious effect upon his well-being. Disease in any part of the body, overwork, lack of fresh air and exercise, insufficient sleep, nervous fatigue and, especially, anxiety and worry increase tinnitus; good health and hygiene, as evidenced by proper balance between work and play, plenty of sleep, fresh air, exercise and good food, and absence of nervous tension and anxiety tend to lessen tinnitus.

Attitude of Physician. The attitude of the physician toward the patient with tinnitus and the reaction of the patient toward his symptom are important. Tinnitus can become so overwhelming that it dominates the entire life of the patient, colors his conscious attitudes and influences his subconscious reactions; fortunately, this is not usually the case, but the symptom is always important enough to assure the patient the sympathetic and understanding attention of the physician. It is a mistake, not only in the science but also in the art of medicine, to ignore tinnitus and to create the impression that the physician is not sufficiently interested in the patient and his problem to make a serious attempt to help him. It is also a mistake to evidence undue solicitude and thus increase the patient's anxious concentration upon his symptom so that he can think of nothing else. Best results will be obtained by making the patient feel that everything possible is being done for his tinnitus while encouraging him to ignore it as completely as possible; this is important because many cases of tinnitus cannot be helped medically and the patient's only relief lies in his control of his own reaction to it.

Study of Patient. Complete study of the patient, comprising not only his physical and psychologic nature but also his hygiene of living, should be made. Any abnormal condition or infection in the ears, nose, throat, or teeth should be corrected. Eustachian tube obstruction, especially that caused by acute head infection, may cause tinnitus but has a definite tendency to spontaneous resolution; it is helped by inflation; the aspiration of the middle ear fluid in acute serous otitis media which does not clear spontaneously may improve the attendant tinnitus. Improvement of the tinnitus following the repeated use of inflation, applicators, or bougies in chronic tubal obstruction is at best limited and temporary but seems to benefit some patients. Infected lymphoid masses in or near the pharyngeal orifice of the eustachian tube should be removed either surgically or by postnasal radiation. Marked retroversion or malocclusion of the lower jaw, the so-called "closed bite," caused by loss of opposing molars, may interfere with tubal function by backward pressure of the ascending ramus of the mandible and should be corrected as far as possible by the use of dentures.

Drugs. Innumerable drugs have been tried, none universally satisfactory. Among these are sedatives such as bromides and the barbiturates which lessen the general nerve irritability and so make the tinnitus more endurable, iodides, calcium, atropine, vasodilators such as histamine and nicotinic acid, in vogue at the present time, caffeine, theobromine, endocrine preparations, strychinine, vitamin B complex, insulin, and intravenous injections of procaine hydrochloride (novocaine); none of these can be relied upon to give relief, but all may be tried.

Surgical Measures. Various types of surgical treatment have been tried with varying degrees of success; lumbar puncture to lower the intralabyrinthine pressure and alcohol injection of the sphenopalatine ganglion and stellate ganglionectomy in an effort to influence the tinnitus by reflex have yielded indifferent results. Obliteration of the membranous labyrinth by alcohol injection or electrocoagulation for the relief of vertigo may also help tinnitus but at the expense of loss of hearing. Section of the vestibular nerve for relief of vertigo in endolymphatic hydrops (Ménière's disease) has been reported as relieving the tinnitus in about 50 per cent of the patients; when it persists, it is attributed to degenerative changes in the central end of the severed nerve. In view of the present concept of this disease, such a procedure does not seem logical.

Resection of the tympanic plexus in the mucous membrane of the promontory of the mesial wall of the middle ear, tympanosympathectomy (Lempert) may bring relief in tinnitus associated with chronic adhesive processes of the middle ear. Fenestration of the horizontal canal for the relief of deafness in otosclerosis and chronic adhesive processes with stapedial fixation but with well-functioning nerve mechanism effects relief of tinnitus paralleling the improvement in hearing.

REFERENCES

Atkinson, Miles: Tinnitus Aurium. Ann. Otol., Rhin. & Laryng., *53:*742, 1944.

Atkinson, Miles: Tinnitus Aurium. Arch. Otolaryng., *45:*68, 1947.

Fowler, E. P.: Control of Head Noises—Their Illusions of Loudness and of Timbre. *Ibid.*, *37:*391, 1943.

Fowler, E. P.: Head Noises and Deafness: Peripheral and Central. Laryngoscope, *49:*1011, 1939.

Fowler, E. P.: Head Noises in Normal and in Disordered Ears. Arch. Otolaryng., *39:*498, 1944.

Fowler, E. P.: Nonvibratory Tinnitus. *Ibid.*, *47:*29, 1948.

Fowler, E. P.: The Emotional Factor in Tinnitus Aurium. Laryngoscope, *58:*145, 1948.

Fowler, E. P.: Tinnitus Aurium in the Light of Recent Research. Ann. Otol., Rhin. & Laryng., *50:*139, 1941.

Haydon, D. B., and Chainski, E. L.: Tinnitus: Etiology and Treatment. *Ibid.*, *48:*443, 1939.

Lempert, J.: A Surgical Technic for the Relief of Tinnitus Aurium. Arch. Otolaryng., *43:*199, 1946.

CHAPTER IX

VERTIGO

CHARLES E. CONNOR, M.D.

Definition. Vertigo is the cerebral sensation resulting from disturbance of equilibrium, the normal relation of the patient to his environment, or his normal position in space.

Incidence. Vertigo is a symptom, not a disease, of a great number of disorders and is a very common complaint. Whatever its cause, character, or intensity, it is the result of disturbed function of the vestibular apparatus, the end-organ, tracts, or cortical centers. Vertigo varies in intensity from the very slight disturbances of equilibrium described by patients as lightheadedness, giddiness, fainting sensation, balloonheadedness, head floating off shoulders, swimming sensation in head, to the severe disturbances of seeming rotation attended by spontaneous manifestations such as nystagmus, past pointing, falling and vasomotor disturbances.

EQUILIBRIUM

Equilibrium is a complex state in which three factors are important; the eyes, because they give visual evidence of any disturbance of the normal relation of the person to his environment; the skin, deep muscle, joint, visceral sense, because it records any disturbance in the normal relationship of these structures; and the vestibular labyrinth itself, always in a state of tonus resulting from constant stimulation from the other two factors and constantly recording linear and rotational movement of the patient himself. Equilibrium can be reasonably well maintained if two of these three functions are active; the blind man with normal labyrinth and intact skin, joint, and deep muscle sense has no trouble and the tabetic person with normal eyes and labyrinth has no disturbance of equilibrium. The patient with dead labyrinths but with good vision and normal joint and deep muscle sensation does very well after compensation for the loss of labyrinthine function has been established. But the blind person who develops tabes or whose labyrinths are nonfunctioning will have trouble maintaining his balance, as will the tabetic person who tries to walk in the dark or the person with dead labyrinths who develops blindness or tabes.

The labyrinths are in constant and very delicately balanced activity, the functional result of which is equilibrium; if the activity of either labyrinth is increased, diminished or destroyed, equilibrium is impossible until the other labyrinth, aided by vision and skin, joint, deep muscle and visceral sense, compensates for the loss and re-establishes equilibrium; such re-established equilibrium is never as stable as that present in the normal person.

ANATOMY OF THE VESTIBULAR APPARATUS

The auditory nerve has two divisions: the acoustic, the function of which is hearing, and the end-organ the cochlea; and |the vestibular, the function of which is the maintenance of equilibrium and the end-organ the vestibular labyrinth. This latter structure is composed of two separate end-organs; the kinetic labyrinth, or semicircular canals, for the perception of angular motion, rotation; and the static labyrinth formed of the utricle and saccule, for the perception of linear motion and of tilting or change of posture.

Each membranous labyrinth consists of three semicircular canals, conforming to the shape of the bony semicircular canals but much smaller, and two sacs in the bony vestibule, the utricle and the saccule. The saccule is joined to the ductus cochlearis by a small canal, the ductus reuniens, and by a duct to a similar structure of the utricle, the two uniting to form the ductus endolymphaticus; this pierces the inner wall of the bony vestibule and terminates in a subdural dilatation, the saccus endolymphaticus, on the posterior surface of the petrous bone. It is considered a drainage outlet for the endolymph. The entire membranous labyrinth is surrounded by perilymph.

Both ends of each semicircular canal, one ampullated and containing the end-organ, the crista and cupula, join the utricle, thus making the canal functionally a complete circle and currents in the contained endolymph possible.

Each vestibular labyrinth consists of three canals, the horizontal, which is actually 30 degrees above the horizontal plane, the superior, roughly bisecting the angle between frontal and sagittal plane anteriorly, and the posterior, bisecting the same angle posteriorly. Each canal is at right angles to the other two so that motion in any plane is perceived; maximal stimulation of any canal is produced by motion in the plane in which it lies.

Nerves. The nerves from the cristae of the semicircular canals and the maculae of the utricle and saccule proceed through the vestibular nerve in the internal auditory meatus, where the vestibular ganglion, Scarpa's, is located, and from thence to the medulla where the fibers either directly or by collaterals enter the vestibular nuclei, the medial, the spinal, the lateral, or Deiters', and the superior, or Bechterew's. From this point, the pattern of distribution of the nerve fibers becomes very widespread, and at some points not too well known. Pathways go to the eye muscle nuclei through the posterior longitudinal bundle for the transmission of afferent and efferent impulses having to do with the recognition and correction of abnormal changes in the posture and movement of the body musculature. There is intimate association with the vagus centers controlling such vasomotor phenomena as syncope, pallor, sweating, nausea and vomiting.

PHYSIOLOGY OF THE VESTIBULAR APPARATUS

Both vestibular labyrinths considered as one unit are composed of three synergistically functioning pairs of canals. These are the two horizontal canals, and the superior canal of each side with the posterior canal of the opposite side; the plane of any pair of canals, as in the case of individual canals of each labyrinth, is at right angles to the planes of the other pairs of canals so that motion in any plane is recorded. It is not possible to stimulate one canal or one pair of canals to the entire exclusion of the other canals.

Each functionally synergistic pair of canals is maximally stimulated by rotation in its own plane when the maximum flow of endolymph occurs; the farther the axis of rotation departs from the perpendicular to the plane of rotation, the less is the flow of endolymph and the weaker the stimulation. It is possible for a canal to be stimulated by rotation about an axis lying in its own plane, a chord or diameter of the physiologic circle constituted by the canal and vestibule; in this case, stimulation of the canal is considered to result from the development of whorls in the endolymph rather than linear displacement.

The three end-organs: cochlea, semicircular canals and utricle and saccule, are anatomically and physiologically similar; each has a hair cell with supporting tissue and a mechanism for stimulating it.

In the cochlea, the terminal hair cell is activated by the overlying tectorial membrane, a plume-like, gelatinous structure which transmits to the hair cell vibrations of the endolymph of the ductus cochlearis in which it floats. In the ampulla of each semicircular canal the hair cells are found in a specialized epithelium, the crista, which is surmounted by a caplike structure, the cupula, floating in the endolymph of the canal; waves in the endolymph move the cupula and so stimulate the hair cells of the crista which are in contact with its lower surface. The macula of the utricle, which is quadrilateral and approximately in the frontal plane, is an area of specialized epithelium containing hair cells and supporting connective tissue cells; these are overlain with the otolith membrane, a gelatinous mass floating in the endolymph and containing small masses of calcium salts, the otoliths (ear stones), or otoconia. The hair cells are in contact with the lower surface of the otolith membrane and are stimulated by its movement or change in position. The sacular macula has a similar structure and is approximately in the sagittal plane.

ACTIVATION

Semicircular Canals. These are normally stimulated by motion and more especially by change in the rate of motion of the contained endolymph, initiated by angular or rotatory motion of the head or by rocking or lateral movements of the head from motion of the body.

Utricle. The utricle is normally activated by any motion which changes the position of the head with relation to the field of gravity, such as tipping or tilting, or by linear motion forward or backward, none of these involving motion of the head with reference to the body.

Saccule. The function of the saccule is not known sufficiently well at the present time to permit a conclusive statement regarding it; its position, approximately in the sagittal plane, suggests that its function might possibly be that of recording lateral motion of the head not involving motion of the head with relation to the body. Many physicians believe that its function is essentially the same as that of the utricle. Such changes in the position of the head may stimulate the maculae of the utricle and saccule by gross displacement of the otolith membrane over the field of hair cells or by changes in the tension or torque existing between each otolith and the hairs with which it is connected. Endolymph currents and centrifugal force have also been mentioned as inciting agents.

The vestibular apparatus, by which we mean the semicircular canals, the utricles and the saccules, is normally stimulated by motion of the endolymph (some physicists doubt the possibility of mass displacement of the endolymph) and, in the case of the latter structures, by the additional factor of gravity changes. Such stimulation, more or less constant in normal daily life, is utilized in exaggerated intensity in the functional examination of the vestibular mechanism by the caloric (irrigation), the turning, or the electric (galvanic) method. Disease processes, either in the end-organ itself or in its central connections, may initiate reactions, probably biochemical in character, which account for the vertigo seen so frequently in systemic disturbances.

FUNCTION OF VESTIBULAR APPARATUS

The vestibular mechanism responds to stimulation by the exercise of one or both of its functions, sensory and motor. The sensory function registers the disturbance in the normal relationship of the body to its environment by the cerebral reaction which we know as vertigo; the motor function initiates the action of extrinsic eye and body musculature designed to correct such disturbance.

Sensory. If the sensory function alone is disturbed, falling may be in any direction, independent of head position; this is seen in long-absent vestibular function, chronic disease of the central nervous system, such as disseminated sclerosis and syringomyelia, and in chronic cerebellar disease without increased intracranial pressure, such as sclerosis and chronic encephalitis; it may occur in certain acute diseases of the central vestibular system and in hemorrhage.

Motor. When the motor function is disturbed so that the compensatory muscular reactions cannot be effected, falling is definitely related to the accompanying nystagmus and usually occurs in the direction of the slow or vestibular component (opposite the quick component); this type of reaction is seen in acute labyrinthitis and neuritis of the vestibular nerve, the more severe types of peripheral lesion. In acute lesions and tumors of the cerebellar lobes, falling is usually to the diseased side; tumors of the vermis may cause forward falling. In cerebral hemorrhage, encephalitis and acute diseases of the central vestibular system, falling may be independent of head position or in the direction of quick component of the nystagmus.

Maintenance of Visceral Tone. A third function of the vestibular labyrinth is the maintenance of general muscle, joint and visceral tone effected by its own state of constant tonus, the result of intrinsic biochemical processes. Vertigo is the subjective symptom, and nystagmus, past pointing and falling are the objective signs of labyrinthine stimulation.

CLINICAL MANIFESTATIONS OF VESTIBULAR STIMULATION

Rotary Vertigo. Vertigo may take the familiar objective rotary form seen in disseminated sclerosis and cerebellar tumor in which objects seem to rotate about the patient, usually in the horizontal plane, or the subjective form, in which the patient himself rotates, also in the horizontal plane.

Tactile Error. It may be manifested in the form of the so-called "tactile error," occasionally seen in acute suppurative otitis media before drainage, chronic adhesive otitis media, disseminated sclerosis and cerebellar tumor, in which there is mass displacement of large segments of the environment, not in rotation; the floor may rise up, the ceiling appear to descend, the foot of the bed or the feet of the chair may go up.

Lateropulsion. A third form of vertigo is lateropulsion, or lateral deviation in progression seen in chronic adhesive otitis media with secondary inner ear changes and in nonsuppurative disease of the central nervous system such as hydrocephalus, tumor, encephalitis and disseminated sclerosis.

NYSTAGMUS

Nystagmus is an involuntary movement of the eyes, almost always synchronous and associated; rarely, dissociation may be present. The movement may be rhythmic (unequal phases) or oscillatory (equal phases) and either quick or slow; in amplitude, it may be large, medium or small; and in character, horizontal, rotary, mixed, oblique, or vertical. It varies in degree of intensity; first degree nystagmus is that elicited by looking in the direction of its quick component, second degree is that present when the gaze is forward, and third degree is that present when the gaze is directed opposite the quick component. The motion may be to the right, left, up, down, or in an oblique direction.

Peripheral Nystagmus. Peripheral, or labyrinthine, nystagmus may be either horizontal or rotary, more frequently the latter, but also vertical if associated with labyrinthine vertigo; it is rhythmic, increased by looking in the direction of the quick component, and is to the side of greatest stimulation, either by turning or disease. It is accompanied by vertigo in the direction of its quick component and by reaction movements, falling, past pointing and swaying, in the opposite direction; direction of fall may be influenced by head position because of change in the direction of the endolymph flow resulting therefrom. Hearing is almost always affected and tinnitus may be present. Vertigo and reaction movements are proportionate to nystagmus.

Nystagmus Due to Central Lesions. Nystagmus due to a central lesion may be vertical, horizontal, rotary, or oblique and may show not only disharmony between its intensity and that of accompanying reactions such as intense nystagmus with but mild vertigo, but even complete dissociation, such as marked nystagmus with slight or absent cochlear symptoms. Marked nystagmus, either vertical or oblique, without vertigo or reaction movements may occur. Prolonged postrotatory nystagmus with normal cochlear reaction is indicative of a central lesion, as is perverted or inverted nystagmus, conjugate deviation and dissociated movement of the eyes. Nystagmus due to cerebellar lesions is characteristically slow, coarse and often diagonal.

Optical Nystagmus. This nystagmus is oscillatory or mixed, rapid, jerky and never accompanied by true labyrinthine vertigo; it may be in any direction, especially horizontal or vertical. Slight dizziness may occur on attempts at fixation, but disappears when such attempts are abandoned or the eyes are closed. It is caused by high refractive error, corneal opacities, or degenerative disease of the retina, especially in the the region of the fovea and by lesions of the visual tracts.

Physiologic Nystagmus. Fixation nystagmus is caused by attempts to center on the fovea objects in the peripheral field of vision or to keep moving objects centered, as in railroad or elevator nystagmus; it may be horizontal or mixed, oscillatory or jerky, is not attended by vertigo, and is not indicative of any pathologic lesion.

REACTION MOVEMENTS

Past Pointing. Past pointing of the arms, either spontaneous or elicited in functional examination, and the falling reaction as manifested in the response of trunk musculature to intrinsic stimuli or external forces which tend to disturb the normal relation of the person to his environment are the conscious attempts of the patient to correct the disturbance in his environmental relationships caused by vertigo and nystagmus; as such, they are of distinctly less diagnostic import than the completely involuntary disturbances upon which they depend. When they are in accord with other manifestations of disturbed vestibular function, they are of limited value; when they are at variance with other findings, the latter receive the greater emphasis.

Past pointing is performed by bringing the extended arm and forefinger from a resting position on the patient's knee up to touch the extended forefinger of the examiner; failure to do so constitutes past pointing. The eyes are closed.

Quantitative variations in the amplitude of past pointing are of less diagnostic significance than changes in the direction of the reaction, such as perverted past pointing, in which the direction is abnormal, or an inverted past pointing, in which the direction is reversed. A perverted past pointing, when associated with other indications of an intracranial lesion and nystagmus, is indicative of a cerebellar lesion.

The Falling Reaction. The falling reaction is elicited by having the blindfolded patient attempt to walk a straight line or by the Romberg test, eyes being closed and feet together or with heel to toe; if the position of the head influences the direction of fall, this being opposite the quick component of the nystagmus, the lesion is in the labyrinth or vestibular nerve; occasionally, in acute lesions of the central vestibular system, encephalitis or bleeding, the falling is in the direction of the quick component. If the falling is consistently in one direction, not being influenced by the position of the head, the lesion is probably cerebellar, an acute process, abscess, or tumor. If there is no consistent direction of the fall, the vertigo is entirely sensory and without motor disturbance, as pointed out previously.

LAWS OF VESTIBULAR PHYSIOLOGY

The intensity of the past pointing and falling reactions is not an accurate gage of the extent of the peripheral causal lesion. Experimental work and clinical observation have shown that the occurrence of symptoms of vestibular stimulation, nystagmus, vertigo, and the reaction movements of past pointing and falling are governed by well-defined laws of vestibular physiology; since an understanding of these laws is essential to the interpretation of experimental and clinical observations they are stated briefly here.

Vestibular reactions elicited by and during the turning test are not used because of the difficulty of their observations; the reactions which ensue when turning is stopped, postrotational, are studied because of ease of observation. Obviously, they are opposite in direction to the rotational manifestations.

1. The semicircular canals are stimulated by movement, especially change in rate of movement, of the contained endolymph. In the horizontal canals, movement of the endolymph toward the canal side of the

crista is twice as effective as movement toward the utricular side of the crista; in the vertical canals, the reverse is true (Ewald's first law).

2. The more strongly stimulated crista produces vertigo and nystagmus toward its own side and reaction movements, past pointing and falling, toward the opposite side. The more weakly stimulated crista produces vertigo and nystagmus to the opposite side and reaction movements to the same side (Ewald's second law).

3. Primary vestibular reactions are vertigo and nystagmus; secondary reactions, depending on vertigo and containing an element of cerebration are past pointing and falling.

4. The plane of nystagmus is the plane of the canal stimulated. Horizontal nystagmus results from stimulation of the horizontal canal, rotary nystagmus (eyes rotate about pupillary axis) from stimulation of the vertical canals (frontal plane) (Flourens' law).

5. Nystagmus due to rotation is always in a plane at right angles to the axis of rotation, irrespective of the position of the head (Arellano).

6. Nystagmus is always in the direction opposite to the rotation.

7. The direction of nystagmus is that of its quick component.

8. Nystagmus and vertigo are in the same direction (except in face-up position).

9. Nystagmus and vertigo are in the same plane.

10. The plane of reaction movements is that of the vertigo.

11. The direction of reaction movements is opposite to that of the vertigo and nystagmus.

12. The intensity of reaction movements is proportionate to that of the vertigo.

13. The duration of postrotatory vertigo is approximately that of postrotatory nystagmus.

VESTIBULAR REACTIONS

After Turning. A patient, with head tipped 30 degrees forward from the erect position to bring the horizontal canals into the horizontal plane and with eyes closed, is turned to the right ten times in twenty seconds; when the chair is suddenly stopped, the patient has horizontal nystagmus to the left, he has a subjective sensation of turning to the left, and he past points and falls to the right.

When the chair starts turning, lag of the endolymph in the canal causes its relative flow to the left in each canal; the canal side of the crista of the right canal will be stimulated, the strong response causing reaction to the same (right side) and the utricular side of the crista of the left canal will be stimulated, the weak response causing reaction to the opposite (right) side. Both canals cause reaction to the side of turning and the patient has nystagmus and vertigo to the right, and reaction movements, falling and pointing, to the left. These are the reactions of rotation.

After a certain number of turns, perhaps ten, the endolymph lag is overcome and endolymph and canal walls move at the same rate: the patient has no nystagmus and no vertigo. He seems to be sitting still in the chair.

When the chair is suddenly stopped, inertia again is responsible for a current in the endolymph in the direction of turning (right). This current stimulates the canal side of the crista in the left canal, the strong stimulus causing reaction to the same or left side; in the right canal, the utricular side of the crista is stimulated, the weak stimulus causing reaction to the opposite, or left, side. The stimuli from both canals produce reaction to the left side and the patient will have horizontal nystagmus and vertigo to the left and reaction movements, past pointing and falling, to the right.

These reactions are reversed in the vertical canals because of the reversal of direction of the reactions caused by stimulation of the canal and utricular sides of the cristae. In the horizontal canals, stimulation of the canal side of the crista by the endolymph current produces a stronger reaction than does stimulation of the utricular side; in the vertical canals, the reverse is true. In both cases, the stronger stimulus produces reaction to the same side, the weaker reaction to the opposite side.

After Douching. The reactions following cold caloric irrigation of the right ear may be explained as follows. It is to be remembered that the superior vertical canal is 45 degrees anterior to the coronal plane passing through the crus commune, the canal common to both the superior and posterior vertical canals; the posterior vertical canal is 45 degrees posterior to the same coronal plane. An understanding of the effects of turning or irrigation upon the vertical canals is facilitated by considering them as one vertical canal lying in the coronal plane.

Cold water irrigation of the right ear, with head erect, causes a flow of the endolymph from above downward, a convection current due to chilling of the endolymph. This causes a current in the endolymph toward the canal side of the crista, which, in the case of the vertical canals, elicits the weak response, with reactions always to the opposite side. The nystagmus will be to the left, in the frontal plane and hence rotary; the vertigo will be to the left and reaction movements, past pointing and falling, to the right.

VESTIBULAR EXAMINATION

There are three methods of vestibular examination: the caloric, the rotation, and the galvanic.

Caloric Tests. Cold water is generally used in the caloric test, as the vasomotor reactions following irrigation with hot water are often disagreeable and hard to control. Water 13° C. (55° F.) may be used in small amounts, 5 and 10 cc., with head erect (Fig. 55), noting the latent period of time required for appearance of the nystagmus, its duration and character. It should be a rotary nystagmus to the opposite side. Vertigo is also to the opposite side and reaction movements to the same side. If results are inconclusive, the head may be tipped back 60 degrees to test the horizontal canals (now in the vertical plane); larger amounts of water, 25 to 100 cc., may be used.

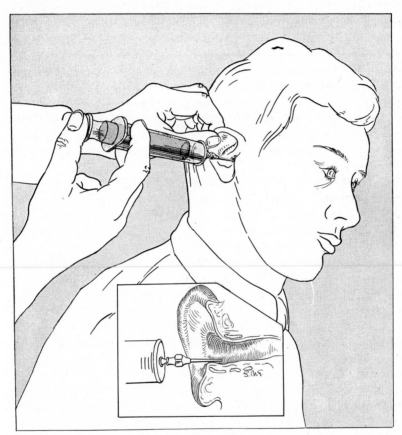

Fig. 55. A simple method of testing the vestibular reaction is accomplished with the use of cold water in small amounts injected against the ear drum. First, 5 or 10 cc. of water at 55° F. are used, with head erect, noting the latent period or time required for appearance of the nystagmus to the opposite side. Vertigo is also to the opposite side and reaction movements to the same side. If results are inconclusive, the head may be tipped back 60 degrees to test the horizontal canals (now in the vertical plane); larger amounts of water, 25 to 100 cc., may be used.

Mass irrigation with large amounts of warmer water, 20° C. (68° F.), may be used; the latent time and duration of response is measured. Vasomotor reactions may be marked.

Reactions are obtained with great regularity when the head is tipped back because the horizontal canals, which are most easily affected by thermal changes because of their anatomical location, are stimulated in this position; the vertical canals, more deeply situated in the petrous bone, are not so easily affected by temperature changes and their reactions are not so regularly induced. The caloric method of testing is the most commonly used because it permits examination of each labyrinth separately; when care is used, vasomotor reactions are not excessive.

Turning Tests. Turning may be carried out with any type of rotating chair, although a chair especially designed for the purpose facilitates the examination. The patient is turned in both directions with the head in various positions, erect, forward, backward, or on either shoulder, and the postrotatory nystagmus, vertigo and reaction movements are studied; in a normal patient, these should all fall within a fairly normal pattern. Turning tests both labyrinths at the same time, and for this reason is useful for determining the degree of compensation which has been established after partial or complete unilateral loss of function; unless performed in a leisurely manner, marked vasomotor symptoms may be produced.

Galvanic Tests. The galvanic tests are less commonly employed, possibly because of the equipment required, but also because the caloric, and if necessary, the turning tests give all necessary information. Each side is examined separately, first with the cathode, which stimulates, and the anode, which depresses, vestibular function. Galvanism tests not only the vestibular end-organ itself but also the vestibular nerve; a positive reaction to galvanism may be obtained in the presence of a dead labyrinth because it comes from the vestibular nerve. A negative galvanic response indicates a nonfunctioning nerve.

Evaluation of the Tests. In evaluating these tests, it is well to remember that vestibular reactions depend on the functioning of a very complex nervous mechanism which is easily influenced by many different conditions and circumstances, both intrinsic and extrinsic. Minor variations in quantitative characteristics, such as duration of nystagmus or extent of past pointing, are common and usually are of no great importance; they may not be present on retesting. Definite qualitative variations from normal, such as wrong type of nystagmus or wrong direction of nystagmus or past pointing, are usually constant and significant of a pathologic lesion in the vestibular system. Final conclusions should not be drawn from one examination, especially if abnormal responses are obtained; only when such responses are repeatedly present and have been correlated with all other findings should their diagnostic significance be determined.

PATHOGENESIS

Vertigo is a symptom which occurs in a great many diseases of the ear itself, of its central nervous system ramifications, or of other organs or tissues; it must be correlated with other physical findings in arriving at a diagnosis.

Lesions of External and Middle Ear. Most of the aural causes for vertigo are in the internal ear, but some are found in both the external and middle ear. Cerumen impacted against the drum may increase middle ear pressure which is transmitted through the oval window to the inner ear. Acute otitis media may cause congestion in the inner ear, or retained secretions may cause pressure with resultant vertigo. Chronic adhesive middle ear processes may interfere with the mobility of the ossicular chain, especially of the stapes, and obstruction of the eustachian tube may cause absorption of the air in the middle ear; both may influence the pressure on the perilymph of the inner ear and so cause dizziness. Otosclerosis, by interfering with the mobility of the stapes, and too vigorous inflation of the ear, by increasing middle ear pressure, may do the same. The compression and decompression of caisson workers, if hurried, may cause dizziness by influencing pressure on the perilymph.

Lesions of Inner Ear. The various types of labyrinthitis, serous, suppurative, acute, chronic, circumscribed, diffuse, latent, manifest, usually develop the symptom of vertigo at some point in their course. Infection may reach the inner ear through the round or oval window, vascular channels and fistulas in the mesial wall of the middle ear, or the internal auditory meatus by extension from a suppurative meningitis. Head injury, concussion and skull fracture through the petrous pyramid, by edema, congestion, hemorrhage, or even laceration and disintegration of the epithelial end-organ, frequently causes vertigo. Degenerative processes in the labyrinth caused by long-continued absorption of toxins or by pressure on the vestibular nerve may do the same. Syphilis, acquired or congenital, may be the causal factor.

Lesions of the Vestibular Nerve. Neuritis from whatever source, toxic or inflammatory, pressure with atrophy and degeneration from tumors in the cerebellopontine angle and syphilis may be mentioned.

Diseases of Central Nervous System. Diseases of the central vestibular tracts may cause vertigo; disseminated sclerosis, syringobulbia, syringomyelia, tabes, encephalitis and syphilis are to be considered, as is pressure transmitted from a space occupying lesion, abscess, tumor, hydrocephalus, or a generalized increase in intracranial pressure.

Systemic Disease. The labyrinth may be affected by changes in blood pressure, by diseases of the blood and by products of disease in other organs and tissues carried by the circulation. Vertigo may be caused by the hypertension of arteriosclerosis, the hypotension of shock, the anemia of syncope, the plethora of polycythemia vera, and by hemorrhage, thrombus and embolus. The toxemia of any severe acute infection, such as scarlet fever, measles, cerebrospinal meningitis, malaria and influenza, or long-continued absorption from a localized chronic infection may cause labyrinthine symptoms. Toxic neuritis due to absorption of drugs and chemicals such as alcohol, tobacco, quinine, the salicylates, mercury, lead, arsenic, caffeine and amyl nitrate often causes vertigo, as do the products of metabolic disturbances attendant on systemic diseases, such as nephritis, diabetes, pernicious anemia, chlorosis, syphilis and intestinal disorders. Leukemic deposits in the labyrinth may cause profound disturbance. Vasomotor changes incident to emotional or psychotic disturbances occasionally cause dizziness.

TREATMENT

The treatment of vertigo may be as simple as removing a mass of cerumen from the external canal or inflating a blocked eustachian tube, or it may present a problem the solution of which calls for complete diagnostic studies and the exercise of experienced judgment.

Pathologic processes in the ear itself should be corrected so far as possible, as should all abnormalities in the nose, accessory sinuses, teeth and tonsils. Any deviation from normal in the patient's general physical condition and his hygiene of living should be rectified and every effort made to bring him into perfect physical condition. This involves treatment of all local or systemic conditions present which are recognized as possible causes of vertigo; the cooperation of those engaged in almost any field of medicine, the internist, the neurologist and the ophthalmologist, may be essential. There is no universally applicable treatment or cure for vertigo; its treatment is that of its cause, whatever that may be.

ENDOLYMPHATIC HYDROPS (MÉNIÈRE'S DISEASE)

Special mention should be made of a disease entity upon which much light has been thrown in the last decade.

In 1861, a French writer named Ménière described the fatal illness, attended by deafness, vertigo, and vomiting, of a young girl in whom postmortem studies revealed a sanguinous fluid that was interpreted as hemorrhage in the semicircular canals and vestibule; he later amplified this report by the addition of nine case histories showing deafness, tinnitus and vertigo. This triad of symptoms became known as "Ménière's disease" or, more properly, "Ménière's symptom complex" and included all such cases in which the pathologic cause was unknown. Only in the last decade have postmortem studies shown the cause of this clinical entity to be a hydrops of the endolymphatic system, especially of the ductus cochlearis (Fig. 56), although the utricle, saccule and ductus reuniens may also be involved. Degenerative changes have been found in the maculae, cristae and spiral ganglion. The term "endolymphatic hydrops" more properly describes the pathologic changes responsible for the symptoms.

Etiology. The cause of the hydrops is not definitely known. Altered permeability of capillary walls owing to intrinsic physical allergy has been advanced in explanation and seems to find some support in the therapeutic results obtained from nicotinic acid and histamine. Evidence points to some type of vasomotor disturbance as the underlying factor.

Incidence. The condition is common. It is characterized by sudden irregularly recurring attacks of vertigo, usually rotatory and, if severe, accompanied by nystagmus and the falling reaction (inability to stand or walk); if of slight intensity, only a swaying sensation or feeling of weakness may be present. Increased hearing impairment and tinnitus or intensification of a pre-existing tinnitus are often present, and vasomotor symptoms, nausea, vomiting and sweating, may occur in severe cases.

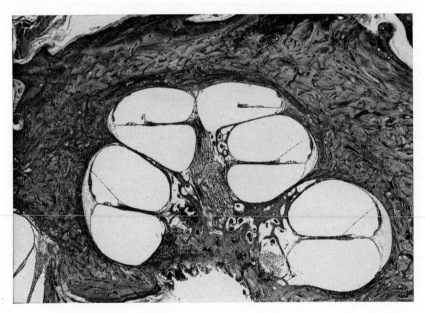

Fig. 56A

Fig. 56. Midmodiolar sections of both cochleas in a case of unilateral Ménière's disease in a man, aged forty-seven. Death from subdural hematoma resulting from a fall during an attack of vertigo.

A. Horizontal section of right cochlea showing a normal cochlear duct. (The defects in Reissner's membrane in the apical coil are artefacts.) The number of ganglion cells and nerve fibers in the spiral ganglion of the basal coil is reduced. Extravasated red blood cells are present in the internal meatus and modiolus, the result of the head injury.

Diagnosis. There are no physical findings pathognomonic of endolymphatic hydrops, and diagnosis may often be based upon a history of attacks. Functional tests usually reveal hearing impairment in the affected ear; vestibular tests may be normal or show depressed or absent function. Before a diagnosis of endolymphatic hydrops can be established, all other causes of vertigo, such as labyrinthitis, cardiovascular disease, or lesions of the central nervous system must be ruled out.

Treatment. Medical treatment based upon the theory of retention of fluid or of sodium ions as the causative factor has taken the form of *restriction of fluids, salt-free* and *low sodium diets,* and the substitution of *ammonium chloride* or a *potassium salt* for sodium chloride; these methods have had some success but often fail. Daily intravenous administration of histamine for three weeks or more and the intramuscular and oral use of nicotinic acid, both treatments based upon the theory of allergenic cause of the physical type, have been reported as giving good results and are the medical treatments of choice at the present time.

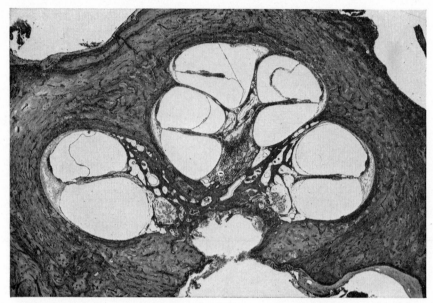

Fig. 56B

B. Vertical section of the left cochlea. The cochlear duct is moderately dilated throughout, almost filling the vestibular scala and extending into the helicotrema.

The spiral ganglion of the basal coil shows a reduction from the normal in number of nerve cells and fibers.

The organ of Corti shows moderate postmortem degeneration in both ears but is sufficiently well preserved to indicate that the antemortem condition was approximately the same histologically in both ears. Remnants of the hair cells are seen throughout all coils in both ears and the stria vascularis is similar in both. (Lindsay, J. R.: Arch. Otolaryng., *39.* Monograph on Ménière's Disease. Published by the American Academy of Ophthalmology and Otolaryngology.)

Surgical treatment should be considered for patients who have not responded to medical treatment and who must have relief from their vertigo. Various procedures have been tried, including *destruction of the saccus endolymphaticus, fractional division of the vestibular portion of auditory nerve, alcohol injection of the labyrinth* through the round window, *avulsion of the membranous labyrinth* through the fenestrated horizontal semicircular canal and, in recent years, *electrocoagulation* of the same structure through the same approach. The latter procedure, permanently relieves the vertigo. Hearing almost always impaired, may be wholly destroyed. Electrocoagulation is the method of choice at the present time in America, but is indicated only in cases in which one ear is involved, medical therapy has failed, and in which the patient is incapacitated by the disease.

REFERENCES

Baumoel, S., and Marks, M. I.: Evaluation of Vertigo Following Head Injuries· Arch. Otolaryng., 33:204, 1941.

Cawthorne, T. E.: Ménière's Disease. Ann. Otol., Rhin. & Laryng., 56:18, 1947.

Cawthorne, T. E.: The Treatment of Ménière's Disease. J. Laryng. & Otol., 58:363, 1943.

Dandy, W. E.: The Surgical Treatment of Ménière's Disease. Surg., Gynec. & Obst., 72:421, 1941.

Day, K. M.: Hydrops of Labyrinth (Ménière's Disease), Diagnosis and Results of Labyrinth Surgery. Laryngoscope, 56:33, 1946.

Furstenberg, A. C., Lashmet, F. H., and Lathrop, F.: Ménière's Symptom Complex: Medical Treatment. Ann. Otol., Rhin. & Laryng., 43:1035, 1934.

Hallpike, C. S., and Cairns, H.: Observations on the Pathology of Ménière's Syndrome. J. Laryng. & Otol., 53:625, 1938.

Lindsay, J. R.: Labyrinthine Dropsy and Ménière's Disease. Arch. Otolaryng., 35:853, 1942.

Lindsay, J. R.: Ménière's Disease. Monograph published by the American Academy of Ophthalmology & Otolaryngology, 1947.

Mygind, S. H., and Dederding, D.: Ménière's Disease as an Indicator of Disturbances in the Water Metabolism, Capillary Function and Body Condition. Ann. Otol., Rhin. & Laryng., 47:55, 1938.

Mygind, S. H., and Dederding, D.: Clinical Experiments with Reference to the Influence of the Water Metabolism on the Ear. Ibid., 47:360, 1938.

Mygind, S. H., and Dederding, D.: The Diagnosis and Treatment of Ménèire's Disease. Ibid., 47:768, 1938.

Mygind, S. H., and Dederding, D.: The Pathogenesis of Ménière's Disease and of Kindred Conditions in the Ear and the Rest of the Body. Ibid., 47:938, 1938.

Northington, P.: Functional Ear Damage in Head Injury. Surg. Clin. North America, 21:357, 1941.

Portmann, G.: The Saccus Endolymphaticus and an Operation for Draining the same for Relief of Vertigo. J. Laryng. & Otol., 42:809, 1927.

Shelden, C. H., and Horton, B. T.: Treatment of Ménière's Disease with Histamine Administered Intravenously. Proc. Staff Meet., Mayo Clin., 15:17, 1940.

Simonton, K. M.: Ménière's Symptom Complex: A Review of the Literature. Ann. Otol., Rhin. & Laryng., 49:80, 1940.

Simonton, K. M.: The Symptom of Dizziness: Its Significance in General Practice. Proc. Staff Meet., Mayo Clin., 16:465, 1941.

Symposium on Vertigo. Tr. Am. Acad. Ophth. & Otolaryng., (Nov.-Dec.), p. 27, 1941.

Talbott, J. H., and Brown, M. R.: Ménière's Syndrome. J.A.M.A., 114:125, 1940.

Vertigo—Symposium Before the American Otological Society. Ann. Otol., Rhin. & Laryng., 56:514, 1947.

Williams, H. L.: Intrinsic Allergy as it Affects the Ear, Nose and Throat: The Instrinsic Allergy Syndrome. Tr. Am. Acad. Ophth., & Otolaryng., 48:379, 1944.

Wright, A.: Ménière's Disease. Results of Treatment of 60 Cases by Alcohol Injection through Foot Plate of Stapes. J. Laryng. & Otol., 59:334, 1944.

CHAPTER X

HEARING AIDS AND SPEECH (LIP) READING

CONRAD J. HOLMBERG, M.D.

The physician's responsibility to his hard of hearing and deafened patients should not terminate with his diagnosis of permanent hearing impairment and with his assurance that he has met the limitations of effective medical and surgical treatment for such a condition. These limitations are well established in the present state of our knowledge, particularly in the case of the perceptive type and congenital forms of deafness.

There are certain services and aids to hearing that can and should be performed or recommended by the physician to his deaf patients in attempts to rehabilitate them after maximum medical and surgical treatment has been rendered. The basic problem is one of proper training and education in the utilization of residual hearing and in the acquisition of a means of free communication with their fellows. Proper education includes speech (lip) reading, auditory training in the use of hearing aids, speech conservation and correction, as well as vocational, psychological, social and personal guidance of the patient. These are the important services rendered by schools and other organizations devoted to the care and training of deaf and hard of hearing people. The physician should know such local and state directed educational facilities through which his patients may receive proper aural rehabilitative guidance and supervision. Every physician dealing with the care, education and guidance of the deaf patient should equip himself with information relative to the agencies through which such services can be obtained.

SCHOOLS FOR THE DEAF

Residential Schools. In most states, there are residential schools for hard of hearing and deaf children, as part of the state educational program. Other institutions, such as the Central Institute for the Deaf in St. Louis and the Lexington School for the Deaf in New York City, are either privately endowed or supported by private tuition. The latter institution receives some children supported by the state. Such schools accept deaf children of all school ages and some preschool children requiring special education and training through the use of amplified speech, hearing aids, speech (lip) reading, auditory training and visual

112

education. The oral method of training the deaf employing these procedures and principles is rapidly replacing the older, and now outmoded,
manual method (sign language).

There are also parochial schools in some of the larger cities receiving
state or local city aid as well as private enrollments.

Day Schools. In most of the larger cities, day schools for the deaf,
which are part of the public school systems, offer the advantages and
opportunities for the hard of hearing child to participate in the same
school environment with normally hearing children as well as remain in
the activities of the home. Here the child goes to the same public school
building and plays and often studies with schoolmates who have normal
hearing, but his education is supervised by teachers expertly trained in
the specialized procedures necessary for teaching the deaf child.

The relative advantages of each type of school must be weighed in
determining the needs of each child. The degree of hearing impairment,
the child's early development in the home, his ability to compensate for
his disability and compete with normally hearing children in social
activities are all factors in choosing a school.

Nursery Schools. This is now recognized as an important phase of
the deaf child's adjustment and preparedness for the later grades. Here
the early learning of speech and speech reading can be gained to the
greatest advantage. Nursery schools for preschool children are now an
addition to the curriculum of the day schools of public systems of many
large cities. The importance of developing speech and speech habits and
utilizing residual hearing in the first three or four years of life of the
deaf child has until recent years been the most neglected and perhaps
most misunderstood phase of educating and developing the deaf child.

Correspondence Courses. Well-established correspondence courses
which offer guidance and education for the parents of the very young
deaf child have fostered the development of parent interest and cooperation in the early speech training and psychological adjustment of the
child, which is so essential during the important years before the age of
nursery school. The John Tracy Clinic in Los Angeles, California, is
perhaps the foremost and the best known institution conducting such
service at the present time.

THE AMERICAN HEARING SOCIETY

This is a national organization, with its headquarters in the Volta
Bureau Building at 1537 35th Street N. W., Washington, D. C. It was
first organized about 1919 as the American Society for the Hard of
Hearing, and in many communities it is still referred to under that
title. There are 118 local chapters of the society now located in the larger
cities of the country. The society promotes a program of education and
guidance for the social and economic rehabilitation of adults and children with impaired hearing. In cooperation with medical groups such

as the Council on Physical Medicine of the American Medical Association, the Society sponsors scientific efforts in the prevention of deafness and conservation of hearing. It has available current lists of the hearing aids declared acceptable by the Council of the American Medical Association. Through its publication service, literature is available at a small cost offering information dealing with hard of hearing children, hearing tests, hearing aids, hearing clinics, speech (lip) reading, speech correction and auditory training. The Society publishes a monthly periodical called "Hearing News," available to its members, presenting up-to-date information on all subjects relating to aural rehabilitation, and helpful current news dealing with the economical aspects of the hearing aid problem. A Children's Hearing Aid Fund has been established by the Society to provide hearing aids for children whose parents cannot afford to buy the instruments.

Local chapters serve as social, recreational and employment centers for the hard of hearing, as well as an information bureau for the general public, schools and the medical profession in problems relating to deafness. Speech (lip) reading and auditory training classes are provided for both adults and children in the local chapters. Hearing aid service for the proper selection and fitting of aids to patients referred by physicians has been introduced into the program of several larger chapters of the society, such as those in New York City and Chicago.

CIVILIAN HEARING AID CLINICS

Hearing and speech clinics or centers are now a contribution of many of our larger universities. Here careful otological studies and hearing tests are made and after a thorough analysis of the patient's need for a hearing aid, the proper selection and fitting of a reliable aid is carried out. Auditory training in the use of the aid then follows, along with any social, educational, or vocational guidance the patient may need or request. Trained technicians in audiometry, acoustic and electronic engineers, teachers in auditory training, speech reading and speech correction, psychologists and social workers all cooperate under the supervision of an otologist to provide a complete and centralized program of aural rehabilitation. Such centers have been patterned largely after the Army and Navy plan and have received tremendous impetus from the accomplishments of the Military Aural Rehabilitation Program in the Second World War.

The American Academy of Ophthalmology and Otolaryngology has urged that every state have at least one such hearing center, preferably in connection with a medical school and university where such service is available to any hard of hearing patient referred by a physician.

Similar facilities for testing and selection of hearing aids are available through some of the private schools for the deaf, such as the Central Institute for the Deaf in St. Louis.

The two most essential features of this broad scope of rehabilitative and educational measures available to the deaf and hard of hearing, as far as the otolaryngologist is concerned, are the proper selection and fitting of a hearing aid and adequate training in speech (lip) reading. The physician who accepts the responsibility for the care and guidance of these hard of hearing patients must acquire some knowledge and adequate information to direct them to these proper channels for acquiring such services. Many otologists prefer to have the proper equipment in the office and give the time necessary to conduct complete audiometric studies including speech reception testing as well as hearing aid service to their patients. Others depend on the experience and supervision offered in the previously mentioned hearing centers. Where such centers do not exist in a community, physicians must depend on the reliable dealers in hearing aids for the selection and fitting of an aid.

In recommending an aid, the otologist must be acquainted with the various makes and models of instruments available in the community and he should know which of these instruments are accepted by the Council on Physical Medicine of the American Medical Association. The choice of an aid should be confined to those that have been accepted by the Council. A list of Council-accepted hearing aids can be obtained from the chairman of this Council, from the nearest chapter of the American Hearing Society, from the County Medical Society or from interested otologists.

HEARING AIDS

A hearing aid is any device used for the purpose of increasing the intensity of sound energy reaching the ears of the hard of hearing listener. The sound coming to the ear can be made louder in several different ways: by collecting more sound energy into the external canal of the ear; by preventing the loss or spread of sound transmission between the source and the listener; or by bringing electrically amplified sound into the ear. The electrical hearing aid is in the latter class. Hearing aids can be classified as nonelectric and electric, or mechanical and electric.

Nonelectric, or Mechanical Aids. *Cupped Hand.* The most primitive and simplest of all hearing devices is as old as man himself and its simple principle probably evolved as an imitative gesture by man in his attempt to attain equality in the hearing sense with lower animals. The use of the cupped hand behind the ear is one of the most effective methods of collecting more sound energy into the ear. The ability of the dog, horse and many other animals with prominent ears to direct them toward the source of sound to augment the hearing sense probably gave man the suggestion of cupping his hand behind the ear to help him hear. This gesture also becomes a signal from the listener to the speaker that he is having difficulty in hearing and the speaker then usually raises his voice. This idea could well have served to develop the early artificial hearing devices, namely, hearing trumpets and speaking tubes.

Hearing Horn. With a hearing horn, or trumpet, placed in the ear, the amount of sound energy collected is increased as with the cupped hand because the open end of the horn is larger than the external auricle and canal of the ear.

Speaking Tube. This is a flexible tube with a bell-shaped mouthpiece on one end, which is held close to the mouth of the speaker and an ear piece, which is inserted into the ear of the listener. This serves to bring the speaker close to the listener and prevents the dissipation of sound as it is directed to the ear. The stethoscope, and speaking tubes in apartment houses between hallway and rooms are examples of this principle of hearing aid. Although seen very rarely, the hearing horn and speaking tube are still used today because of their simplicity and low cost and are probably preferred by some elderly people who because of their type of hearing loss may find the adjustment to a more complicated electrical device too difficult.

Bone Conduction Aids. Many bone conduction devices of a mechanical nature have been utilized to collect and increase the vibrations of sound transmitted to the nerve of hearing through the bones of the skull. An ingenious fan with a flaring piece of metal to collect the sound and a mouthpiece to transmit the sound through the teeth to the skull and inner ear was one of the early developments. The modern bone conducting receiver is a small, encased, vibrating magnet and diaphragm assembly shaped to fit snugly against the mastoid bone behind the ear.

Artificial Middle Ear. Mechanical devices developed with the idea of replacing diseased and absent middle ear structures with an artificial drumhead and ossicle have long been attempted in the treatment of hearing impairment caused by chronic otitis media and mastoiditis. Only recently, however, have the efforts to employ such a device shown evidence of producing useful improvement in hearing in a few selected cases. The principle of the so-called artificial ear is based on the idea of replacing the destroyed sound conduction mechanism with a flexible slender probe attached to a thin membrane on a cylindrical cuff inserted into the inner bony canal and middle ear. The idea was patterned after the ossicular chain of the bird's middle ear which is represented by a single sticklike structure instead of three ossicles (Pohlman).

Electrical Aids. In construction and principle, the modern electrical hearing aid is similar to any form of electrical communication system for speech, such as the telephone, radio and loud speaker systems. By such a device, sound energy is converted into electrical energy which is carried along a system of wires to a receiver. The electrical energy is here reconverted into sound energy to reach the ear. This transformation is accomplished at the expense of the batteries producing the electrical power rather than at the expense of the voice of the speaker. In this way, more sound is actually received from the communication system than is put into it.

Components. In general, the fundamental components of any electrical communication system are quite similar. These are:

1. Microphone or transmitter, which picks up the sound and changes sound energy into electrical energy.

2. Amplifier, which increases the amount of sound energy or loudness by increasing the electrical energy derived from the battery.

3. Receiver, which reconverts the electrical energy into sound energy and directs it into the ear.

4. Batteries, which supply the electrical power for transforming sound into electrical energy and transmitting it to the receiver.

There are two types of electrical hearing aids in use today which differ largely in their transmitting and amplifying principles. These are the carbon type and vacuum-tube type, but the latter has largely displaced the carbon instrument, particularly for use with severe hearing loss.

Carbon Type. In the carbon type of aid, the principles used in the transmitter, amplifier and receiver are very similar to those of a standard telephone system. In the transmitter, carbon particles are agitated by sound vibration striking a moving diaphragm. As the pressure on the carbon particles changes, the electrical resistance between them also changes, which in turn varies the flow of electrical current in the system. The receiver is very similar to the telephone receiver, in which a thin magnetic diaphragm is agitated according to the strength of current passing through magnetic coils. The sound produced by these vibrations of the diaphragm is the electrical equivalent of the sound pulsations striking the transmitter. Some carbon instruments are a simple system of only transmitter and receiver. Others used for severe hearing loss have a carbon amplifier similar in principle to that used in long-distance telephone systems. It contains a magnet, diaphragm and carbon block and is a combination of a magnetic receiver and carbon microphone.

Vacuum-Tube Type. The vacuum-tube aid differs from the carbon type instrument largely in its type of amplifier in which small vacuum tubes similar to those in a radio are utilized. It requires two batteries of different voltages, an A battery to heat the filaments of the tubes and a B battery to produce the electric current for the speech frequency power. Most vacuum-tube instruments employ a crystal microphone, as compared with the magnetic carbon microphone of the carbon aid and either a magnetic or crystal type air conduction receiver. These receivers are now made small enough to be worn in the ear and are supported by a molded plastic earpiece which permits closer contact of the receiver to the external auditory canal and prevents dissipation of the sound. (Fig. 57.)

In the newer, single-pack models of vacuum tube instruments, the microphone amplifier, batteries and volume and tone control devices are all concentrated in one small compact unit, as compared with the carbon instrument and older vacuum tube models requiring a separate carrier for the batteries. Tubes and batteries have been reduced in size and weight to make some of the newest single unit models not much larger than a cigarette package. The use of a printed circuit principle to replace much of the wiring system now employed in most modern aids will further decrease the size and weight of these instruments. To meet the vanity of many users of hearing aids who are self-conscious about the instrument, a refinement has been made in air conduction receivers. The latter can be concealed in the ladies' hair or placed below the collar in the clothing. A flesh-colored plastic tube leads from the receiver to the molded ear piece in the folds of the external auricle. (Fig. 58.)

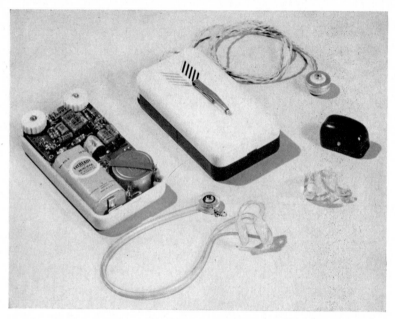

Fig. 57. The component parts of a modern hearing aid.

ADVANTAGES. The uniform amplification with respect to frequency, giving superior quality of sound, as well as the greater acoustic output of the vacuum-tube instrument are the chief advantages of this type over the carbon type. Because of the newer developments and improvements in the vacuum-tube amplifiers in hearing aids, the popularity and efficiency of the modern instruments have increased in proportion to the improvements in radio. It is estimated that 800,000 are now in use, but it is also estimated that 2,000,000 people in the United States are still in need of hearing aids and do not have them. In 1946, the number purchased was more than double the number purchased in 1943. The average age of the users is 55.

PRICES. Prices of the newer modern instruments vary from about $75 to $200. This difference in price is partially accounted for by performance characteristics of the instruments, such as tone control, type of frequency response, but primarily is owing to the maximum acoustic gain that the particular aid can deliver. The size, weight and style of instrument with various refinements in adjustments for control of volume and tone, devices for reducing intrinsic noises, as well as the follow-up service on the instrument provided by the dealers, are other factors that account for difference in quality and price. Some of the lower priced aids are sold in over-the-counter fashion without the benefit of preliminary audiometric testing and study of the patient's needs. Upkeep costs vary from $30 to $75 a year or more depending largely upon the amount of use

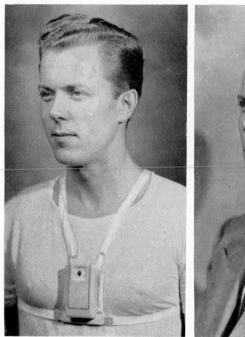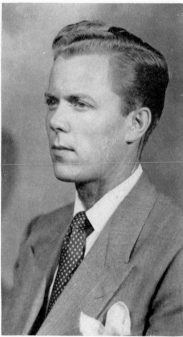

Fig. 58. One manner in which the modern, all-in-one type hearing aid is worn, and the appearance of the concealed receiver.

(battery consumption) of the instrument, also the need for new accessories, such as receiver cords and other parts that tend to wear out.

Relation of Aids to Hearing Impairment. The decision as to who should wear a hearing aid or who should have the benefit of a trial with an aid is probably the most important problem for the otologist who has been consulted for treatment and advice to hard of hearing patients. Anyone who has presented the complaints and any other evidence of having difficulty in understanding speech in his occupational as well as everyday conversation, should be considered a possible candidate for a hearing aid. This may be the best general rule to follow. Need for an aid varies with many different personal situations, such as occupational and social requirements, the type of noise environment at work and at home, and whether the need for amplification is largely for recreational purposes in the movies, lecture hall, church and large social gatherings, or for business and professional reasons where accurate hearing in every-day conversation is usually more essential. An elderly person who is unemployed obviously has less need for hearing amplified sound and speech than the business man or the young socially minded person.

Older people unfortunately present greater problems in their adjust-ment to a hearing aid and in adapting themselves to the auditory train-ing needed to help them use the aid. This is due largely to perceptive type of impairment in which high-frequency loss predominates and which is more common with advancing age. It may also be due to their variable temperaments, superstitions and ways of living. Sometimes poor health leads to lack of patience, concentration and mental energy necessary in adjusting themselves to mechanical things and new ideas.

Confusion Deafness. Hearing impairment for the higher frequencies above 1000 cycles, measured audiometrically, which is characteristic of nerve or perception deafness is often called confusion deafness because the higher frequencies convey the consonants in speech and loss of ability to hear consonants interferes with intelligibility more than does loss for the vowels. In nerve deafness, there is also an intolerance for loud speech and noise which is not present in conduction deafness. Faint, high tones may not be heard at all, but when the loudness is increased only slightly where it would normally be considered just audible and comfortable the sound becomes annoying and seems too loud to the nerve deaf patient. This abnormally rapid increase in loudness is called recruitment. It is a distinguishing feature of perception or nerve deafness and accounts for most of the difficulty encountered by older people in using an aid. It also explains the annoyance expressed by older deaf people when they complain that the speaker is shouting at them with his voice only slightly raised.

Good auditory training in the use of the aid and encouragement to practice speech reading may often bring the nerve deaf patient over the hump to where he can better use his aid with benefit and comfort.

Conduction Deafness. This type is more suitable to treatment with a hearing aid, largely because the frequency response of most good hearing aids can compensate for the low and middle frequencies characteristic of this form of hearing impairment. With this condition, there is usually normal nerve function unless the impairment has progressed to become a mixed type with accompanying perceptive changes. Where nerve function remains good, the effect of recruitment with annoyance of loud noises is not a disturbing factor to the user of an aid.

Every hard of hearing patient who seeks advice from the otologist with reference to his suitability for and the procurement of a hearing aid deserves a complete otological study. This should include all the available and acceptable hearing tests that aid in determining the type and degree of hearing impairment. Physical findings with reference to diseases of the conductive and perceptive mechanism in each case may reveal factors that are more important to a candidate for a hearing aid than the mere determination of type and extent of hearing loss. Defects or anomalies of the external auricle, canal and drumhead, a discharging middle ear or the presence of a chronic otitis externa may preclude his using an air conduction receiver in favor of the less suitable bone conduction receiver, if nerve function is adequate. No one but the physician or otologist is qualified to make such determinations.

Tests for Selection of Hearing Aids. The audiometric studies should include pure tone audiometer readings, tuning fork tests, and speech reception testing. Until recently, most hearing tests have been used to measure purely the sensitivity of the hearing mechanism or at what intensity level the ear is capable of detecting sound or speech. The reponse to such tests also helps to determine whether the loss of hearing is due to fault of the conduction or the perception apparatus of the ear. Conversational voice, whisper and watch tick tests performed in ordinary office surroundings have long been used to determine sensitivity of hearing and they will continue to have their place in routine office testing, but because of the difficulty in standardizing such tests and because they do not produce exact frequencies of sound at even intensities, they cannot be used as true measurements of hearing.

Audiometer. By means of the audiometer we can get accurate and reliable measurements of hearing loss for pure tones at threshold level and from the audiogram we get a picture of the type of hearing loss curve which represents the frequency areas (low, middle or high) that are most affected. This is essential information in the selection of a hearing aid as well as in making the diagnosis. Bone conduction response audiograms aid in the evaluation of nerve function.

The auditory deficiencies as shown by the audiogram of each hard of hearing person may vary to the extent that different people may require instruments with different response characteristics to meet their needs. Attempts have been made to control the frequency response in various instruments and thus amplify the areas of depressed hearing in the patient's audiogram to satisfy their requirements. This has been the commonly accepted principle of "selective amplification" which has been often featured in the advertising of some aids. This principle overlooked such factors as speech intelligibility and tolerance for loud sounds which produce too many response characteristics requiring compensation. Attempts now by instrument makers to give amplification to fit the audiogram are limited to two or three adjustments which give high or low tone emphasis or a flat response. A recent report from studies made at Harvard University shows that regardless of the nature of the hearing loss, most patients would get the best results with an instrument amplifying a wide range of frequencies uniformly or with a moderate emphasis on the higher frequencies. In other words, a flat-type of frequency response will usually compensate for most of the common types of hearing loss.

Threshold Level. With newer developments in audiometers, tests have been directed toward measurements of ability to hear at intensities above threshold level; that is, in the middle and upper regions of the auditory area (around 50 or 60 decibels above threshold) where ordinary conversational speech is heard. Equal loudness curves, matching one frequency with another at high intensities, are now used to determine how well the hearing aid candidate hears loud sounds. This measurement matched against his threshold curve gives valuable information as to the effectiveness of a hearing aid. Threshold audiograms alone can be helpful in merely determining the need for a hearing aid, and the following general rule can be used: if hearing loss in the better ear averages more than 30 decibels in the speech range (250 to 2048 double vibrations per second), a hearing aid is indicated. Effective compensation for this range of hearing loss by an aid will vary depending on such factors as recruitment and the severe losses for high tones with only moderate loss for middle and low tones. Correlation between threshold tests for pure tone and for speech suggest that a hearing loss for speech of 35 decibels in the better ear represents the level at which a hearing aid is needed for average social needs.

Speech Testing. The average hard of hearing patient who seeks improved hearing by means of a hearing aid is interested primarily in hearing and understanding ordinary conversational speech. The need for hearing pure tones or musical sounds is usually a secondary one. For this reason, speech reception testing or speech audiometry should play just as important a role in the tests for selection of a hearing aid and in auditory training as our time-honored pure tone audiometer tests. Electrical methods of directly measuring the threshold of speech are now available and are based somewhat on the principle of the pure tone audiometer. Standardized recorded speech tests are delivered through a loudspeaker in sound-treated rooms, or the monitored voice can be delivered through a microphone and into earphones on the listener or into a loudspeaker. Volume control meters determine the intensity or loudness of the speech delivered. More practical speech testing can now be performed by the otologist in his office using small portable turntables attached to and calibrated with the pure tone audiometer. The air conduction receiver delivers the speech produced by the recorded tests and the attenuator dial is used to control and measure the intensity of speech sound delivered.

Speech Understanding. Along with these standardized methods of testing the threshold for speech have come other systematic tests for measuring the ability to understand speech. Word lists and sentence tests which evaluate certain auxiliary functions related to the interpretation of speech such as sentence intelligibility, ability to identify words (articulation scoring), sound discrimination, tolerance for loud sounds and others, are now available and in use in hearing centers to give better evaluation of hearing loss and for better selection of hearing aids. The otologist who has the equipment for conducting speech testing can obtain these phonographic recordings of word and sentence lists from the Central Institute for the Deaf in St. Louis, Missouri.

Where hearing centers are available in the community, the physician and otologist can best serve his hard of hearing patients who are candidates for a hearing aid by referring them to such a clinic for an auditory survey and selection of an aid. Here most of the approved and accepted aids are available to be tried and examined and a selection made with the unbiased assistance and guidance of qualified technicians under the medical direction of a department of otolaryngology.

SPEECH (LIP) READING

Lip reading is now more appropriately called speech reading and is defined as an art of understanding the thoughts of another by observing the movements of the lips. Regardless of whether we possess normal or impaired hearing, we can understand the speech of another by attentively observing not only the speaker's lips, but his gestures and facial expressions. The help and information we gain through such observation can be fully appreciated, however, only when our hearing is impaired or when we are unable to see the speaker's face.

It is customary and essential to recommend speech reading very early in any case of severe hearing impairment, but in all probability, the need for such training should begin as soon as permanent or progressive type of hearing loss is severe enough to prevent normal participation in conversation. Training in speech reading is acquired more readily in the early stages of hearing impairment when the speech reader can still employ his residual hearing to good advantage in association with seeing speech to assist in word discrimination. Training should not be postponed until a hearing aid is essential to meet conversational needs, and by the same token, the use of a hearing aid by the hard of hearing child or adult should not be deferred until speech reading becomes a necessity. The common notion that the use of an aid will interfere with learning the art and also hinder the natural ability to use some degree of speech reading unconsciously has been disproved. The two functions should be employed together toward the same purpose. The value of speech reading has not been sufficiently stressed for the partially deaf or hard of hearing person, but the results attained with hard of hearing children in the modern schools and with adults in the Service Hearing Rehabilitation Programs have laid the foundation for better understanding and appreciation of this aid to hearing. The modern oral method of teaching the deaf, using the principle of combining amplified hearing with seeing and feeling speech has disproved the idea that use of an aid lessens the skill in speech reading or eliminates the need for learning it.

Teachers. Although everyone possesses some degree of natural ability to understand a speaker's thought by observing the movements of his lips, practical skill in lip reading must be attained by formal instruction from teachers well trained in the basic principles of education and psychology. Many teachers of speech reading have impaired hearing and therefore possess a more sympathetic understanding of the methods of teaching and the personality problems of the students. However, it is not essential that good teachers have impaired hearing if they are well trained in both hearing and speech theory. There are many available training schools for speech reading teachers among the speech and hearing clinics of universities, schools for the deaf, and the Army and Navy Aural Rehabilitation Centers. The challenge in this educational field to qualified candidates for teaching has been made more attractive and vital as a result of the increased emphasis given to aural rehabilitation in civilian and service hearing centers. However, there still exists a need today for competent teachers.

Methods of Teaching. These have varied from the early principle established by different schools of thought in some of the European countries and later in this country as new schools developed. However, the principles of all modern methods are based on the utilization of hearing, sight and feeling of sounds developed by the speaker. The combination of hearing by the unaided ear, or by amplification with an aid, and seeing is a great advantage over mere visual observation of the speaker. This is true even when an aid gives a severely deafened person just enough help to allow him to hear some sounds but no words. Feeling the muscle action of the face, mouth, and larynx and also the force of the breath produced by the sounds of words as they are spoken, help in developing the mental image of the words on the listener's mind. For example, consonants are grouped into categories, depending on the part of the mouth where the sounds are felt, such as those felt on the lips; in the front of the mouth as they are made by the tip of the tongue, teeth and palate; and in the back of the mouth as they are made by the back of the tongue against the palate. The student soon learns that the first group is more visible than the others.

The hard of hearing student must first develop the proper attitude toward his handicap and the future problems it imposes on both himself and his associates. He must then attempt to meet these problems by using every available means to attain social communication and develop a normal life. He should first attempt to use all his residual hearing by means of an aid and then master speech reading as early as possible in the progress of his deafness.

REFERENCES

Berry, G.: The Evaluation and Practicability of Hearing Aids. Ann. Otol., Rhin. & Laryng., *57*:500, 1948.

Carhart, R.: Hearing Aids—Tests for Selection. Laryngoscope, *56*:780, 1946.

Carhart, R., and Thompson, E. A.: Hearing Aid Fitting. Tr. Am. Acad. Ophth., & Otolaryng., 354 (Mar.–Apr.), 1947.

Davis, H.: Hearing and Deafness. New York, Murray Hill Books, Inc., 1947.

Davis, H., Hudgins, C. V., Marquist, R. J., Nichols, R. H., Jr., Peterson, G. E., Ross, D. A., and Stevens, S. S.: Selection of Hearing Aids. Laryngoscope, *56*:85 and *56*:135, 1946.

Ewing, A. W. G.: Hearing Aid Clinics in England. *Ibid.*, *57*:41, 1947.

Ewing, A. W. G.: Hearing Aids for the Deaf. Practitioner, *158*:129, 1947.

Fee, G. A.: The Use and Limitations of Hearing Aids. Canad. M. A. J., *56*:366, 1947.

Nichols, R. H., Jr.: Physical Characteristics of Hearing Aids. Laryngoscope, *57*:31, 1947.

Pohlman, M. E.: Artificial Middle Ear. Ann. Otol., Rhin. & Laryng., *56*:647, 1947.

Part II

The Nose

CHAPTER XI

APPLIED ANATOMY AND PHYSIOLOGY
OF THE NOSE

Anderson C. Hilding, M.D.

The chief purpose of the nose is the preparation of air for use in the lungs.

EXTERNAL NOSE

The upper part of the external nose is formed by the nasal bones and the frontal process of the maxillae, and the lower, larger part is formed by a group of cartilages, with skin and connective tissue covering the whole ensemble (Fig. 59). The cartilages are the lateral nasal cartilages,

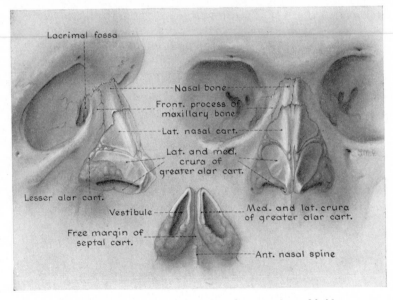

Fig. 59. The structure of the external nose and nasal bridge.

the major and minor alar cartilages, the anterior margin of the septal cartilage and certain sesamoid cartilages. The nostrils and tip of the nose are shaped by the major alar cartilages. Each of these cartilages is a thin, flexible plate bent upon itself in such a manner as to form both the medial and lateral wall of the naris of its own side. The columella which separates the nares is formed by the lower margin of the septal cartilage, the medial portions of the two major alar cartilages and the anterior nasal spine, together with a covering of skin.

INTERNAL NOSE

The internal nose is the air conditioning chamber and is lined by a thick, red, moist lining. It contains the septum and turbinates. Its walls and floor are rigid. It measures about 3 inches (7.5 cm.) in length and 2 inches (5 cm.) in height. The roof is arched from front to back, but the floor is about level. The internal nose opens posteriorly into the pharynx through the two choanae which are considerably larger than the nares. They are oval in shape and measure about 1 inch (2.5 cm.) in height and $\frac{1}{2}$ inch (1.25 cm.) in transverse diameter. The transverse diameter of the internal nose is variable, being narrow above and wider below, and wider in the middle than either anteriorly or posteriorly. These are, however, not the most important dimensions. The internal nose is largely filled by the septum and the turbinates. The irregular air spaces left between these structures form the flues for the flow of air streams. They are all narrow and of such shape as to cause the air to flow in thin sheets. The septum divides the internal nose into approximately equal halves. The vertical air spaces adjacent to the septum are approximately straight and parallel to its surface. Those lying about the turbinates are about the same thickness as the vertical air spaces and follow the shapes of the turbinates. The widest portion of the nasal air space is probably in the inferior meatuses. The combined volume of these flues is about 15 to 20 cc., or half this on each side. The flues are generally only a few millimeters in width.

The sinuses are irregular air cavities lying adjacent to the internal nose with which they connect through their ostia.

SEPTUM

The septum is a rather thin, centrally placed wall which divides the internal nose into two halves. It is often somewhat irregular in thickness and not infrequently is more or less warped.

The skeletal portion of the septum is composed of the septal cartilage (quadrangular) anteriorly, the perpendicular plate of the ethmoid above, the vomer and rostrum of the sphenoid posteriorly and a ridge below made up of the crest of the maxillae and the crest of the palatines (Fig. 60). Ridges and spurs which sometimes require removal occur not infrequently. Warping of the septum may be so great that it interferes with air flow and must be corrected surgically. Warping may be due to growth factors or less commonly to trauma. The adjacent turbinates commonly compensate for irregularities in the septum (if these are not too great) by increasing in size on the concave side and decreasing on the other side in such a way as to maintain the optimum width of the air spaces.

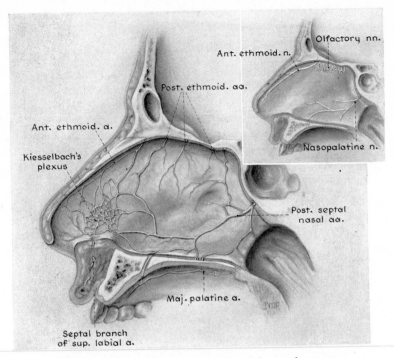

Fig. 60. The blood and nerve supply of the nasal septum.

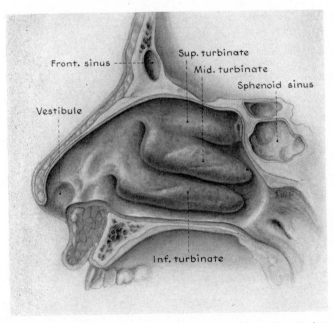

Fig. 61. The shape, position and relationships of the turbinates on the lateral nasal wall.

There are swell bodies of erectile tissue on both sides of the septum which serve to adjust its thickness under varying atmospheric conditions.

TURBINATES

There are two large turbinates on each side (middle and inferior conchae) and usually one and sometimes two rudimentary ones (superior and supreme conchae) (Fig. 61). The middle, superior and supreme conchae are parts of the ethmoidal labyrinth. The inferior concha is a separate bone which is attached to both the ethmoid labyrinth and to the maxilla.

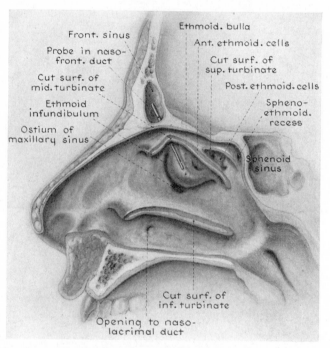

Fig. 62. The lateral nasal wall with turbinates removed, showing the position of the sinus orifices.

The middle and inferior turbinates are long, fleshy bodies hanging downward from the lateral wall and extending horizontally almost the full length of the lateral wall. They are fairly well streamlined, being almost bulbous anteriorly and decreasing in diameter to the posterior ends which are rather slender. Like the septum, these turbinates are supplied with swell bodies or cavernous venous spaces which serve to adjust their size. They are the radiators of the nose and are served by a rich blood supply.

BLOOD SUPPLY

The sphenopalatine branch of the internal maxillary artery supplies the conchae, the meatuses and septum. The anterior and posterior ethmoidal branches of the ophthalmic artery supply the ethmoidal and frontal sinuses and roof of the nose. A branch of the superior labial artery and the infra-orbital and alveolar branches of the internal maxillary supply the maxillary sinus, and the pharyngeal branch of the same artery is distributed to the sphenoid. The veins form a close cavernous plexus under the mucous membrane. This plexus is especially well marked over the middle and inferior concha and the lower portion of the septum, where it forms the so-called swell bodies. Venous drainage is principally through the ophthalmic, anterior facial and sphenopalatine veins.

LATERAL WALL

The lateral wall of the internal nose is rather irregular and in general inclines laterally from above downward. The spaces between the inferior and middle turbinates and the lateral wall are called the inferior and middle meatuses. The space just beneath and lateral to the superior turbinate is called the superior meatus. The ostia of the frontal, maxillary and anterior ethmoids lie in the middle meatus. Those of the posterior ethmoids and the sphenoid lie in the superior meatus (Fig. 62).

SINUSES

The sinuses are irregular air cavities which lie adjacent to the nose. Many theories as to their function have been advanced, but none is supported by sufficient evidence to be tenable.

There are about twelve sinuses on each side. The number is somewhat variable and is not always the same on the two sides. They are divided into anterior and posterior groups. The anterior includes the frontal, the maxillary and the anterior ethmoids, while the posterior ethmoids and the sphenoid comprise the posterior group. The ostia of the anterior group open into the hiatus semilunaris in the middle meatus. The posterior group drain into the superior meatus.

The sinuses are located in bones, the names of which they carry. The frontal sinus lies between the outer and inner tables of the frontal bone (Fig. 63). The lower portion also extends backward under the cranial cavity for a short distance. The floor of the frontal sinus forms a portion of the roof of the orbit. The maxillary sinus fills a large part of the maxilla. It extends from the orbit, where it forms a part of the floor, down to the apices of the teeth, some of which may protrude into the cavity (Fig. 64a). The ethmoidal sinuses occupy much of the ethmoidal labyrinth. The sphenoid sinus occupies the sphenoid bone and may extend into the wings of the sphenoid, the pterygoid plates and even into the clinoid processes (Fig. 64b).

At birth, the maxillary and ethmoid sinuses are present, but the sphenoid is very rudimentary and the frontal has not yet begun to develop.

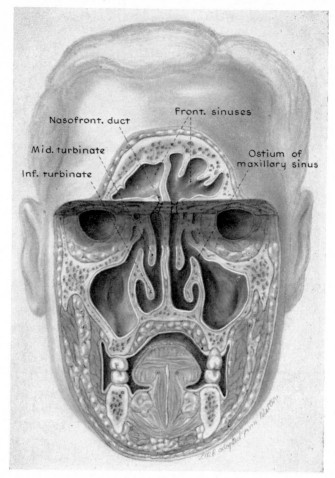

Fig. 63. A frontal section through the head showing the relative position of the sinuses

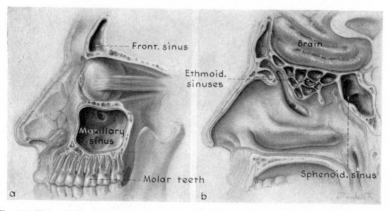

Fig. 64. The relative positions of: a, The maxillary sinus (antrum) in relation to the teeth, and b, the frontal, ethmoid and sphenoid sinuses in relation to the cranium.

All of the sinuses vary a great deal in size and configuration. They have no obvious physiologic function and are of importance principally because of the complications of nasal disease which arise in them.

Theory of Development. Proetz has advanced the theory that the sinuses are developmental accidents and are without function. They form as the facial bones grow away from the cranium, which is comparatively stationary. For instance, as the maxilla grows inferiorly and laterally in order to form strong supports for the alveolar process, the nasal mucosa is sucked, as it were, into the space thus left vacant, where it lines the cavity which is formed. This would account for the position of the ostium in the upper, medial portion of the sinus. Similarly, the frontal sinus opens as the outer table of the frontal bone grows away from the stationary inner table to accommodate itself to the rapid growth of the facial bones.

This manner of development of the sinuses is still theory, but there is considerable evidence to support it and it seems more plausible than any yet advanced.

RESPIRATORY MUCOSA

The mucous membrane of the respiratory tract is a highly specialized tissue (almost an organ) which lines the entire tract from the nasal vesti-

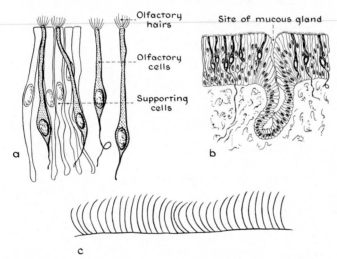

Fig. 65A. The important elements of the nasal mucosa are: a, The olfactory cells. b, The ciliated, columnar, pseudostratified type of epithelium containing mucous glands, which are more abundant in some areas than others. c, The cilia. The actual amplitude of the beat is greater than is depicted here.

bules to the bronchioles, with the exception of the pharynx. Both the epithelium itself and the submocosa vary markedly in various portions of the tract. Their thickness is more or less proportionate to the force of air flow. Both are comparatively thick on the turbinates and septum,

thinner in the more protected meatuses and thinnest of all in the sinuses.
Typically, the respiratory epithelium is a columnar, pseudostratified,
ciliated epithelium. The columnar cells are ciliated and lie next to the
surface (Fig. 65). Beneath them lie four or five irregular layers of replacement cells. Such typical epithelium is found in the meatuses. In the more

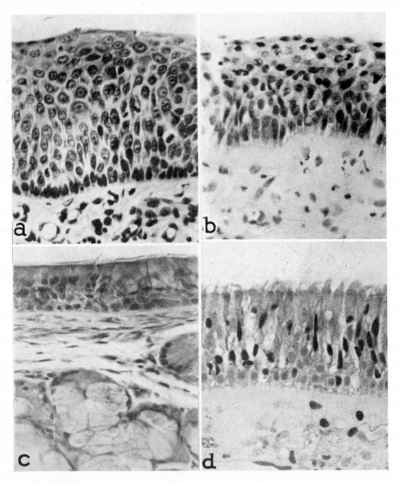

Fig. 65B. Photomicrographs of respiratory epithelium as related to the impact of
respired air: a. pre-turbinal area: b. anterior end of inferior turbinate: c. inferior
meatus showing glands containing serous and mucous cells: d. middle one-third of
inferior turbinate. Within the sinuses, the epithelium is of a cuboidal form.

exposed portions, as on the anterior end of the middle turbinate, the
cells may lie ten or fifteen deep. The cilia are absent, as though blown
away by the blast of inrushing air, and the surface cells look more like
squamous cells than columnar. On the other hand, the epithelium in
the sinuses is only two or three layers deep and the well-ciliated surface

cells are short and cuboidal. The mucous glands and blood vessels in the stroma of the submucosa similarly are abundant or scanty in proportion to the force of the air flow over the surface. The swell bodies mentioned before are cavernous venous spaces lying in the stroma over the middle and inferior turbinates and lower portion of septum.

NERVE SUPPLY

The nerve supply of the nasal space is derived from the first and second divisions of the trigeminal nerve. In front and above, branches of the first (ophthalmic division) of the trigeminal nerve carry the sensory afferent impulses. Posteriorly and below, the second (maxillary division) of the trigeminal nerve provides the nerve supply to the lower and posterior portions of the nasal mucosa and septum by way of the

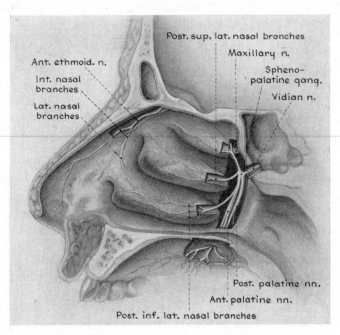

Fig. 66. The nerve supply of the lateral nasal wall.

sphenopalatine ganglion. This ganglion is of considerable clinical importance to the nasal space. In addition to sensory fibers from the maxillary division of the trigeminal nerve, it receives parasympathetic fibers from the great superficial petrosal nerve which comes from the geniculate ganglion of the facial nerve and sympathetic fibers from the deep petrosal nerve. These petrosal nerves join to form the vidian nerve before reaching the ganglion (Fig. 66).

The position of the ganglion in the pterygopalatine fossa close to the sphenopalatine fossa makes it accessible for the application of topical anesthesia or an astringent or a caustic. The sphenopalatine foramen lies just behind and above the posterior tip of the middle turbinate.

The sinus mucosa receives its sensory supply from the nerve fibers which pass through the ostia.

FUNCTIONS OF THE NOSE

The functions of the nose may be classed as both primary and secondary. The two primary functions are sense of smell and air conditioning.

PRIMARY FUNCTIONS

The Sense of Smell. This function is comparatively unimportant clinically. Years ago, much more attention was given to it. Bawden in 1901 collected a bibliography of 885 articles from the second half of the last century, and Proetz has recently reviewed the subject in his essays on "Applied Physiology of the Nose."

The olfactory area consists of modified respiratory epithelium and lies in the roof of the nose and extends downward somewhat both on the septum and the lateral wall.

The olfactory sense cells lie rather deep in the epithelium, supported by sustentacular cells. They send out a peripheral process which terminates on the surface in a bulb upon which are numerous olfactory hairs. The axones are collected together in nerve filaments which pass through the cribriform plate into the olfactory bulb, there to form a synapse with the dendrites of the mitral cells. The axones of these cells form the olfactory tract, which passes to the brain to make connection with numerous nuclei, fasciculi and tracts. The central olfactory apparatus is highly complex. A good diagram and brief discussion of it may be found in Rasmussen: "The Principal Nervous Pathways."

The inspired air during olfaction is directed to the area by the upper, narrowed portion of the vestibule, usually in small sniffs. Man's sense of smell is comparatively rudimentary, yet the sensitivity of the organ of smell is truly startling. McKenzie states that vanillin is perceptible by us as a smell when it amounts to no more than 0.000000005 gm. in a liter of air. The process by which odors are perceived has not been certainly determined. There are two theories: the chemical and the undulation theory. According to the former, the particles of odorous substances are distributed by diffusion through the air and initiate a chemical reaction when they reach the olfactory epithelium. According to the undulation theory, waves of energy similar to light impinge upon the olfactory nerve endings.

Some of the lower animals—dogs, deer, mice, buzzards—are dependent upon the sense of smell for safety or food or both. They have this sense developed to a remarkable degree, as anyone who has watched a hunting dog follow the trail of a pheasant will realize. Quantitatively, ours is in no way comparable.

Air Conditioning. This is the other primary function of the nose. The inspired air stream passes through the nose in the form of an arc which rises as high as the middle turbinate and then descends into the pharynx. Most of the air flows through the vertical nasal spaces, but some passes through the meatuses. The streams of air are in the form of thin sheets, and the flow is very smooth, with a minimum of turbulence and friction. The expired air follows much the same course, but breaks up into turbulent eddies under the bridge of the nose before flowing out through the vestibules. The variations in pressure are comparatively slight during quiet respiration, being of the magnitude of 10 mm. of water, or about 1/1000th of an atmosphere. The pressure in the nasal spaces is slightly reduced during inspiration and slightly increased during expiration. The direction of air flow to and from the sinus, therefore, is just opposite to that of the lungs. During inspiration, air flows into the lungs, but out of the sinuses and vice versa. The exchange of air through the ostia is, however, very light and is probably of little physiologic importance.

CHANGES IN INSPIRED AIR

The inspired air during the brief passage through the narrow flues of the internal nose is cleaned, moistened and adjusted as to temperature. The journey of 4 inches from the nares to the choanae requires not over a quarter of a second of time and perhaps only a fraction of that. Yet the relative humidity when it reaches the pharynx is 75 per cent or more. The temperature is about 36° C. (96.8° F.), no matter what the temperature was a quarter of a second previously just off the tip of the nose. All dust, bacteria and other particulate matter have been removed and the air is ready to be received into the lungs.

The variability in the demands for heating and humidification and other preparation of the inspired air is met partly by means of changes in the width of the spaces through which the sheets of incoming air must flow. The volume in these spaces is adjustable according to atmospheric conditions through increase or decrease in the size of the swell bodies or erectile tissue.

Humidification. The amount of water evaporated in the nose is said to be about 1000 cc. each twenty-four hours. This is about 1/25 cc. per breath. Of course, the amount evaporated would vary inversely with the humidity of the air outside. When the hot summer air is almost saturated with moisture, there probably is comparatively little evaporation from the nasal surfaces. When the air is dry, as in homes in the winter, the evaporation required at the mucosal surface must be considerable. This evaporation takes place from the surface of the mucous blanket which lines all of the air passages, and the necessary water must be furnished by the mucous blanket.

This blanket is supplied by the mucous glands (and if need be, goblet cells) which are found in the mucosa. Both serous and mucous cells are present in the glands and the relative amount of water in the secretion and its viscosity are determined by the relative amounts of water and mucus produced by these cells. It must follow that there is a delicately adjusted secretory control which is responsive to atmospheric conditions. Enough water must be present at all times to humidify the air, but there must not be an excess or the tip of the nose would drip. This does occur occasionally when the temperature is subzero and one is hurrying home for dinner. Drops collect on the tip of the nose, forcing one to make a decision as to whether to be inelegant and allow them to drip, or to get one's hands cold hunting for a handkerchief.

Temperature Adjustment. The temperature of the inspired air is adjusted at the same time as the humidity. The necessary heat (the

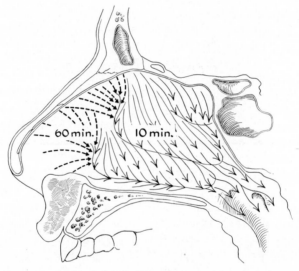

Fig. 67. A diagrammatic sketch of the direction and relative rate of flow of nasal mucous.

temperature must be raised usually) is radiated from the rapidly flowing blood which courses through the stroma of the subepithelial tissue over the turbinates and the septum. The temperature of the inferior turbinate is about 32° C. (89.6° F.), as compared with 36° to 37° C. (96.8° to 98.6° F.) in the pharynx. The reduced temperature is due not only to the lower temperature of the atmosphere but to the rapid evaporation of water at the surface. Consider for a moment what that means. In our subzero winter weather, the air is very dry. If heated to body temperature, the relative humidity would probably not be over 5 per cent. During the fraction of a second in which the air passes through the nose, it is brought almost to body temperature and at the same time the relative humidity is raised to 75 or 80 per cent. The cooling effect of such rapid evaporation must be truly great when added to a starting temperature of $-32°$ C. $(-25°$ F.), as not infrequently occurs in some parts of the United States.

To warm the 500 cubic feet of air which we breathe each twenty-four hours, about 70 large calories of heat are required when the outside temperature is 20° C. (68° F.). This amounts to about 2.5 per cent of the total heat produced in the body. At $-32°$ C. $(-25°$ F.), the heat loss through the nose would be at least four times seventy, and probably much more because of the greater evaporation.

It is to be remembered that the expiratory flow of air restores a little heat to the nasal mucosa or at least stops the heat loss during this cycle of respiration. In addition, a small amount of water is condensed at the surface, since the temperature of the expired air is slightly above that in the nose.

Air Cleaning. The cleansing of the air in the nose is accomplished by the mucous blanket. (Fig. 67). Particulate matter which comes in contact with the secretion adheres to it and becomes incorporated. It is probable also that the electric potential at the surface causes adsorption of bacteria and particulate matter, resulting in adherence to the mucous blanket. Practically all dust and bacteria, therefore, are transferred to the mucous blanket. If the material is too irritating to be disposed of in the usual manner, it is removed by sneezing. A tickling sensation which initiates a series of muscular reflexes develops and the irritating substance together with a varying amount of secretion is removed in a sudden mighty blast.

SECONDARY NASAL FUNCTION

The secondary functions consist in the safe disposal of the material collected from the inspired air, and are of tremendous importance. In addition to all of the foul and noxious material which is deposited upon the lining of the nose, bacteria and viruses, pathogenic and otherwise, find their way into the nose in enormous numbers. They must be disposed of safely. The central factor in these secondary functions is the mucous blanket.

Mucous Blanket

This blanket is a highly viscid, continuous sheet of secretion which extends into all of the spaces and angles of the nose, sinuses, eustachian tubes, pharynx and entire bronchial tree. As Proetz states, "it has not received a tithe of the attention which it deserves." It is exceedingly thin dimensionally, but has some tensile strength. It is in continuous motion, being pushed along by the cilia. From those areas which are not ciliated, it is pulled away by remote traction of cilia in other areas. Its physical qualities of tensile strength and slipperiness make this possible. It is so sticky that particles which come in the slightest contact adhere promptly. The pH is about 7, or neutral, and is maintained fairly constant. This is important because cilia do not function well if the pH varies much. Neither does lysozyme, the contained enzyme which destroys most air-borne bacteria. Lysozyme was first described by Flemming, the discoverer of penicillin. It is an antiseptic enzyme which not only kills bacteria but breaks them up and causes them to dissolve. Its action can be observed under the microscope by exposing sensitive bacteria in suspension. The bacteria swell up, grow fainter, fragment as though exploded and the fragments fade from view. Most air-borne bacteria are almost instantly destroyed when they come into contact with the mucous blanket. So effective is this action that the posterior half of the nose is practically sterile, and usually a culture cannot be grown from this part of the nose by ordinary technics. Although there are some exceptions, practically none of the myriads of bacteria which enter the nares ever reach the back part of the nose alive.

The mucous blanket in the nose and sinuses is moved to the pharynx by cilia and renewed by the glands at least two or three times an hour. In the pharynx it is swallowed and carried into the stomach where the gastric juices destroy residual living bacteria.

Respiratory Epithelium. The respiratory epithelium which carries the cilia is typically a pseudostratified columnar epithelium composed of long columnar cells surmounted by cilia and underlain with three or four layers of replacement cells. It lines the entire respiratory tract from the vestibule of the nose to the alveoli, with the exception of the pharynx. It is not uniform in structure, however, through the entire tract. In general, its character seems to be determined by the impact of streams of air which flow over it. Where the impact of cold, dry contaminated air is most severe, namely, in the anterior third of the nose, the respiratory epithelium carries no cilia. Neither are the surface cells columnar in form. In fact, the respiratory epithelium in this locality is very much like a deep squamous epithelium without cornification at the surface. The nuclei are large and oval. The epithelium in the middle third of the nose, which covers the medial aspect of the turbinates and the adjacent surface of the septum, is a deep columnar type with very long surface cells and many layers of replacement cells. The cilia are inclined to be short and somewhat irregular at the surface.

The middle and inferior meatuses, where the air flow is much more subdued, are lined by short columnar cells with two or three layers of replacement cells beneath, and the cilia are very well developed. They are evenly spaced, uniform and longer than in the common meatus. The sinuses, which normally receive only expired air and this in minute quantities, are lined by a very thin epithelium composed of cuboidal cells at the surface and containing only one or two layers of replacement cells. The cilia are uniform in length and evenly spaced.

The submucosa varies in thickness, as does the epithelium. It is thickest in the most exposed area and is thin almost to the vanishing point in the sinuses.

The mucous blanket is supplied by tubular and racemose glands composed of both serous and mucous cells. In addition, there are varying numbers of goblet cells among the ciliated surface cells, which supply a portion of the secretion.

The respiratory epithelium can be altered as to form by changing its relation to air flow. For instance, the nonciliated, squamous-like epithelium in the anterior portion of the nose can be made to extend more deeply into one side of the nose in experimental animals by closing the other nostril surgically. The percentage of goblet cells can also be altered radically. To what extent the different forms of epithelium in man can thus be influenced by altering the ventilation is not known.

Ciliary Movement. Ciliary movement is a primitive function and its history extends far back in biologic evolution to the unicellular forms. Some bacteria like *Escherichia coli* are ciliated, as are many of the marine forms. The movement is more or less of an automatic one inherent in single cells. That is, it is not dependent upon nerve impulses initiated at distant points in nerve tissue.

Ciliary movement is used in man for the purpose of draining the respiratory tract. It is essential to our very lives that the mucous blanket on the walls of the air passages be exchanged and removed frequently. There is progressive movement of their contents in many other tubular systems in the body, but none of the principles used in the other systems is applicable to the respiratory tract. The contents of the intestinal tract are moved by peristalsis. Hydrostatic pressure, gravity and peristalsis combine to move urine through the ureter to the bladder, The blood is forced through the tubes which contain it by a pump. In the respiratory tract, there is an entirely different situation, since here is a set of tubes which transmit gases and must be held widely patent at all times. Pump action, peristalsis and hydrostatic pressure would be effective on a material like mucus only if the mucus filled the tubes—obviously an impractical arrangement. Hence the cilia.

Cilia. The cilia are about 5 to 7 μ in length and are located on the end-plates of the surface cells in the epithelium. There are twenty-five or thirty on each cell. The cilia seem to work almost automatically. For instance, it is possible to tear a cell into small bits without stopping the contraction of the cilia. A single cilium will continue to stroke as along as a tiny bit of cytoplasm remains attached to it. All of the cilia in an area of epithelium are coordinated in a marvelous manner. Each, as it strokes, is timed in such a way as not to strike the cilium in front or get in the way of the one behind. As one observes them stroking, the ranks bow in unison and the files in sequence. Not only are the strokes of adjacent cilia coordinated as to time, but the directions of untold millions in a sinus are so coordinated as to carry the mucus accurately to the ostium.

6

The strokes of the individual cilia are not just a waving back and forth like wheat stalks in a grain field. Each stroke has a powerful, rapid phase in the direction of flow with the cilium straight and stiff. This is followed by a slower movement of recovery in which the cilium bends. The stroke is not unlike the arm stroke of a swimmer. The cilia in man's respiratory tract stroke about 250 cycles a minute.

Rate of Mucus Flow. The rate of the flow of mucus as motivated by the cilia varies in different portions of the nose. It averages perhaps 5 to 10 mm. per minute on the septum and adjacent surfaces of the turbinates. It is much slower, only a few millimeters an hour, on the nonciliated areas in the anterior portions of the nose, where the mucous blanket is dragged off by remote traction. It is more rapid in the inferior and middle meatuses where the cilia are not so exposed. There is a speed gradient in the sinuses. The rate of flow increases as the ostium is approached. The rate varies from 2 to 4 up to 15 or 20 millimeters per minute.

Direction of Mucus Flow. The direction of streaming in the nose is generally backward. Since the cilia are more active in the protected inferior and middle meatuses, they tend to drag the mucous blanket from the common meatus into these recesses. The direction of flow on the septum is back and somewhat downward toward the floor. On the floor, the direction is back, with a tendency to flow under the inferior turbinate into the inferior meatuses. On the medial aspect of the turbinates, the flow is back and downward to pass under the inferior margin into the corresponding meatus. The drainage from the nonciliated areas in the anterior third of the nose is practically all through the meatuses. This is the area that collects most of the air-borne filth.

The direction of the flow in the sinuses is spiral, beginning, in man, at a point remote from the ostium. The rate increases progressively as the ostium is approached, and in the ostium the mucous blanket passes out in the form of a whirling tube at 15 to 20 millimeters per minute.

The trachea is also said to present spiral streaming. This has not been noticeable in my experience. It has seemed to me that the direction of flow is about axial. The rate in different parts of the trachea seems to be fairly uniform.

The power of the ciliary mechanism is amazing. The conveyor system, or "escalator," as it has been aptly called, will move loads of viscid mucus several hundred times as deep as the cilia are long with apparent ease. In fact, load acts as a stimulant to the cilia. It has been determined by measurement in a frog's mouth that 5 grams per square centimeter is the optimum load. This is probably greater than in man.

Diseases of Epithelium. Most of the diseases of the nose among patients who seek the rhinologist's aid are diseases of the epithelium. Briefly, some of the changes which occur in the epithelium with the diseases that cause them follow:

The ciliated cells may go through metamorphosis and become squamous-like throughout the nose. This is accompanied by atrophy of the turbinates and drying of secretion. The result is extensive crusting throughout the nose with continuous discomfort to the patient and annoyance to his friends, because this is the disease called atrophic rhinitis or "stink nose."

The ciliated cells may change to goblet cells so extensively that the escalator function ceases. Instead, the erstwhile ciliated cells all begin to secrete a heavy viscid mucus which accumulates, since there is nothing to move it away. Moreover, the cells do not completely extrude it. The secretion produced by each cell protrudes from the end of the cell and fuses with the mass in the lumen but remains anchored within the cells. The coughing and straining of the patient in an effort to dislodge the mass of mucus in the lumen sometimes stretches these cells to many times their original length. This condition is found in asthma, and the accumulation of mucus can become so great that the unfortunate sufferer finally dies of asphyxia.

When the epithelium is attacked by pus-producing bacteria, the cells become necrotic and extensive areas may become ulcerative. Such conditions obtain in acute laryngotracheobronchitis, and tracheitis resulting from exposure to poison gas.

Goblet cell formation and swelling of the submucosa results from allergy. The asthmatic condition described is probably due to allergy.

The virus of the common cold and of influenza attack the ciliated cells primarily. The injured epithelium loosens and the ciliated cells break off proximal to the nucleus and float free in the secretion, where they can be observed under the microscope, stroking vigorously. The copious thin secretion with which we are all familiar follows attack by either cold or influenza virus. In the case of the latter, it may become so copious that the patient drowns in his own secretion.

REFERENCES

Butler, D., and Ivy, A.: Effect of Nasal Inhalers on Erectile Tissues of the Nose. Arch. Otolaryng., *38*:309, 1943.

Colson, W.: Bernoulli's Theorem and Upper Respiratory Drainage. Laryngoscope, *55*:444, 1945.

Colson, W.: An Experiment Showing the Bernoulli Action in Emptying the Nasal Sinuses. *Ibid.*, *55*:587, 1945.

Dixon, F., and Hoerr, N.: Lymphatic Drainage of Paranasal Sinuses. *Ibid.*, *54*:165, 1944.

Hilding, A.: Direction and Rate of Drainage of Mucus Secretions from the Internal Surfaces of the Nose. Proc. Staff Meet., Mayo Clin., *6*:285, 1931.

Hilding, A.: Experimental Surgery of the Nose and Sinuses. I. Changes in the Morphology of the Epithelium Following Variations in Ventilation: Arch. Otolaryng., *16*:9, 1932. II. Gross Results Following Removal of the Intersinus Septum and of Strips of Mucous Membrane from the Frontal Sinus of the Dog. *Ibid.*, *17*:321, 1933. III. Results Following Partial and Complete Removal of the Lining Mucous Membrane from the Frontal Sinus of the Dog. *Ibid.*, *17*:760, 1933.

Lierle, D., and Evers, L.: Effect of Certain Drugs on Ciliary Activity of Mucous Membrane of the Upper Respiratory Tract. Laryngoscope, 54:176, 1944.

Post, W.: Nasal Psychosomatic Syndromes Accompanying and Following Acute Anxiety. Ann. Otol., Rhin. & Laryng., 54:747, 1945.

Proetz, A. W.: Applied Physiology of the Nose. Annals Pub. Co., St. Louis, 1941.

Proetz, A.: Physiology of the Nose from Standpoint of the Plastic Surgeon. Arch. Otolaryng., 39:514, 1944.

Proetz, A. W.: The Displacement Method. St. Louis, Annals Pub. Co., 1931.

Rasmussen, A. T.: The Principal Nervous Pathways. New York, The Macmillan Co., 1932, pp. 48–50.

CHAPTER XII

EXAMINATION OF THE NOSE

Anderson C. Hilding, M.D.

History. As in other fields of medicine, a carefully taken history is of first importance in the examination of the patient. In rhinology, it is sometimes difficult to get a clear statement from the patient regarding his complaints. This makes specific questioning valuable.

A majority of patients with nasal disease have one or more of the following symptoms: discharge, nasal obstruction, colds, headache, or pain. Epistaxis would be included under discharge, and the symptom of sneezing attacks are often identified with a complaint of a head cold. Rarely, a complaint of external swelling without other symptoms is encountered.

Examination Form. The following specific details in the questions for history taking are valuable:

DISCHARGE

Character: watery, mucoid, purulent, crusts, bloody
Amount: slight, moderate, profuse
Duration: ....wks. ....mos. ....yrs.

Is the discharge blown out of the right or left nostril or does it go back down the throat? Is there a tendency to clear the throat of excess secretion on arising? Describe the secretion thus expectorated.

NASAL OBSTRUCTION

Degree: slight, moderate, complete block. Side: right, left, both, alternating. Duration: ....wks. ....mos. ....yrs. Is it worse when indoors?...... or out-doors?...... at night when lying down?...... Are you a mouth breather?.... Do you snore?...... Is your throat dry or sore on arising in the morning?......

COLDS

Number per month.... year.... Duration of an attack...... Does your cold start with a sore throat or in the nose?...... Is there any association in your mind between the onset of the cold and fatigue?...... exposure to changes in weather? ...... contact with others who have colds?...... anything else?...... Are the attacks accompanied by sneezing?...... Do your eyes itch or water?.... Have you ever had "hay fever"?.... asthma?.... hives?.... eczema?.... Is there any history in your family (father, mother, brothers, sisters, uncles, aunts, grandparents) of "hay fever," asthma, hives, eczema?............

HEADACHE—PAIN

Location:............... Number of attacks per day............ week....... month......... Is the ache or pain located above your eyes?...... on top of

head?...... over temples?...... in back of head?...... over face or near ears?
...... Is there any characteristic time of day for the onset of the headache or
pain?...... How many weeks, months, years, have you been subject to headaches?
.... Is the ache or pain dull?...... throbbing?...... "shooting"?...... a
sensation of pressure or a tight band?...... What is the average duration of an
attack?.......... hours, days. Are the aches or pains continuous or intermittent?
.... Grade the severity of the discomfort as slight, moderate, severe
.... Is the attack accompanied by nausea or vomiting?........ Visual
disturbances?........ Do you know in advance that you are going to have a headache?........ Is there any relationship in your mind between the headache and eye
trouble?........ sinus disease?...... fatigue?...... other ailments?...... What
relieves the headache?...............

EXTERNAL NOSE EXAMINATION

The examination of the nasal space should be preceded by a careful
inspection of the external nose. It is well to scrutinize the general facial
appearance of the patient, noting any abnormalities of color of the skin,
swelling, and external expression of pain, worry, apprehension, etc.
Then abnormality of shape of the nose should be noted, particularly as
this may be a factor in nasal obstruction. Inspect the contour of the
bridge, tip and base, noting any deviation from normal. Note also the
size and shape of the upper and lower lateral cartilages and the position,
size, and shape of the nostrils.

The nostrils should be oval or pear-shaped and symmetrically placed.
The columella should lie in the midline and should not exceed the diameter of either nostril in width. The alae should be fairly firm when dis-
tended and should not collapse upon inspiration. The flow of air should
be free through both nostrils and about equal on the two sides. This
can be simply tested by having the patient breathe against a mirror
held horizontally under the nose against the upper lip. The areas described by the condensation of moisture serve as an index to the flow
of air. Another method of judging is to close each nostril alternately as
the patient breathes forcibly. The pitch of the tone given off by the
column of air will be the same if both sides are freely open. If one side
is partially constricted, the pitch will be higher on that side.

Mouth breathing usually indicates nasal obstruction. If it has existed
since childhood, the entire face, as well as the external nose, may be
narrowed. The upper teeth are apt to be crowded and displaced and the
roof of the mouth may and often does arch very high.

INTERNAL NOSE EXAMINATION

Anterior Rhinoscopy. The examination of the nasal space from an
anterior approach is known as anterior rhinoscopy. The most important
instrument for this is the nasal speculum (Fig. 68), through which light
is reflected from a head mirror.

The vestibule is first inspected. Its common diseases are furuncles
and fissures, and a not uncommon abnormality is a deformity caused by

dislocation of the septal cartilage at the columella, or a deformity created by the shape of the alar cartilages.

Beyond the vestibule one visualizes the interior of the nose. The air channels are normally about equal in size on the two sides and are

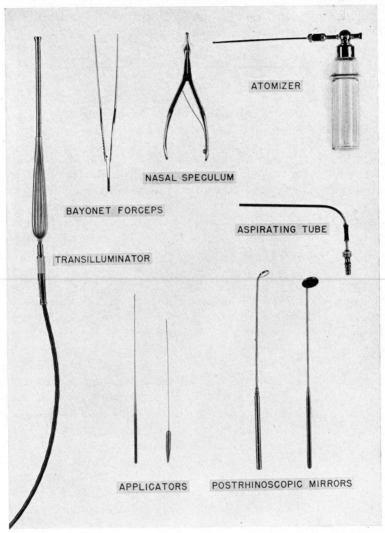

ATOMIZER

NASAL SPECULUM

BAYONET FORCEPS

ASPIRATING TUBE

TRANSILLUMINATOR

APPLICATORS   POSTRHINOSCOPIC MIRRORS

Fig. 68. Instruments usually necessary for the study of the nasal space.

only a few millimeters wide. The lower and middle turbinates should be readily visible on each side but should not impinge upon the septum. The spaces are wide in a negroid type of nose and very narrow in the case of a chronic mouth breather. If mouth breathing has persisted since childhood, it is not uncommon to find a nose in which the bony nasal framework is too small in all dimensions. To borrow a term from the obstetrician, one might call it a "generally contracted" nasal space. That the air channels are narrowed laterally can be determined readily by looking into the nose or even by inspecting the pyramid externally, but the degree to which the nasal space is compromised by elevation of the floor is appreciated best by looking at the roof of the mouth.

The following details are important to record:

Mucosa: injected, pale, congested, dry, hypertrophied, atrophied. *Secretion:* slight, moderate, profuse, watery, mucoid, purulent, crusts. *Origin:*............ *Septum:* normal, irregular, spurs, deviation (describe)............. *Obstruction:* from septum? (grade 1, 2, 3, 4)........... from hypertrophied mucosa or turbinates?........... Describe any abnormalities of the turbinates:.............. Note presence and location of polyps.........................

Mucous Membranes. The condition of the nasal mucosa can be determined by noting, among other things, the color. The normal color is a deep pink. If inflammation is present, it becomes red, and if the patient is suffering from nasal allergy it may be pale or bluish gray in color. A Tallqvist hemoglobinometer is a help in determining and recording color. In addition to color, all swelling, hypertrophy or atrophy, and the quantity, character and position of secretion should be noted. If a bacterial study is to be made, smears and cultures should be taken before any intranasal instrumentation.

Septum. The septum is almost never of uniform thickness and exactly in the midline. Some degree of irregularity is normal. The cartilaginous portion in the anterior third is thicker than the posterior bony portion, especially just between the anterior ends of the middle turbinates. There may be a ridge on one or both sides close to the floor where the septal cartilage joins the ridge of the palatine bones and vomer. However, these normal contours may be exaggerated into sharp ridges and spurs or marked thickening, crumpling, or deflections which may interfere with breathing or even close one or both sides more or less completely.

Turbinates. The turbinates should be inspected especially for hypertrophy, swelling, or atrophy. Any deviation from normal size, shape, position, or color should be noted. Sometimes the turbinates extend too far into the nasal space and must be fractured back into position. They are frequently enlarged or reduced in size to compensate for a deflection of the septum. Not infrequently such a large turbinate filling in a concavity of the septum contains a small air cell. If the color of a turbinate is a deeper red than that of the remainder of the mucosa, there may be an infection in one of the adjacent sinuses.

The middle and inferior meatuses are not visible normally to direct inspection, but the entrance into each under the corresponding turbinate can be seen. If there is a considerable purulent secretion from any of the

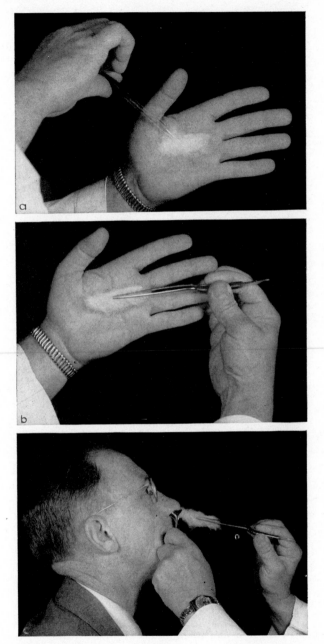

Fig. 69. The making of a cotton pledget for the use of medication for vasoconstriction and the application of a medicament. A fine grained piece of cotton is smoothed out in the palm of a hand, wetted with the medication, and inserted gently and easily into a nasal fossa. This method of introducing a medication is superior to the use of applicators (sticks) wound with a cotton tip, because these pledgets are more comfortable for the patient and the medication reaches more of the surface mucosa.

sinuses opening into the middle meatus, it will show as a wet, yellow streak at the anterior end of the middle meatus. Absence of such a streak does not mean that there is no purulent secretion, because the ciliary flow in the meatus is backward and may be sufficiently rapid to carry away all of the secretion. Hypertrophies of the inferior margins or pos-

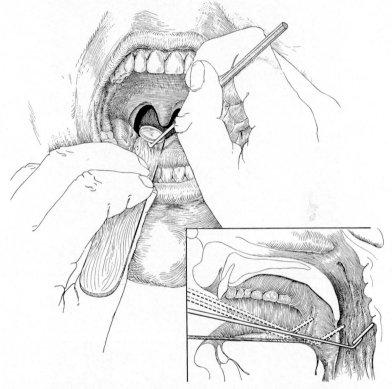

Fig. 70. Examination of the nasopharynx by means of a mirror introduced through the mouth. The figure shows the various positions in succeeding portions of the examination. A tongue blade is gently introduced and the tongue pushed downward. The mirror is slipped along the tongue blade and in many cases does not even touch the tongue itself. The mirror is slightly warmed to prevent fogging during exhalation. The mirror is held exactly as one holds a pen during writing. The handle is lowered as the mirror is introduced into the mouth until light is reflected from the mirror into the nasopharynx. This light returns to the mirror and to the observer's eye. The mirror is rotated by moving the thumb on the handle so that the handle turns on its long axis. This permits a "panorama" view of the nasopharynx.

terior ends of the turbinates can often be better inspected and studied by passing a probe into the corresponding meatus and pushing the hypertrophic part medially into the common meatus where it can be visualized better.

Shrinkage of Nasal Mucosa. The inspection of the nasal space by anterior rhinoscopy is facilitated by a mild shrinkage of the nasal

mucosa. This can be done with any of the vasoconstrictors, such as
1 per cent cocaine introduced on pledgets of cotton (Fig. 69) with a
bayonet forceps. Cocaine in this strength produces a light surface
anesthesia and a probe may be used without discomfort to test the consistency of the mucous membrane to determine the character of thickening, and so on. The shrinkage may also reveal abnormalities such as
scars, ridges, spurs, and polyps which were hidden at first.

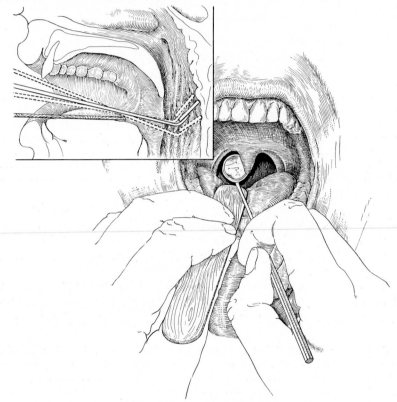

Fig. 71. See caption for Figure 70.

Secretion for study may be obtained by a swab and smeared on a
slide. When making swabs, care should be made to wind them in such
a way that the tip of the wire applicator is well covered with cotton.
Wooden applicators should not be used in the nose unless it be just in
the vestibule. A differential count of the cells in the smear often indicates whether the condition is due to infection or allergy.

POSTERIOR RHINOSCOPY

The next maneuver after inspecting the nasal space by anterior rhinoscopy is to study the space from the posterior aspect; that is, to visualize
the choanae through the nasopharynx (Figs. 70, 71). Since as all com-

plete rhinoscopic studies are supplemented by an examination of the pharynx, and the latter examination of necessity trespasses the oral cavity, the routine check of the oral cavity and nasopharynx should follow at this point. In examining the oral cavity, the condition of the following should be recorded:

Mucosa:............ *Duct orifices:* (parotid, submaxillary, sublingual).........
Teeth:......... *Hard palate:* (describe shape)......... *Occlusion:*.........
Tongue:......... *Soft palate:*...........

Tonsils. The most important structures in the posterior part of the oral cavity are the tonsils. The following aspects concerning these should be noted:

Size (grade 1, 2, 3, 4):...... Color......... Recessed?......... *Crypts:* (prominent or sealed)............ *Expression obtained by the pressure or suction:* (describe)............ *If the patient has had a tonsillectomy and there is some suspected tissue in the fossae:* Is the tissue definite faucial tonsil?............ lymphoid buds?......... lingual hypertrophy?......... remains of plica?......... Is there definite evidence of infection?......... Are the pillars intact?......... *Lingual tonsils:* (grade 1, 2, 3, 4)........... Evidence of infection?.............

Oropharynx and Nasopharynx. Beyond the oral cavity, the clinician next inspects the oropharynx and the nasopharynx. These are two of the three important areas which are usually referred to as the throat. This third area included in the throat is the hypopharynx, or laryngopharynx.

The oropharynx usually can be visualized with reflected light through the open mouth. This examination and that of the nasopharynx which is made with a postnasal mirror should record notations as follows:

Appearance: normal, injected, hypertrophic changes, dry. *Secretion:* mucoid, purulent, adherent, crusts. Are the hypertrophic changes in the nature of granular lymphoid patches?........... lateral pharyngeal bands?........... (grade 1, 2, 3, 4). Size and amount........... Is there any other swelling? (describe) .... Mirror view of the nasopharynx: Adenoid tissue?............. Hypertrophied or atrophied?......... prominent crypts?........... secretion? (describe)........... Fossae of Rosenmüller:........... Eustachian orifices: .... adhesions?............

Pharynx. Very little of the pharynx can be seen through a normal nose. There is usually a space close to the floor where one can look back into the pharynx. If the patient is asked to speak some words such as "twenty-five," the palate can be seen to rise and fall as the words are formed. If it fails to do so, or if the amplitude is diminished, there probably is an adenoid mass in the way. This is an especially valuable test for children in whom a posterior rhinoscopy is not possible. Sometimes the adenoid mass can be seen directly.

Technic

Posterior rhinoscopy is accomplished by means of a postnasal mirror which has been warmed enough to prevent condensation of moisture from the respired air. Some little practice is required to make this examination without causing the patient to gag. One plan is as follows: Depress the tongue, pushing it back and down gently, asking the patient to breathe through the mouth meanwhile. Place the mirror into the throat, avoiding contact with the pharynx and tongue, directing it toward the nasopharynx. Then ask the patient to breathe through his

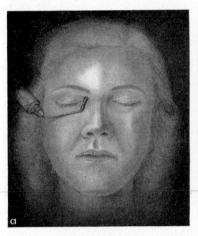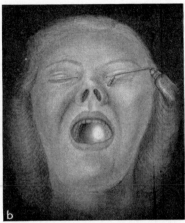

Fig. 72. Transillumination has a limited value in the diagnosis of sinus disease, but is a useful adjunct to the usual steps in the study of the nasal space. Several types of transilluminators are available. The one shown above is a transilluminating tip fitted to a battery handle that can also be used for an otoscope or ophthalmoscope.

The chief value of transillumination is for the frontal and maxillary sinuses. The tip is placed (a) below the floor of the frontal sinus and (b) just within the lower margin of the orbit or over the superior portion of the maxilla below the orbit. The effect of this latter light penetration is noted through the open mouth as the illumination through the hard palate is observed. The physician who employs transillumination should be mindful of the fact that a frontal sinus may be absent, especially on one side, and that thickness of soft tissue and type of bony facial development may affect light penetration.

nose with his mouth open. The palate will drop, permitting a view of the nasopharynx. The patient should be told immediately, "That's just right. Keep trying." If not, he is apt to pull his head away and explain that he can't breathe through his nose with his mouth open. The nasopharynx should be inspected for secretion and color of mucosa. The shape and size of the choanae, the posterior margin of the septum and the turbinates can all be seen. Mulberry hypertrophies of the posterior ends and of the septum are not uncommon and may be the source of postnasal drip. If the adenoid is hypertrophied, this can be determined readily, as can the condition of the eustachian orifices.

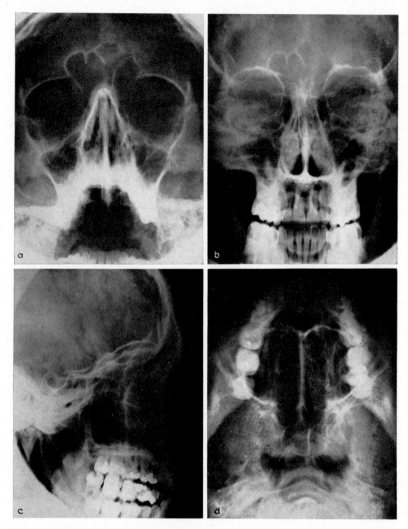

Fig. 73. Photographs of x-rays taken in the various positions used to study the sinuses. It is important to correlate x-ray findings with clinical manifestations.

When a single view is used (a) a relatively good view of the frontals, maxillaries and the sphenoid sinuses (projected through the mouth) is obtained. This is known as the Waldron-Waters position. The tip of the nose and the end of the chin are against the plate, and the direction of the ray is from above the occiput directed anteriorly. This brings the petrosal position of the temporal bones below the level of the maxillaries.

When additional special information is desired relative to the sinuses, an anterior-posterior view (b) is used to determine the possibility of a fluid level in the frontal sinuses, a lateral view (c) depicts the anterior and posterior margins of the frontal sinuses and the sphenoid sinus in relation to the sella turcica, or the sphenoid (d) is projected through the floor of the mouth.

NASAL ACCESSORY SINUSES

After the nasal space has been studied through both the anterior and posterior approaches, additional information is usually desirable regarding the condition of the nasal accessory sinuses. This information is obtained by palpation, transillumination and x-ray to supplement the information already obtained from the history and inspection of the nose. The frontal areas and canine fossae should be palpated and percussed for tenderness. External swelling and inflammation are rare, but tenderness over the frontals and maxillaries frequently occurs in acute sinusitis.

Transillumination has limited value, especially in the case of the frontal sinuses, but often demonstrates maxillary sinusitis very well (Fig. 72). It is useless in ethmoidal and sphenoidal disease. The transilluminator should be in circuit with a rheostat in order that the current may be reduced to the lowest point at which the light passes through the sinuses. Intrasinus disease shows much better with low illumination than with high.

When sinusitis is suspected and it is important to obtain more accurate studies of the sinuses, x-ray studies are made. A single view may be entirely practical in which the contents of all the sinuses are revealed with considerable accuracy. This view, known as the Waters-Waldron position or nose-chin position, is shown in Fig. 73a. The patient's mouth is opened and his nose and chin placed in contact with the film. The rays are then projected through the occiput. Added information may be obtained regarding the frontal sinuses by a posterior-anterior projection in which the patient's nose and forehead are against the film with the head in an upright position. The rays are projected through the occiput (Fig. 73b). A lateral view (Fig. 73c) will give information concerning the sphenoid, ethmoid and frontal sinuses. Additional information on the sphenoid sinus may be determined by a special projection of this sinus through the floor of the mouth (Fig. 73d).

CHAPTER XIII

THE COMMON COLD

ANDERSON C. HILDING, M.D.

Causative Virus. The common cold is a widespread contagious epidemic disease which occurs in all climates especially in the autumn and spring months. It is caused by a filterable virus, as was demonstrated by Kruse in 1914 and corroborated since then by the work of Dochez and his group. The cold has been reproduced experimentally in the chimpanzee under adequate experimental controls both by direct exposure to patients with colds and by the filtered nasopharyngeal washings of sufferers. The virus has been cultured and subcultured, and the disease has been transmitted from one ape to another by means of the passage of this virus. It has been successfully cultured up to eighty times.

The virus grows upon chick embryo medium under anaerobic conditions. It becomes inactivated at 56° C. (132.8° F.) after a short exposure. It remains active at icebox temperature for two weeks and if frozen and desiccated has retained activity as long as four months.

This virus promotes the growth of pathogenic bacteria in the pharynx. The normal bacterial flora of the pharynx is much the same the world over, with some variation from season to season. When the cold virus attacks, the growth of pathogenic bacteria is enhanced and complications are apt to arise from these secondary invaders. The common complications are suppurative rhinitis, sinusitis, otitis media, laryngitis and bronchitis. Epidemics of colds are characterized by their complications, and these in turn depend upon the strains of pathogenic bacteria which happen to be abroad in the community at that time. A study of the children in an orphanage was made by Smillie in 1940. He found that pneumococcus type 14 was present in all the children, but all were well. Then an epidemic of colds went through the institution. The number of pneumococcus type 14 increased in the throats of the children. Several developed otitis media and two developed pneumonia. Pneumococcus 14 was recovered from the sputum of the two with pneumonia and from the ear discharge of those having otitis media.

External Causes. It has long been held that exposure to sudden changes of temperature, especially if chilling and wetting are involved, causes colds. This is such a universal experience that it cannot be disregarded. There have been several controlled studies which indicate definitely that exposure is at least a factor in the causation of colds. Gahwyler made controlled observations on two different occasions upon rather large bodies of troops. The first observation was made on 2700 men sent into the wet trenches, compared with 5300 kept in the barracks; and the second was made on 4500 men kept out in a sharp wind for three days, compared with 3500 kept in their quarters. In both instances, the incidence of colds was about four times as great in the exposed groups as in the protected ones. In both instances, apparently there was chilling from wind and dampness. On the other hand, extreme dry cold, as in subzero weather, does not seem to have this effect of promoting colds.

Chilling seems to bring about this effect by reduction in the temperature of the nasal mucosa. A drop of as much as 6° C. has been measured when the surface of the body, at a distant point, was chilled.

Contagiousness. It has been quite thoroughly established by a number of studies that colds are contagious. Contagiousness begins, according to some workers (Olitsky and McCartney), a few hours before the onset of symptoms and lasts for about two days; that is, the virus will actively transmit the disease if removed during this time. On the other hand, according to Paul and Freese, there is evidence that the carriers may harbor an active virus for many weeks during which the carriers have no symptoms. One of the most striking studies was carried out by Paul and Freese at Spitzbergen where they lived for a year. During the winter months, the cold virus seemed to die out. Immunity from a cold lasts about a month and the virus, in order to survive, must be passed frequently to susceptible persons. In the isolated community at Spitzbergen, everyone has colds during the short shipping season of the summer and then after shipping ceases, the immunity is so universal that the virus dies out. By the time the first ship arrives in the spring, however, everyone is again susceptible and within forty-eight hours after the arrival of the first ship, some 75 per cent of the inhabitants develop colds. This happens whether anyone on board the ship has a cold or not. Apparently there are always one or more carriers on board.

Control. The spread can be controlled by isolation, theoretically, since the spread is due to droplet infection. But people will not submit to isolation. For some strange reason, cold sufferers consider themselves to be self-sacrificing good sports when they remain at work instead of going home. This has two effects. They spread the virus to others and they pick up bacteria from others upon their damaged and susceptible mucous membranes, thereby doubtless enhancing their chances of developing complications.

Incidence. There are three peaks in the incidence of colds in most communities. They are September and October, January and February, and April and May. The incubation period is about twenty-four to thirty-six hours. The patient is most contagious during the first day.

PATHOLOGY

The pathologic picture seen in the nose during colds is that of an inflammatory reaction of the mucous membrane. It is swollen, red, and covered with profuse discharge. The air passages are frequently occluded by swollen nembrane or secretion, or both.

The microscopic changes which take place according to a study which we made some fifteen years ago are about as follows: First, there develops an edema of the submucosa, followed by an infiltration of macrophages and a few cells of the granulocytic series (granulocytes). The first change to appear in the epithelium is a separation of the cells as though a fluid formed between them. They loosen and the surface cells begin to slough off. Some become vacuolated or foamy in appearance; and a necrotic zone may form next to the surface of single cells or groups of cells. This necrosis may extend deep. Then almost the entire epithelium disintegrates; it looks as though it had been exploded. Many and sometimes all of the columnar cells are gone by the third day. Some of the stellate cells close to the basement membrane also slough out. During this stage, the nasal secretion may contain many epithelial cells, many of which are surmounted by vigorously active cilia. Sometimes there may be only a single layer of cells left on the basement membrane. The cells that remain proliferate after the most acute stage has passed until they are many layers deep. A syncytium forms at the surface. Finally the surface cells begin to lengthen until they again look like columnar cells. The cellular infiltration of the submucosa is largely composed of variously shaped lymphocytes and monocytes (mononuclear cells) with a scattering of band and segmented cells (polymorphonuclear cells) and some eosinophils. The edema soon decreases, but the cellular infiltrate increases. By the second or third day, many cells of the granulocytic series (granulocytes) and macrophages are found in the epithelium on their way to the surface. They increase in number as the purulent stage develops.

Repair seems to take place even while there is still much secretion in the nose. A many-layered epithelium full of cells of the granulocytic series was found on the eighth day, and on the tenth day, the surface cells showed elongation and on the fourteenth day, definite columnar form.

In our study, no bacteria were ever found in the epithelium or submucosa, only in the secretion. Neither were any inclusion bodies found.

CLINICAL FEATURES

The outstanding clinical feature of a cold is the profuse, thin secretion. The physical differences between this and the normal secretion are obvious. The secretion of the cold is thin, watery and has a very low viscosity. The chemical differences have not been well worked out. The lysozyme content seems definitely to be reduced beginning before the onset of symptoms. It increases again about the time that symptoms grow better. The pH remains essentially unchanged or becomes slightly alkaline.

PREVENTION

There has been an impressive amount of effort expended upon preventing colds. The results on the whole have been disappointing.

Vaccines. Vaccination by bacterial vaccines has been given thorough trial by the subcutaneous and oral routes and even locally in the mucous membrane. Reports have been both favorable and unfavorable. One author who presents strikingly good results from subcutaneous vaccination writes, "No control series was used, as the primary purpose of the inoculations was to do something for the students and not to test the vaccine. It did not seem fair to exclude students wishing vaccination simply to provide a control group for statistics." Another author, Dr. Harold S. Diehl, using the same method, reduced the incidence of colds in a group of students equally successfully—in fact, by 55 per cent. However, he vaccinated a control group with normal saline solution and obtained even more favorable results in this control group, namely, 61 per cent reduction.

Vaccination by bacterial vaccines both by mouth and subcutaneously appears at this time to be valueless for reducing either the incidence or severity of colds.

Vaccination by nasal spray looked very promising for a time, but studies at Minnesota gave negative results.

Unfortunately, both the cold virus and the group of pathogenic organisms usually found in the nasopharyngeal flora are very weak producers of antigens. One would scarcely expect any notable results from vaccination. The immunity following an attack of coryza lasts only three or four weeks. Likewise, infections by micrococci (staphylococci) and streptococci in general produce no lasting immunity in patients who recover.

Dochez tried vaccination with heat-killed virus by hypodermic injection The results were promising in apes, but negative in man. Vaccination by influenzal virus, on the other hand, appears to be very promising and it was hoped that the cold virus also would produce an effective immunity, but such does not seem to be the case.

Vitamins and Drugs. Attempts to prevent colds by vitamins have proved fruitless. Sulfonamides have been tried and most reports have given negative results. More recently there have been some studies in the military service which seem to indicate that small doses of sulfonamides reduce the incidence, but this is yet to be corroborated. On the other hand, there is fairly good evidence that these drugs prevent complications by bacteria.

Air Conditioning. As now practiced in office buildings and theaters, air conditioning is of no value as a preventative.

There is, however, another type of air conditioning which is aimed at destruction of bacteria and viruses floating in the atmosphere, which seems to be very effective in stopping the spread of infection. The purification can be accomplished either by aerosols, antiseptic chemicals, or by ultraviolet light. The latter seems to be very promising. It can be used either by subjecting the whole room to ultraviolet rays, or just the source of air, or it can be used in the form of barriers of light. Wells states that the foundations for efficienctly purifying air and checking its purity are as well established as the control of the purity of the supply of drinking water. He believes that such control and purification of air supply is necessary to free us from air-borne infection. He likens the contamination of air supply by the nasopharynx to the contamination of water supply by the excreta from the intestinal tract. Perhaps in this we have an effective method of preventing colds in schools and factories.

Hardening Process. The hardening process has long been advocated as a cold preventative; that is, cold baths, outdoor exercise and calisthenics. It may have some value, but has not been subjected to enough well-controlled studies to have established a value. People who spend most of their time outdoors do have fewer colds, but they also have fewer contacts with infection.

TREATMENT

In general, treatment has been as disappointing as prevention and it is just as difficult to determine the value of the suggested remedies. Colds are self limited unless complicated. Some are abortive and are over in a few hours. Some last only twenty-four or forty-eight hours. And others, when complicated, run a course covering several weeks. When symptoms disappear after the exhibition of some remedy, it is difficult to know if the remedy exerted some beneficial influence, or if the attack was about to subside anyway.

Codeine and *papaverine* seem to have some definite value in aborting a cold. This was brought out in a study at Minnesota. The combination is known commercially as Copavin. One tablet containing $\frac{1}{4}$ grain each of codeine and papaverine is prescribed every four hours or after each meal, with a double dose at bedtime.

Steaming often gives symptomatic relief.

If serious complications threaten, then the *sulfonamides* or *penicillin* are indicated.

Isolation should be practiced whenever feasible. It not only prevents spread of the cold virus, but protects the sufferer from bacterial infection of his damaged epithelium by droplets from other persons. If bacterial infection can be prevented, the attack will soon be over because the virus stage is so short.

Of all the many nasal drops that have been advocated, simple *ephedrine in saline solution* seems to give about as much relief from nasal obstruction as anything else. This is of course purely symptomatic treatment. The question might be raised, why do we want to open the nasal passages when nature has closed them? Perhaps the closure is purposeful. I have tried the following: As soon as there is any sign or symptom of an approaching cold, the patient has been instructed to block the nostril (or nostrils) with clean cotton, tightly enough to reduce materially the inflow of air. The cotton must be changed frequently. It has seemed that the irritation is greatly reduced by this simple measure and often the swelling does not become great enough to obstruct the air passage.

Much treatment has been directed toward the cilia, generally with a view toward stimulation. But do we know if the cilia need stimulation during a cold? Perhaps they are working at capacity as it is. In some cases, they are largely destroyed. Under such circumstances, stimulation would seem to be irrational.

If stimulation is desired, it can be had by means of a mildly alkaline solution (8 to 8.5) which contains *magnesium* and *calcium* salts. At pH 8.5 in Tyrode's solution, the cilia will continue to be active for twenty-four hours. Acids, on the other hand, paralyze ciliary action. It ceases entirely if the pH drops to 6.4 or less. If magnesium or calcium ions are omitted, the tissue breaks up and action ceases. The sodium ion, according to Negus, is the strongest inhibitor of ciliary action.

One of the reasons so many testimonials can be found concerning the efficacy of some particular remedy in the control of a cold is the fact that nasal obstruction from other causes is common and the onset of nasal obstruction is often interpreted as the onset of a cold. Vasomotor congestion of a temporary nature is common and is caused by fatigue, chilling, alcohol and so on. Its duration is usually short. Almost any remedy taken at the onset may coincide with the early subsequent relief, since the condition would normally persist for a very brief period. Thus whatever remedy is taken may be credited with the relief.

REFERENCES

Diehl, H. S.: Medicinal Treatment of the Common Cold. J.A.M.A., *101*:2042, 1933

Diehl, H. S., Baker, A. B., and Cowan, D. W.: Cold Vaccines, A Further Evaluation. J.A.M.A., *115*:593, 1940.

Hilding, A.: Summary of Some Known Facts Concerning the Common Cold. Ann. Otol., Rhin. & Laryng., *53*:444, 1944.

Kler, J.: Analysis of Colds in Industry. Arch. Otolaryng., *41*:395, 1945.

Proetz, A. W.: Nasal Physiology in Relation to the Common Cold. Ann. Otol., Rhin. & Laryng., *55*:306, 1946.

Research on the Common Cold. Foreign Letters, J.A.M.A., *131*:935, 1946.

Ruskin, S. L.: The Vascular Dynamics of the Common Cold and Allergic Rhinitis. Arch. Otolaryng., *55*:904, 1946.

Schall, L.: Pathology of Nasal Mucous Membrane and Suggestions as to Treatment. Ann. Otol., Rhin. & Laryng., *53*:390, 1944.

Walsh, T. E.: Prophylaxis of the Common Cold. Arch. Otolaryng., *34*:1093, 1941.

CHAPTER XIV

NASAL ALLERGY

ROBERT E. PRIEST, M.D.

Allergy is a state of hypersensitivity to certain substances in the environment. The nonallergic person suffers no discomfort when he meets these substances, but the allergic person possesses certain tissues which become sensitized to the substance in question. These are called "shock tissues." The sensitizing agents are called "allergens." Shock tissues may be found anywhere within the body. Although we are particularly concerned here with allergy of the tissues lining the nose and paranasal sinuses, we must also consider allergic manifestations elsewhere in the body. A history of eczema, urticaria, asthma, or gastrointestinal allergy is good corroborative evidence when a diagnosis of nasal allergy is being considered. Most allergic persons have more than one allergic manifestation.

The exact mechanism involved in the production of allergic reactions is not known. The process is thought to be similar to immunity formation. A person with an hereditary tendency to become easily sensitized is brought into somewhat prolonged contact with a potential allergen. Certain tissues become sensitized. The person again comes into contact with the allergen and the tissues previously sensitized react, each in its own peculiar way. The clinical reaction depends upon what tissues and organs are affected. Vasodilatation and increased vascular permeability allowing transudation of lymph probably occur in these lesions. The formation of a toxic substance to account for the vascular changes has been postulated.

DIAGNOSIS OF NASAL ALLERGY

Patients with nasal allergy often complain of frequent head colds. They say that they are scarcely over one cold when another begins. Their symptoms differ from those occurring in infectious rhinitis. The allergic cold is usually characterized by profuse, watery nasal discharge. The patient does not have fever during the invasive stage; the secretion does not progress from thin at first to thick and purulent later, as in infectious rhinitis. Some patients with nasal allergy have infrequent attacks, since their allergen is seldom encountered.

The diagnosis of nasal allergy should be established by systematic investigation. This may include history, nasal examination, a study of

164

the cytology of nasal secretions, paranasal sinus examination, skin tests and elimination regimens. In some cases, all these methods of examination may be needed, while in others only a few will be necessary. Schemes for the elimination of suspected allergens are used as diagnostic procedures as well as for treatment.

HISTORY

The diagnosis of allergic rhinitis is made largely by the characteristic history. In addition to the allergic cold symptoms detailed previously, inquiry into family history is important. Many allergic persons have allergic relatives. Questions concerning childhood may disclose food idiosyncrasies, previous asthma, hay fever, eczema, or hives. Detailed queries as to onset of the present illness are most important. The association of the onset of symptoms with a change in occupation or residence may furnish a significant clue. The best method of obtaining an accurate history is to follow a definite plan of inquiry.

In history-taking in cases of seasonal hay fever, certain special points are worth noting. The exact date of onset of symptoms should coincide with the pollination time of the suspected plant. A history of previous treatment should include the pollens used, dosage and degree of freedom from symptoms produced by the therapy.

HISTORY FORM FOR NASAL ALLERGY

Family History:

Did father . . . . have	1) hay fever
mother	2) asthma
sister	3) asthma coincidental with hay fever
brother	4) urticaria
uncle	5) eczema
aunt	6) migraine
cousin	7) chronic nasal or sinus disease

Past History:

As a baby, did you have: eczema . . . . . ., gastrointestinal disturbances? . . . . . . As a child, did you have: hay fever? . . . . . . urticaria? . . . . . . eczema? . . . . . . migraine? . . . . . . chronic nasal or sinus disease? . . . . . . gastrointestinal disorders? . . . . . . Did certain foods trouble you? . . . . . . Which foods? . . . . Have you had any nose or throat operations? . . . . . . List them: . . . .

Present Illness:

How does your nose bother you? Sneezing . . . . . ., itching . . . . . ., discharge . . . . . . (character: thin . . . . . ., watery . . . . . ., profuse . . . . . ., scanty . . . . . ., purulent . . . . . ., thick . . . . . .) anosmia . . . . . ., obstruction to breathing . . . . . ., other symptoms . . . . Right side only . . . . . .; left side only . . . . . .; both sides . . . . . . Constantly . . . . . .; intermittently . . . . Is there seasonal variation: Worse: summer . . . . . ., fall . . . . . ., winter . . . . . ., spring . . . . . . Worse: night . . . . . ., forenoon . . . . . ., afternoon . . . . . ., evening . . . . . ., Worse: dry . . . ., or damp . . . . weather. Do eyes swell . . . . . ., itch . . . . . ., burn . . . . . .? Do any foods disagree with you? . . . . . . Which ones? . . . . Do you eat them often?

.... How long have they disagreed?........... What is your occupation?
.... Where do you work?................ How long have you
done this work?.......... Did your trouble begin with any change in your work?
.... Where do you live?................ How long have you lived
there?.......... Do you live near grass, weeds, flowers, trees?.......... What
ones?.. Did your trouble begin with
any change in residence?....... Did your trouble begin with change of life?....
.... Pregnancy?............ Do you come into contact with: cats......,
dogs......, horses......, cattle......, poultry......, other house pets......
Of what materials are the following articles in your possession made? Pillows......
.........., blankets................, mattresses................., rugs....
.... Do you have house plants?.......... Do you use face powder?
....

NASAL EXAMINATION

The nasal mucosa in most nasal allergies is pale, grayish-pink, moist and swollen (Fig. 74). The secretion is thin or mucoid rather than thick

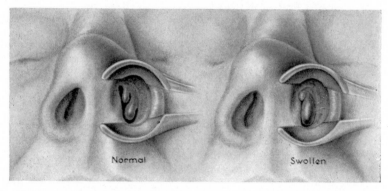

Fig. 74. A comparison of the anterior rhinoscopic views in the normal nose with one in which the turbinates are swollen as in acute allergic rhinitis.

and purulent. Purulent secretion may indicate the presence of infectious rhinitis or sinusitis superimposed on an allergic state. Polyps are commonly present in noses of persons with chronic allergy. Experienced rhinologists recognize the moist allergic-type of nasal interior at a glance.

NASAL SMEARS

Microscopic examination of stained smears of nasal secretion is useful in the diagnosis of nasal allergy. The typical smear in nasal allergy contains large numbers of eosinophilic leukocytes (Fig. 75). Sometimes these cells fill the field. They may be clumped and enmeshed in blue-staining debris.

When eosinophilic leukocytes appear in combination with segmented (polymorphonuclear) neutrophilic leukocytes, allergy is not ruled out. The presence of both infection and allergy may be indicated. Sometimes one can follow the disappearance of neutrophilic leukocytes as infection recedes, and the reappearance of eosinophils as the pre-existing allergic state resumes prominence.

Why eosinophils occur in the nasal secretions of allergic persons is not understood. The significance of nasal smear examinations is still debated. It is believed that the finding of a high proportion of eosino-

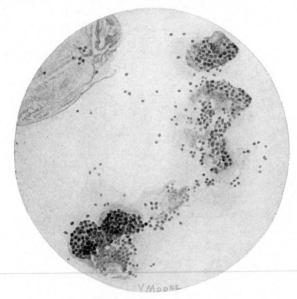

Fig. 75. Illustration of material from nasal smear stained as described in text. The granules in the cells stain with eosin and therefore are pink. The cytoplasm is blue. The cells are broken up in the average nasal smear and they do not have the uniform morphology of eosinophils in a blood smear. Sometimes the granules are found outside the broken-up cells as well as in the cytoplasm. This is shown in the illustration.

phils among the cells present in a stained smear of nasal secretions is evidence that the patient's nose shows an allergic reaction. When only a few eosinophils are found, the diagnosis is in doubt. The nasal smear must be evaluated as part of the general diagnostic problem.

Procedure for Staining Slides

A satisfactory method for staining nasal smears is as follows:

Stains:

1. Eosin Y (yellowish) USP, 0.3 gm. in 60 cc. methyl alcohol.
2. Methylene blue, 0.3 gm. in 60 cc. methyl alcohol.

Staining procedure:

1. Fix slides with heat.
2. Cover slide with eosin for one minute.
3. Cover slide with distilled water and leave on for one more minute.

4. Rinse slide off with distilled water.
5. Decolorize very quickly with 95 per cent alcohol.
6. Cover slide with methylene blue and leave for ten seconds.
7. Wash with distilled water.
8. Decolorize with 95 per cent alcohol and allow to dry.

Use oil immersion lens to examine.

SKIN TESTS

Skin tests are performed by applying suspected allergens to the patient's skin. The reaction of the skin about each point where test material is applied is observed and recorded. A reaction indicating sensitivity is similar to a mosquito bite in appearance. It consists of a central area of edema surrounded by an erythematous wheal which may have irregular projections called pseudopods at its periphery. The violence of the skin reaction does not necessarily indicate the degree of nasal mucous membrane sensitivity. Skin tests are more accurate with inhalants than with foods.

Skin tests are carried out in several different ways. *Intradermal tests* are made by injecting enough test material between the layers of the skin to raise a small wheal. *Scratch tests* are made by applying the suspected allergens to short scratches made in the skin by a needle or a knife. One allergen is rubbed into each scratch. *Pressure puncture tests* are made with an ordinary sewing needle held nearly parallel to the skin surface. From four to eight oblique punctures are made through the epidermis in the same manner as in making a smallpox vaccination. A little allergen is carried in with each puncture. *Patch tests* are done by holding some of the suspected allergen against the skin by means of bandage, tape, or transparent material such as cellophane. The latter permits continuous observation of the reaction.

Skin testing is not without danger. In very sensitive persons, severe allergic reactions may be precipitated, particularly by intradermal tests. Death has resulted from such reactions. A syringe filled with 1:1000 epinephrine should be at hand when tests are made. This medication counteracts the allergic reaction. As soon as a definite systemic allergic reaction is known to be occurring, $\frac{1}{2}$ cc. should be injected subcutaneously. The untoward reaction precipitated by the test may be an ordinary attack of allergic rhinitis or asthma. Severe reactions resemble traumatic shock. The patient grows cold, perspires, becomes pale, feels faint. The pulse is thready and the condition is obviously grave. The patient's general health should be carefully evaluated before skin testing may be safely undertaken.

ELIMINATION REGIMENS

The elimination of a particular substance from the patient's environment would seem to be simple, but in reality it may be difficult. Common allergens occur in unexpected places. For example, soybeans are used to make flour, and may occur in salad dressings, sausage, milk substitutes, ice cream, shortenings, butter substitutes, cheeses, printer's ink, massage cream, soap, coffee substitutes, plastics and elsewhere. As another example, consider cottonseed and cottonseed oil. One or both are found in mattresses, upholstering, house dust, fertilizers, salad oil, shortening, candies and cosmetics. Cottonseed oil has been fed to cows and has caused eczema in cottonseed-sensitive babies given the milk of those cows. Corn is another common substance which causes symptoms as either a food or inhalant. It is found in canned fruits, candy, sausage, sugar, bread, starch, syrup, grape juice, chewing gum, baking powder, ice cream and elsewhere. Other very common allergens with wide distribution are wheat, milk and eggs.

A perusal of these lists makes clear the extreme difficulty of knowing just where a particular allergenic substance may be encountered. Yet such knowledge is essential to the proper application of any elimination scheme.

Elaborate plans have been worked out to enable patients to avoid completely certain items of food. The diets of Rowe are an example. They supply sample menus, recipes and instructions concerning application of the regimen. Elimination of contact with inhalants may be necessary in addition to removal of foods from the diet.

TREATMENT

Treatment of nasal allergy requires well-balanced judgment. It is easy to be overenthusiastic in judging the results of treatment. Most physicians have seen dramatic results from elimination of allergenic substances and desensitization therapy, but it is well to remember that no adequate experimental control exists in any one allergic patient. At least part of any patient's apparent improvement may be due to suggestion. One should keep in mind the results obtained by Diehl and his associates in their cold prevention studies. Members of their statistically significant control group reported 61 per cent reduction in number of colds after administration of completely inert medications. Jensen and Stoesser have demonstrated that the psychic factors must be recognized and treated in some cases to obtain satisfactory therapeutic results.

It is often impossible to separate the results due to suggestion and those due to biochemical influences. An editorial in the Journal of Allergy says that: "The many curious coincidences following therapeutic measures and dietetic restrictions must not be interpreted and reported as cause and effect unless supported by repeated trials. Etiological diagnoses must have the ring of common sense and not wishful thinking."

LOCAL NASAL TREATMENT

Any therapeutic procedure which diminishes the ability of the nasal mucosa to swell but does not produce undue dryness and crusting increases the patient's nasal breathing space. Topical application of 1 per cent *ephedrine sulfate*, or 1 per cent *ephedrine sulfate* and 1 per cent *cocaine hydrochloride* gives temporary relief. One must be cautious about the use of cocaine for fear of addiction. Pharmacologically there is advantage in the mixture, since the curves of mucous membrane shrinkage for the two substances are reciprocal. *Tuamine sulfate* 2 per cent, and *phenylephrine hydrochloride* (neo-synephrine) $\frac{1}{4}$ per cent, are also good vasoconstrictors. One must bear in mind the necessity for approximating the nasal *p*H when selecting a vasoconstrictor. The effect of the medication on nasal ciliary action must also be considered.

Permanent reduction in the volume of the nasal mucosa can be obtained by *cauterization* of the inferior and middle turbinates with an actual cautery, an electrocautery (high frequency) needle, or by injection of a *sclerosing solution* into the submucosal tissue. The guiding principle here is to avoid destruction of the nasal epithelium.

Removal of Nasal Polyps. This is often necessary in the treatment of allergic rhinitis. This procedure is not difficult, but accurate diagnosis is essential. Physicians unaccustomed to examination of the interior of the nose may mistake swollen turbinates for nasal polyps. Examination after shrinkage of the lining membrane with 1 per cent ephedrine solution, together with the use of a cotton-tipped probe for palpation, helps in identification of nasal structures.

Polyps have narrow pedicles. They are gray, round, and resemble moist white grapes in appearance. Their size varies from a few millimeters to 4 or 5 cm. in diameter. Mirror examination of the nasopharynx may show that polyps project into the nasopharynx, occluding one or both choanae.

Anesthesia for polypectomy may be obtained by proper topical application of local anesthetic agents to the nasal mucosa. One must know the limitations of any such medication and be informed as to its potential dangers. Cocaine is the most effective, as well as one of the most toxic local anesthetics. It is safe not to use over 2 grains (0.128 gm.) at any one time, whether in solution or crystalline form. It is safest to precede its use by oral administration of the usual bedtime dose of a barbiturate such as phenobarbital or pentobarbital sodium. Barbiturates are antidotes for cocaine. Severe cocaine reactions can be controlled by intravenous injection of barbiturates.

The actual removal of a nasal polyp is accomplished by looping the wire of a standard nasal snare around the polyp, sliding the wire up onto the pedicle, and nearly closing the snare. The polyp is then avulsed so that the pedicle is torn off near its point of origin. Recurrence of polyps is common in allergic noses. The rate of recurrence varies greatly. Some patients must have polyps removed every six months; others only every few years. The rate of recurrence of nasal polyps decreases when proper allergic management is instituted. All tissues removed from the nose should be studied histologically.

SYSTEMIC TREATMENT

Rational systemic treatment of allergic reactions depends either on removing suspected allergenic substances from the patient's environment or on increasing the patient's tolerance to them.

Removal from contact is the method of choice when feasible. Animal emanations, feathers, wool, silk and similar substances are handled in this way. Foods are eliminated from the diet.

Desensitization by injection of progressively increasing doses of allergens which cannot be removed from the environment may be necessary. Increased tolerance to pollens and house dust are secured by this means. Desensitization to histamine is supposed to increase the tolerance to allergens generally. Histamine is theoretically destroyed by the enzyme histaminase. Claims that this agent reduces allergic reactions have been advanced by some investigators and denied by others. Certain drugs are supposed to be antihistaminic and therefore are thought to be of value in treating allergic persons. Diphenhydramine hydrochloride (benadryl) and tryphennamine hydrochloride (pyribenzamine) are examples of such drugs. Members of this family of drugs vary in the degree of relief they confer, and also in their tendency to produce asthma while relieving nasal congestion. They cannot be used indiscriminately. Their asthma-producing qualities must be taken into account.

REFERENCES

Diehl, H. S., Baker, A. B., and Cowan, D. W.: Cold Vaccines, a Further Evaluation. J.A.M.A., *115*:593, 1940.

Diehl, H. S.: The Common Cold. Proc. Interst. Postgrad. M.A. North America, p. 252, 1943.

Editorial: Allergy at the Crossroads. J. Allergy, *16*:109, 1945.

Elimination Diets. San Francisco, J. W. Stacey, Inc., Distributor.

Fabricant, N. D.: Significance of the *p*H of Nasal Secretions in Situ. Arch. Otolaryng., *34*:150 and 297, 1941.

Fabricant, N. D.: Effect of Silver Preparations and Antiseptics on the *p*H of Nasal Secretions in Situ. *Ibid.*, *34*:302, 1941.

Fishof, F. E.: The Treatment of Vasomotor Rhinitis and Allied Conditions with Sodium Morrhuate. *Ibid.*, *27*:413, 1938.

Goodhill, V.: Pyribenzamine in Allergic Rhinitis. Laryngoscope, *46*:687, 1946.

Hansel, F. K.: Principles of Diagnosis and Treatment of Allergy as Related to Otalaryngology. *Ibid.*, *53*:260, 1943.

Healy, J. C.: Evaluation of Allergen Diagnosis. Ann. Otol., Rhin. & Laryng., *55*:871 1946.

Jensen, R. A., and Stoesser, A. V.: Emotional Factor in Bronchial Asthma in Children. Am. J. Dis. Child., *62*:80, 1941.

Proetz, A. W.: 2-Amino-Heptane Sulfate as a Vasoconstrictor. Ann. Otol., Rhin. &
    Laryng., *51*:112, 1942.

Proetz, A. W.: Effects of Drugs on Living Nasal Ciliated Epithelium. *Ibid.*, *43*:450,
    1934.

Rowe, A. H.: Elimination Diets and Patient's Allergies. A Handbook of Allergy.
    Philadelphia, Lea & Febiger, 1944.

Shambaugh, G. E., Jr.: Nasal Allergy for the Practicing Rhinologist. Ann. Otol.,
    Rhin. & Laryng., *54*:43, 1945.

Stoesser, A. V.: Recent Observations on Hay Fever in Children. Journal Lancet,
    62:174, 1942.

Thacker, E. A.: Treatment of Chronic Obstructive Rhinitis with Injections of Sodium
    Psylliate. Ann. Otol., Rhin. & Laryng., *49*:939, 1940.

CHAPTER XV

CHRONIC NASAL OBSTRUCTION

George M. Tangen, M.D.

Nasal obstruction occurs in all age groups, and children are apparently affected as frequently as adults. Patients with this complaint make up a

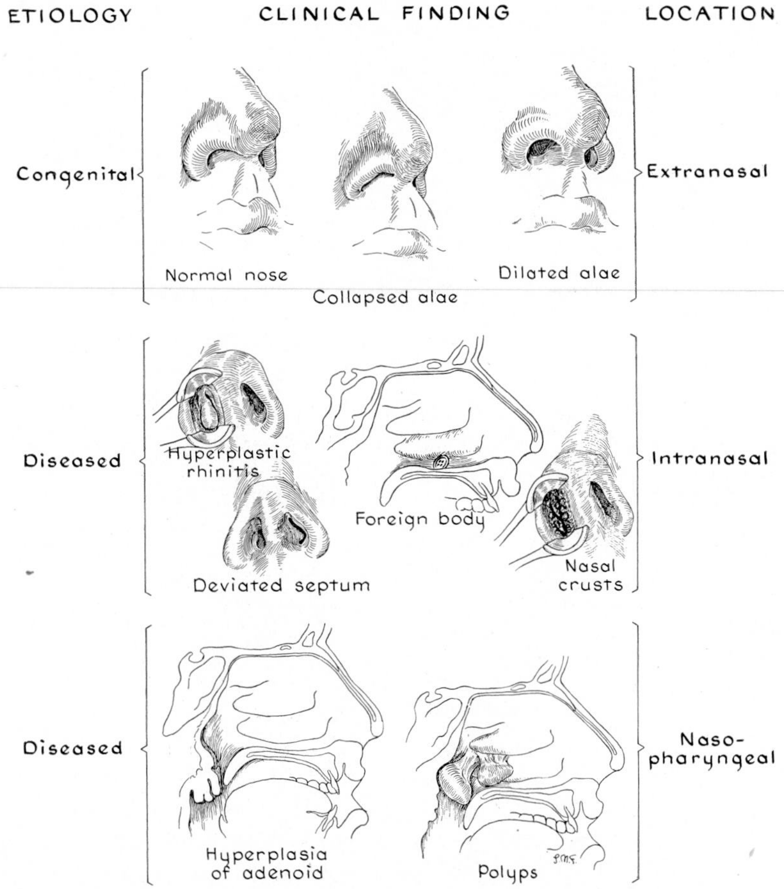

Fig. 76. A chart depicting the causes of nasal obstruction.

large percentage of a rhinologist's practice. This seems understandable when one reviews the numerous causes of nasal obstruction (Fig. 76). There are three types of nasal obstruction: acute, intermittent and chronic. The degree of distress complained of by any patient seems to bear an inconstant relationship to the extent of the obstruction actually visualized in the nasal passages. The suddenness of the onset of the obstruction is apparently the determining factor in the degree of discomfort produced. Many patients with marked blockage of both nares of a chronic nature complain of very little discomfort. This may be due to the gradual onset of the trouble and the ability of the nasal passages to compensate for the obstruction. On the other hand, the obstruction

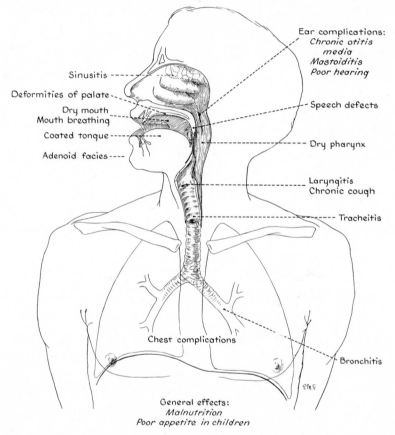

Fig. 77. A chart depicting the effects of nasal obstruction.

produced by acute allergic rhinitis, or coryza, may be very uncomfortable because of the suddenness of the attack, and the inability of the nasal chambers to compensate for the congestion within a short period of time.

Obstruction of the nasal passages produces physiologic changes and interferes with the normal functions of the nose. The main processes interfered with are: (1) respiratory, (2) olfactory and gustatory, (3) phonatory, and (4) ventilation of the paranasal sinuses, eustachian tubes and middle ear.

In addition to these local processes, there are changes elsewhere in the respiratory tract (Fig. 77). Most patients with marked nasal obstruction mouth breathe and as a result have dryness of the mouth and pharynx, a tendency to coated tongue, and an odor to the breath. The larynx and trachea may even be affected by this dryness.

Children with chronic nasal obstruction seem more subject to attacks of colds, sinusitis, pharyngitis, laryngitis and bronchitis. They may also suffer from congestion and inflammation of the eustachian tubes and middle ear, and mild but potentially serious hearing loss.

The average child with persistent nasal obstruction tends to sleep poorly and show evidence of impaired nutrition because of a poor appetite. This is particularly noticeable in cases of large, obstructing adenoids. The "adenoid facies" has long been recognized as a mark of chronic nasal or postnasal obstruction.

ETIOLOGY

Nasal obstruction may be produced by *extranasal, intranasal,* and *nasopharyngeal* defects, and miscellaneous causes.

1. Extranasal defects involving:
   The bone
       Depressed nasal fractures
       Narrow bridge
   The cartilage
       Upper lateral cartilage
       Lower lateral cartilage
   The anterior nares
       Depressed nasal tip
       Collapsed alae
       Thick columella
       Atresia

2. Intranasal defects involving:
   The septum
   The lateral nasal walls
       Chronic allergic rhinitis
       Nonallergic rhinitis
       New growths
   The posterior nares
       Choanal atresia
       Choanal polyps

3. Nasopharyngeal defects:
       Hypertrophied adenoids
       Fibroma

EXTRANASAL DEFECTS

The external supportive framework of the nose is formed by the nasal bones and the frontal processes of the maxilla above and by the upper and lower lateral cartilages below. The external nares are created by the flaring wings of the lower lateral cartilages and the central strut, or columella, which is formed by the medial crura of the lower lateral cartilage. Extranasal deformities of these parts, whether congenital or acquired, have not received the attention they deserve. The plastic surgeon has readily corrected the deformed nose for cosmetic reasons but unfortunately has often given very little consideration to the functional factors involved.

ETIOLOGY

Bone. Excess narrowing of the nasal bones over the bridge may reduce and impair the function of the nasal chambers. Depressed nasal fractures may produce similar results.

7

Cartilage. The lower cartilaginous vault is subject to abnormalities which may produce nasal obstruction. The upper and lower lateral cartilages are important from a functional standpoint. The upper lateral cartilages may well be considered the lateral upper wings of the quadrangular cartilage of the nasal septum. A lateral dislocation of these cartilages, which is a common traumatic deformity of the nose, may involve the nasal septum. Congenitally thin, weak, upper lateral cartilages may be unable to support the alar openings and "suck in" uring nasal inspiration. This defect may be simulated if one places his fingers lightly over the lateral sides of the nose just above the alar cartilages. The simple weight of the finger pressure will produce considerable nasal obstruction. The same effect may be produced by a saddle nose deformity as a consequence of injury and subsequent absorption of the upper lateral cartilage and septum. This may also occur after a submucous resection operation, when insufficient quadrangular cartilage is left at the junction of the bony and cartilaginous bridge. The retraction accompanying healing depresses the bridge. Excessive narrowing of the lower lateral cartilage or collapse of the alar wings likewise causes inspiratory obstruction.

Anterior Nares. The anterior nares are subject to several structural defects. The nasal tip may be excessively long and depressed. The columella may be thick and broad, the alae thin and weak, and in a common deformity, the anterior end of the septum projects into and occludes an alar opening. Of chief importance are the cases of thin, collapsed alae and depressed nasal tip. Simple elevation and inspection of the nares will reveal these obstructive factors. Rarely the anterior nares may also be found occluded by a membrane, owing to faulty development. This congenital atresia is seen in the newborn; it is due to a persistence of an embryonic membrane closing the orifice during intra-uterine development. The anterior nares may also be occluded by scarring and contraction of the nostrils following trauma.

DIAGNOSIS

Inspection and Palpation. This part of the nasal examination is frequently overlooked or given little attention. The external contour and shape of the nose may give a hint as to the type and cause of the internal obstruction. For example, a patient may have a very thin narrow bridge and poorly developed and weak upper and lower lateral cartilages; palpation of the sides of the nose and elevation of the nasal tip reveals these causes for nasal obstruction. Regardless of the type of intranasal obstruction, it would be useless to correct internal obstructions without giving due consideration to external deformities.

TREATMENT

Rhinoplastic Surgery. For the relief of nasal obstruction, it may be necessary to correct a displaced nasal bridge, a saddle nose, a long nose with depressed tip, a weak or deflected upper lateral cartilage, or nasal alae that collapse on inspiration. The obstruction produced by a dislocation of the anterior end of the septum into one nostril often requires surgical treatment.

The maneuvers in these rhinoplastic procedures usually necessitate intranasal incisions through which the skin and subcutaneous tissue covering the dorsum and sides of the nose are elevated, thus exposing the bony and cartilaginous vault of the nose for correction. Then saw or chisel cuts are made laterally and medially through the nasal bones and frontal processes of the maxilla, thereby freeing the displaced bones for proper correction. When the anterior end of the septum is transfixed by a suitable, through and through incision, repair of obstructive defects of this partition may be made coincidently with the rhinoplasty. If the nose is too long, or the nasal tip depressed, it may be shortened and elevated by the removal of a wedge-shaped piece of the projecting end of the septal cartilage. Resuture of the columella to the septum allows for further tip elevation. The framework of the nostrils, alae and columella are likewise exposed through excisions which leave no external scar and allow wide exposure for surgical correction. The insertion of cartilage along the nasal bridge or as support for the nasal tip is frequently necessary to correct saddle deformities or loss of columella support. In many cases of rhinoplastic surgery, a combination of the above corrective procedures including submucous resection are necessary for a proper cosmetic and functional result.

INTRANASAL DEFECTS

The nasal cavity extends on each side from the nostril to the posterior choanae through which it opens into the nasopharynx. The two nasal chambers are separated normally by a more or less straight septum From the lateral wall of each nasal cavity spring the inferior, middle and superior turbinates. These irregular turbinate swellings project into the normal air stream. Thus the passageways may be obstructed in many of these areas. The bony turbinate projections and the bony septum may be deformed and produce mechanical blockage. The mucous membrane covering these areas has the unique property of greatly increasing in size when mechanically or chemically irritated. The greatest swelling occurs over the inferior and middle turbinate bodies and the adjoining septal surfaces. Seldom is a nasal obstruction produced by one defect within the nose.

DIAGNOSIS

An evaluation of the cause of a chronic intranasal obstruction may involve several procedures (Fig. 78). The diagnostic steps may be outlined as follows:

Examination of the Nasal Passages with the Head Mirror and Reflected Light. Anterior rhinoscopy is not difficult, but practice with the head mirror and the nasal speculum is necessary for satis-

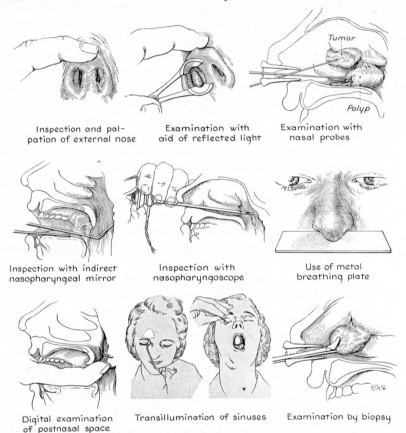

Inspection and palpation of external nose

Examination with aid of reflected light

Examination with nasal probes

Inspection with indirect nasopharyngeal mirror

Inspection with nasopharyngoscope

Use of metal breathing plate

Digital examination of postnasal space

Transillumination of sinuses

Examination by biopsy

Fig. 78. A chart depicting the procedures used in a routine examination to determine the causes of chronic nasal obstruction.

factory results. The beginner has difficulty coordinating the reflected spot of light and properly focusing it within the nasal cavity. Usually, he expects to see too much in one view. Without efficient shrinkage of the nasal mucosa, only the anterior one-third of the nasal cavity can be seen. After the application of vasoconstrictors (1 per cent ephedrine in isotonic saline solution or 1 to 4 per cent cocaine hydrochloride solution) about two-thirds of the cavity may be inspected. The lower part of the nasal chamber and floor of the nose are best visualized with the head held in a horizontal position. To inspect the central, upper and posterior portions, the head is tilted progressively farther back. Successively, the nose should be observed for septal deformities, excessive secretions, mucosal swelling, fleshy overgrowths, or any other cause of nasal obstruction.

Palpation by Probe. Small cotton-tipped metal or wooden applicators are used to palpate the mucosa. This procedure has limited value to anyone but an experienced rhinologist. The nasal mucous membrane is sensitive and any intranasal manipulation should be gentle. It is possible to distinguish between simple vasomotor changes or actual hyperplasia of the mucosa.

Mirror Examination of the Nasopharynx. Next to anterior rhinoscopy, this is the most important examination to determine the cause of chronic nasal obstruction. For details of technic, see Figs. 152, 153. In this examination the choanae, the vault of the nasopharynx, Rosenmüller's fossae and the eustachian orifices can be seen.

Nasopharyngoscope. The nasopharyngoscope is comparable to the electrically lighted cystoscope. The nasal passages are usually treated with a weak cocaine solution before the instrument is passed. The passage is easily accomplished. However, considerable experience is necessary to interpret what is seen.

Metal Breathing Plate. This provides a simple and fairly practical test for determining the relative degree of breathing space through each nasal fossa.

Digital Examination. Palpation of the postnasal space with or without general anesthesia may occasionally be found useful in children. In adults, a similar palpation of the nasopharynx may be carried out under local anesthesia.

Transillumination of the Sinuses. This will give a possible indication of a sinus factor in chronic nasal obstruction (Fig. 72).

X-ray Studies. A lateral view of the nasopharynx may be helpful in outlining a mass or swelling in the nasopharynx as a cause of chronic nasal obstruction (Fig. 73).

Nasal Biopsy. In doubtful cases of tumor mass which show an evident cause for chronic obstruction, a biopsy should be made of the tissue. This can be done under local anesthesia supplied by cocaine.

THE SEPTUM

Malformation of the nasal septum is a common cause of nasal obstruction. This partition is a composite structure. Its skeleton is formed from before backward by the columella, the quadrangular septal cartilage, the perpendicular plate of the ethmoid, the vomer and the septal crests of the palatine processes of the maxillary and palatine bones. This dividing wall which the combination of these bones and cartilages make should be straight and divide the nasal fossae into two equal chambers. This ideal is seldom seen. Most people have some irregularity of the septum which often produces little obstruction.

Etiology

Two factors, one developmental, the other traumatic, produce most of the deformities of the septum. The posterior defects are caused by an improper rate of growth between the palate and the base of the cranium. This causes a buckling of the partition between the two opposing forces. The anteriorly placed deformities involving the septal cartilage usually result from trauma. It is common for small children to injure the anterior portion of the nose by frequent falls, thereby displacing the septal cartilage from its groove on the maxillary crest and vomer along the floor of the nose. This anterior dislocation of the septum projects into the fossa on one side and may produce considerable obstruction. Most of these injuries are overlooked in childhood and do not receive consideration until symptoms of nasal obstruction are observed as the child grows older. It should be emphasized that minor or seemingly trivial nasal injuries in childhood should receive examination and treatment at the time of the accident. Immediate reduction of these fractures is always indicated. The difficulty of reduction increases rapidly after the first twenty-four to forty-eight hours. After this period, healing and fibrosis make reduction difficult to maintain.

Treatment

Submucous Resection. When an irregularity of the nasal septum prohibits normal nasal function, the skillfully performed correction of this obstruction offers a very satisfactory improvement. The degree of relief obtained by surgery is in direct proportion to the obstructive distress experienced by the patient. The indications for surgery should be carefully considered. In general, slight defects rarely interfere with the normal physiologic functions of the nose, namely, respiratory, olfactory, gustatory, phonatory, and ventilation of the sinuses and middle ear. When it can be shown that these functions are affected, surgery should be considered. The patient with nasal allergy may have a considerable proportion of his obstruction caused by hypertrophy of the nasal mucosa and not by the irregularity of the septum. This surgery is performed under local anesthesia, except in the occasional instances when it is done on a child.

The mucous membrane is incised on the convex side of the deflection and is elevated freely from the cartilage and bone of the septum (Fig. 79). After this elevation is complete, extending from the roof to the floor of the nasal space, an incision is made through the cartilage near the original mucosal incision and the mucous membrane is elevated in a similar manner on the opposite side of the septum. Then by means of the proper instruments, the obstructing portions of the quadrangular cartilage, the perpendicular plate of the ethmoid and the vomer are removed. The ultimate goal of the operation is to have the two septal mucous membranes hang in a perpendicular plane in the center of the nasal space. When these heal together, a thin, membranous septum results. The original incision through the mucous membrane is sutured with one or two approximating silk sutures, and some type of intranasal splint or packing is applied for support and prevention of the

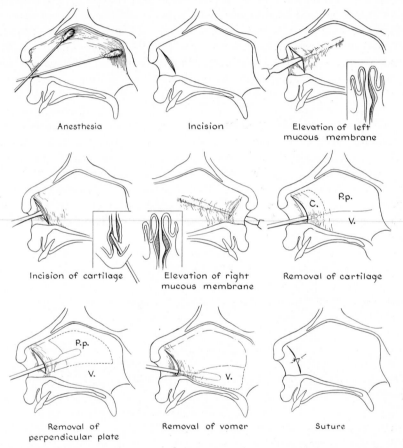

Fig. 79. The important steps in the performance of a submucous resection.

formation of a postoperative hematoma. This packing is removed in twelve to twenty-four hours and a bland, oily vasoconstrictor solution is prescribed to relieve the postoperative nasal congestion. The patient is cautioned against forcibly blowing his nose and excessive exercise for several days. Hospitalization is usually necessary for only twenty-four hours. Septal perforations result when the septal mucosa is torn or lacerated in corresponding areas on both sides.

THE LATERAL NASAL WALLS

The nasal chamber has a triangular form, wide below and gradually narrowing towards the top. It was intended that this space should be separated by a median partition, the septum, into two equal halves. This is uncommon, however, owing to the high incidence of irregularities of the septum, caused by developmental factors or trauma.

The anatomy and physiology of the lateral nasal wall have been previously described. The turbinates with their venous spaces subject to engorgement and the mucosa which reacts acutely to inflammatory and allergenic factors play an important role in acute obstructions. Repeated attacks of this swelling seem to lead to permanent hypertrophy or hyperplasia with resulting enlargement of the turbinal bodies and the mucosa, thus causing chronic obstruction.

Chronic Allergic Rhinitis

There are several conditions which may produce temporary or permanent swellings of the mucous membrane lining the nasal passages. The most common cause for acute temporary occlusion of the nose is an acute rhinitis in the form of the common cold. Next in frequency, and invariably a cause of chronic obstruction, is the nasal condition produced by an allergenic substance. In chronic cases, there are invariably episodes in which evidence of suppuration is prominent. This results from a superimposed infection.

At the beginning, the victim of allergic rhinitis suffers from attacks of sneezing, watery and mucoid discharge, and intermittent or continuous nasal blockage which may be unilateral or bilateral. There may be increased lachrymation, excessive postnasal discharge, a tendency toward a dry pharynx and symptoms of bronchitis.

Symptoms and Signs. The nasal mucous membrane presents a characteristic appearance. Its color is usually pale and the tissue is edematous and boggy. There is an excess of clear, tenacious mucus covering the membrane. Touching the mucosal surface, especially that of the inferior turbinate, results in a deep indentation of the tissue. Upon the release of pressure, the tissue immediately fills out and resumes its smooth, edematous contour. This simple test reveals at once if the intranasal swelling is due to venous stasis in the submucosal vascular spaces or to an actual hyperplasia of the mucous membrane, such as is found in chronic hypertrophic rhinitis. This chronic edema of the nasal mucosa frequently results in the formation of nasal polyps in the region of the middle meatus or anterior ethmoid region. These fleshy overgrowths, resembling moist white grapes, hang from the middle meatuses, and in many cases completely fill the nasal passages. If they project posteriorly into the nasopharynx, they are called choanal polyps. Nasal and choanal polyps are the most common types of tumor mass found in the nasal passages.

Diagnosis. The diagnosis of chronic nasal allergy is made by evaluating the symptoms, the appearance of the nasal mucous membrane, the examination of the nasal smears, the analysis of properly made skin tests and elimination regimens. Recently, with the introduction of such drugs as diphenhydramine hydrochloride (benadryl) and tripelennamine hydrochloride (pyribenzamine), these may be helpful as therapeutic tests.

Treatment. There are various medications for relief of allergic rhinitis. The *vasoconstrictors*, such as ephedrine, phenylephrine hydrochloride (neo-synephrine), naphazoline hydrochloride (privine), and so on, are not advised except for temporary relief. In the acute phase of hay fever, the following nasal spray is effective in relieving the congestion and irritation:

	Gm. or cc.
Cocaine hydrochloride	0.26
Phenol	0.0036
Antipyrine	0.45
Ephedrine sulfate solution, 3 per cent	14.0
Isotonic saline	q.s. ad 30.0

(Not to be refilled)

For rest at night, these capsules are helpful:

Ephedrine with amytal or seconal āā ⅜ grain.

Taken internally for relief of allergic symptoms:

Diphenhydramine hydrochloride (benadryl) capsules. . . . . . . 50 mg.
or Tripelennamine hydrochloride (pyribenzamine) tablets. . . . 50 mg.
One capsule or tablet is taken three or four times daily (adults).

Nasal Polyps

Nasal polyps are the most common growths found within the nose. They are usually attached by pedicles to the upper posterior part of the nasal cavity in the region of the middle meatus or within the antra. In prolonged allergic conditions, marked edema within the mucous membrane causes a prolapse of the tissue with the resulting characteristic grape-like masses producing annoying symptoms of nasal obstruction, pressure, excess secretion and so on. Polyps have a characteristic appearance. They look like glistening, moist, white grapes hanging from the roof of the nose. Palpation with a probe reveals that they are freely movable, attached by pedicles, and arise from the surfaces of the middle turbinates, the hiatus semilunaris, or the ostea of the ethmoid and maxillary sinuses.

Treatment. The removal of nasal polyps is a procedure common to general practice. If skillfully and carefully performed, it gives great relief. The nose is first anesthetized locally by cocaine. The points of origin of the polyps are then ascertained and the loop of a small nasal

snare is threaded over each polyp from below (Fig. 80). The snare
loop should be carried upward as close to the site of origin as possible.
The base of the polyp should not be cut through, but rather the snare
wire should be gradually tightened on the base of the polyp and the
growth evulsed with a gentle tug on the closed snare. If small polyps are
present, they may be removed with a small ring or biting forceps. A

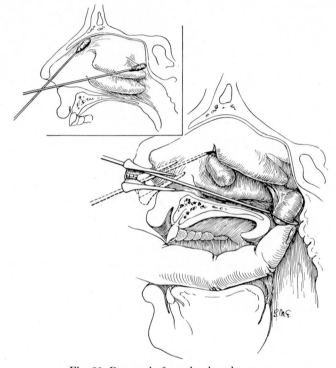

Fig. 80. Removal of nasal polyps by snare.

small anterior nasal pack is usually inserted to control any excessive
postoperative bleeding. Nasal polyps, which are the result of some form
of allergy, will promptly recur if this factor is not eliminated.

Nonallergic Chronic Rhinitis

Chronic inflammation of the nasal cavities, other than simple rhinitis
and allergic rhinitis, may occur in three forms. They are: (1) chronic
hypertrophic rhinitis, (2) chronic rhinitis sicca, and (3) atrophic rhinitis.

Chronic Hypertrophic Rhinitis. Chronic hypertrophic rhinitis
results from repeated acute nasal infections, from recurrent attacks of
suppurative sinusitis, which produce a chronic state, and from vasomotor
states independent of local disease. Hypertrophy of nasal mucosa is
known to occur in some persons from constitutional factors which are
not clearly defined. It is seen in a temporary form at puberty, during

menses and in the course of pregnancy. This suggests an endocrine factor. It is known that the administration of thyroid substance has a beneficial effect in some cases of mucosal hypertrophy even though metabolic tests do not indicate a definite hypothyroidism.

Symptoms. This type of rhinitis is characterized by soft tissue swelling, excessive secretion, and in longstanding cases by actual hypertrophy of the mucosa, thickening of the periosteum and new bone formation. These changes produce annoying symptoms. The nasal obstruction is characteristically intermittent. It is worse on the dependent side when lying down. The secretions may be thick and sticky and may produce a chronic irritation of the nasopharynx and pharynx which causes hawking and clearing of the throat. Hypertrophy of the posterior ends of the inferior turbinate may occur. Long continued nasal and sinus infections may produce polyps and prolapsed antral cysts which block one side of the nose and nasopharynx.

Chronic Rhinitis Sicca. Chronic rhinitis sicca occurs often in women during and after menopause, owing to some ill defined endocrine or metabolic disturbance. Diabetic, nephritic and other debilitated patients are similarly affected. It is characterized by chronic congestion, diminution of the nasal secretions and abnormal dryness of the nose and pharynx. There is crusting over the turbinate bodies, which bleed easily when the crusts are removed. The secretions have a musty odor. There is no atrophy of the mucosa or bony tissue which distinguishes it from atrophic rhinitis.

The treatment consists in attention to matters of general health and the local application of a medication that will stimulate secretion, such as the formula of Proetz:

	Cc.
Alcohol	0.6
Glycerin	0.6
Isotonic saline	120.0
Spirits of cologne	M 5.0

One-half dropperful in each nostril every three hours.

Atrophic Rhinitis. Atrophic rhinitis, which is a chronic disease, is described in Chapter XX. The obstruction is produced by crusts which may fill each nasal cavity almost as a cast.

Hypertrophy of Turbinates

Treatment. When chronic nasal obstruction is the result of hypertrophied turbinates in the instances in which suppurative and allergenic factors have been eliminated, this obstruction can be relieved by shrinkage of the turbinate with the use of cautery or sclerosing solution.

Anesthesia is obtained with cocaine when cautery is used and butacaine sulfate (butyn sulfate), which does not cause shrinkage, when injections are employed.

Cauterization is performed with a red hot cautery blade, the edge of which is inserted deeply to the bony framework in the middle of the turbinate from posterior to anterior tip. This does not destroy an important amount of nasal mucosa.

The solutions used for injection are "sylnasol" or 5 per cent sodium morrhuate injection. A solution of 0.25 to 0.50 cc. is injected into the submucous layer of the inferior or middle turbinate (Fig. 81). A long needle is inserted through an anterior puncture the length of the turbinate. As it is withdrawn, small amounts of the sclerosing solution are deposited. Vasoconstriction is then maintained for several days by the use of ephedrine nose drops. Only one side of a nose is treated at a time,

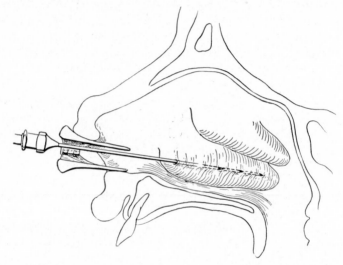

Fig. 81. Injection of sclerosing solution to shrink an inferior turbinate.

but several injections are usually needed in each turbinate at weekly or longer intervals to accomplish the desired results.

New Growths

Benign new growths, with the exception of nasal polyps, are not commonly found in the nasal passages. Angioma, fibroma, papilloma, enchondroma and osteoma may occur at any age, but are more common near middle life. These growths are painless and the chief symptom is progressive nasal blockage. An angioma usually arises from the septum as a soft, red, granular mass. It bleeds freely on palpation. Fibromas may arise from any area. They are smooth and rather firm to touch. Papillomas usually are found growing in the region of the nasal vestibule, originating in the squamous epithelium covering this area. Malignant new growths are not uncommon in the nasal space. Squamous cell carcinoma and transitional cell carcinoma are the types most often encountered. Carcinoma of the maxillary sinus is usually of the squamous cell type, and nasal obstruction is not encountered until a relatively late stage when the tumor actually invades the nasal fossa, or infection supervenes, causing edema and discharge. Transitional cell carcinoma when diagnosed in the nasal space has usually arisen from the ethmoids or turbinates. Squamous cell carcinomas are found on the septum. Sarcomas may be encountered in the nasal space. Cancer arising in the posterior ethmoids and sphenoid usually invades the orbit or cranial cavity.

Treatment. Benign new growths in the nasal fossae are safe to remove surgically with adequate control of the bleeding. Malignant growths should be handled only by those doctors experienced with the indications for the proper use of surgery, x-ray and radium, since a combination of these is needed to obtain the best results. Exposure of the growth may require technical skill. Occasionally it is necessary to perform a lateral rhinotomy and turn the external nose to the side to to expose the nasal fossae adequately.

THE POSTERIOR NARES, OR CHOANAE

The posterior nares, or choanae, may be chronically blocked by hypertrophy of the posterior ends of the inferior turbinates, choanal polyps, or congenital choanal atresia.

Choanal Atresia

This is an uncommon congenital defect producing incomplete or complete obstruction of one or both posterior nares. The closure may be by membrane, cartilage, or bone. These tissues persist, owing to failure of absorption or regular development of the buccopharyngeal membrane during the embryonic period.

The membranous obstruction extends upward from the soft palate at its juncture with the hard palate, closing the posterior openings just behind the choanae. The bony overgrowths are located about one millimeter anterior to the openings into the nasopharynx so when viewed from behind in the postnasal examination a slight indentation is noted.

Diagnosis. Diagnosis is made at or shortly after birth. When the obstruction is bilateral, the infant nurses poorly or not at all because the nursing act with the infant's mouth closed over the nipple requires nasal respiration. Evidence of dehydration and malnutrition develops quickly if the obstruction is not relieved. The obstruction may be demonstrated by failure to pass a small catheter or probe through the nose into the pharynx.

Treatment. The only adequate treatment is *surgical removal* of the occluding membrane or bony tissue. It is usually necessary to remove a portion of the posterior border of the nasal septum to ensure a permanent opening. In bilateral atresia, prompt surgery is required, while in the unilateral cases, operation may be done at any time. The membranous cases readily respond to surgical excision, but those having a bony obstruction require more radical treatment. The bony overgrowth is removed with a rasp or bone-cutting forceps. To ensure against contracture and closure, it is important to remove a good portion of the posterior end of the vomer. Tubes made from acrylic substance may need to be kept in the nasal spaces during the healing period to keep the new choanal openings patent.

Choanal Polyps

Nasal polyps often form in the posterior part of the nose and block one or both choanae. The cyst formed from antral membrane which prolapses through the ostium in the middle meatus has all of the characteristics of a solitary large nasal polyp except for the fluid content.

Treatment. Choanal polyps and cysts, which prolapse into the nasopharynx, are somewhat more difficult to remove, but in general may be removed in the same manner as nasal polyps. The nasal snare is passed into the nose along the nasal floor well back into the nasopharynx. With a finger passed up behind the soft palate, the loop of the snare is directed over the body of the polyp. The loop is then tightened and the mass is evulsed with an anterior pull on the nasal snare. The method of removal just described is the method of choice, but if the mass is extremely large and prolapses deep into the nasopharynx, the tumor may well be removed intraorally. Local anesthesia usually suffices, but occasionally general anesthesia is necessary. Intratrachial anesthesia allows uninterrupted manipulation and work in the nasopharynx.

THE NASOPHARYNX

The nasopharynx is often overlooked as a site of chronic nasal obstruction. The common cause occurs in childhood and is due to adenoid hypertrophy. A relatively rare cause is found in a nasopharyngeal fibroma.

Hyperplasia of Adenoid

The occurrence of lymphoid tissue in the nasopharynx is discussed in Chapter XXVI. In children, this obstruction often produces a more or less classical picture, the so-called "adenoid facies," characterized by obvious mouth breathing, a dull facial expression, a high arch palate, malocclusion of the teeth, particularly the anterior teeth and a nasal speech. The treatment is also discussed in Chapter XXVI.

Nasopharyngeal Fibroma

This is a peculiar tumor which occurs in the adolescent age. It occurs almost exclusively in males and arises from fibrous tissue in the spheno-ethmoidal recess, the base of the sphenoid, or in the nasopharynx. It is pathologically benign, but may destroy from pressure necrosis.

The histological structure of the tumor may suggest fibroma, fibro-angioma, or fibromyxoma. It tends to be very vascular with large venous structures devoid of a contractile coat. For this reason, surgical removal by the inexperienced physician may be hazardous because of accompanying hemorrhage. Fibromas have been mistaken for adenoids. Some cases should be treated with x-ray and radium or radon implants. Others can be safely removed by surgery in which surgical diathermy is employed. The constitutional changes incident to growth favor the involution of this tumor.

MISCELLANEOUS CAUSES

Foreign Bodies. Foreign bodies as a cause of chronic nasal obstruction are practically always encountered in children. Children at play

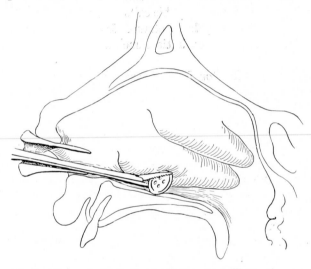

Fig. 82. Removal of a foreign body by use of alligator forceps.

are prone to place small objects in the nasal passages. Usually they do this on the right side. The common foreign bodies found in children are beads, buttons, erasers, marbles, peas, beans, stones and nuts. Unless sharp or very large, recently inserted objects give little or no discomfort. Unsuspected foreign bodies cause unilateral obstruction, and discharge with odor. The majority of foreign bodies are either found in the anterior part of the vestibule or in the inferior meatus along the floor of the nose. No object should be allowed to remain in the nasal passages because of the danger of producing necrosis and secondary infection, and aspiration into the lower respiratory tract.

Treatment. Foreign bodies may be rather easily removed if co-operation of the child can be obtained, or general anesthesia may be required to permit inspection and instrumentation of the nasal fossa without trauma or fright and pain on the part of the patient. An alligator forceps, an instrument with a small curved hook and a suction tip, is usually all the armamentarium that the surgeon needs (Fig. 82). Topical anesthesia with cocaine is often all that is needed. If general anesthesia is used, the patient's head should be lowered so that the sudden passage of the foreign body into the nasopharynx will not offer the added risk of aspiration into the larynx or trachea. A mouth gag, palate retractor, tongue depressor and tonsil suction tip should be part of the equipment so that the foreign body can be extracted in case it falls or is pushed into the pharynx.

Rhinoliths

These are sometimes seen as a special form of foreign body. They are usually found in adults. Insoluble salts of the nasal secretions form a calcareous mass about any long-retained foreign body or blood clot. A chronic sinus discharge may initiate such a mass to form in the nasal passages.

Treatment. An alligator forceps usually is sufficient for removal under local anesthesia. The mass may have to be crushed and removed piecemeal.

Nasal Synechia

Adhesions between the nasal septum and lateral walls of the nose may give obstructive symptoms. The adhesive connective tissue bands result from the loss of the epithelium of two adjacent mucosal surfaces. This injury to the mucosa may result from nasal fractures, operations, or intranasal lacerations. Cautery of the septum or turbinates may produce such an obstruction.

Treatment. Synechia causing chronic nasal obstruction should be removed by excising the connecting tissue, but it is not always easy to prevent reformation of the synechia. A non-irritating mold of rubber or acrylic substance may be needed between the opposing surfaces, but foreign substances of this type in the nose are not well tolerated. In some cases, electrocoagulation may be used to advantage. Rubber finger cots or dental wax splints should be inserted, well lubricated, between the raw surfaces and kept in place until the parts are well healed.

Local Medication

The temporary and reversible edema and swelling of the nasal mucous membrane, resulting from attacks of acute rhinitis, chronic vasomotor rhinitis, and other chronic infections, may be momentarily relieved by numerous vasoconstrictor drugs. Most victims of chronic nasal obstruction are using local medication, usually nose drops, or inhalers, when the physician is consulted. Millions of dollars are spent each year for this ill-advised self medication. Obviously, the condition causing the obstruction cannot be cured by this treatment. Only a transient relief is obtained. Prolonged use of local medication disposes to a chronic congested state called "rhinitis medicamentosa."

Numerous investigators have studied this problem. They have shown that caution must be used in prescribing "nose drops" promiscuously. This applies particularly to an allergic individual. The nasal mucous membrane is extremely sensitive to any irritant, especially when it is intermittently applied. After an initial vasoconstriction, a secondary vasodilatation occurs, which makes the nasal obstruction even worse than the original insult. Moreover, the mucous cells may be unduly stimulated and increase the nasal blockage by excessive secretion. The delicate cilia are injured at the same time and thus evacuation of the mucous collection is impaired, which aggravates the nasal blockage. These factors warrant consideration when prescribing intranasal medication. If used judiciously, vasoconstrictors may be of benefit in acute cases of infection, in preoperative anesthesia, and for adequate inspection of the nasal chambers. However, when used in chronic conditions causing nasal obstruction, secondary ill effects may result.

REFERENCES

Beck, A. L.: Abscess of the Nasal Septum Complicating Acute Ethmoiditis. Arch. Otolaryng., *42:*275, 1945.

Bolotaw, Nathan A.: Surgical Treatment of Nasal Obstruction. *Ibid., 40:*198, 1944.

Brown, J. M.: The Surgical Treatment of Nasopharyngeal Fibroma. Ann. Otol., Rhin. & Laryng., *56:*294, 1947.

Cinelli, Albert A.: Nasal Atresias. A Surgical critique. *Ibid., 49:*912, 1940.

Formon, S., et al: Plastic Repair of the Obstructing Nasal Septum. Arch. Otolaryng., *47:*7, 1948.

Fox, S. L.: Chronic Vasomotor Rhinitis in Pregnancy. Bull. School Med. Univ. Maryland, *31:*104, 1947.

Gelfand, Harold H.: The Allergic Aspect of Vasomotor Rhinitis. Arch. Otolaryng., *37:*1, 1943.

Kaplan, S.: Combined Septal Resection and Rhinoplasty for Restoration of Nasal Respiratory Function. *Ibid., 47:*395, 1948.

Kazanjian, V. H.: The Treatment of Congenital Atresia of the Choanae. Ann. Otol., Rhin. & Laryng., *51:*704, 1942.

Kully, B. M.: Use and Abuse of Nasal Vasoconstrictor Medications. J.A.M.A., *127:*307, 1945.

Lake, C. F.: Rhinitis Medicamentosa. Proc. Staff Meet. Mayo Clin., *21:*367, 1946.

Marks, M.: Vasomotor Rhinitis: Treatment by Submucous Injections of Phenol. J. Laryng. & Otol., *6:*282, 1946.

Proetz, A. W.: Physiology of the Nose from the Standpoint of the Plastic Surgeon. Arch. Otolaryng., *39:*514, 1944.

Robison, J. Mathew: Physiology and Functional Pathology of Lymphatic System Applied to Allergy of the Nose and Paranasal Sinuses. J. Allergy, *17:*53, 1946.

Ruddy, Lorenz W.: Transpalatine Operation for Congenital Atresia of Choanae in the Small Child or Infant. Arch. Otolaryng., *41:*432, 1945.

Salinger, S.: Traumatic Deformities of the Nasal Septum. Ann. Otol., Rhin. & Laryng., *53:*274, 1944.

Schall, LeRoy A.: Malignant Tumors of the Nose and Nasal Accessory Sinuses. J.A.M.A., *137*:1273, 1948.

Shea, J. J.: The Pathology of Nasal Polyps and Related Growths. Ann. Otol., Rhin. & Laryng., *56*:1029, 1947.

Sooy, Francis A.: Naso-alveolar Cysts. Laryngoscope, *54*:18, 1944.

Stauffer, H. B.: Rhinolith. Ann. Otol., Rhin. & Laryng., *52*:190, 1943.

Tamari, A., and Busby, W.: Evaluation of Submucosal Shrinking Methods for Chronic Nasal Obstructions. Arch. Otolaryng., *39*:331, 1944.

Thacker, E. A.: Value of Fatty Acid Derivatives in Treatment of Chronic Obstructive Rhinitis. *Ibid.*, *37*:699, 1943.

Thacker, E. A.: Value of Fatty Acid Derivatives in Treatment of Chronic Obstructive Rhinitis. *Ibid.*, *36*:336, 1942.

Thacker, E. A.: Chronic Nasal Obstruction; Its Causes and Treatment. J.A.M.A., *131*:1039, 1946.

Wachsberger, A.: The Deviated Septum. Arch. Otolaryng., *37*:789, 1943.

Wright, W. K., Shambaugh, G. E., Jr., and Green, L.: Congenital Choanal Atresia. A New Surgical Approach. Ann. Otol., Rhin. & Laryng., *56*:120, 1947.

CHAPTER XVI

ACUTE AND CHRONIC SINUS DISEASE

CHARLES E. CONNOR, M.D.

The nasal accessory sinuses are cavities in the bones of the skull and face produced by the outpouching of the embryonic respiratory epithelium into the surrounding cartilaginous nasal capsule; their size, shape and anatomical relationships depend upon the extent of pneumatization, which is controlled by factors not definitely known; variations in intrasinous pressure incidental to respiration and early infection in the sinus cavities, just as in the cell systems of the ear, may limit their development.

The variations in the size, shape and relationships of the sinuses are improtant because upon them depend the signs and symptoms of sinus disease, the development of complications, the surgical accessibility of the cavities and, in part, the development of chronicity. These factors will be discussed in the consideration of each sinus.

DEVELOPMENT OF SINUSES

Frontal Sinus. The sinuses are formed, assume clinical significance and reach maturity at different times. The first rudiments of the frontal sinus may be seen as early as the fourth month of fetal life in the pits and furrows of the anterior portion of the middle meatus, the frontal recess; the frontal sinus will develop from one of these pits (primitive anterior ethmoidal cell), rarely from a furrow (infundibulum ethmoidale) or from the frontal recess itself. These structures are well developed at birth, but the sinus is not topographically frontal at that age, and its exact point of origin may not be indicated until the eighteenth or twentieth month of life when it enters the vertical portion of the frontal bone; the age at which it reaches full development varies from the eighth to the fifteenth year. It acquires clinical significance as a frontal sinus only after it enters the frontal bone; prior to that time it is clinically an anterior ethmoidal cell.

Ethmoidal Sinus. The development of the ethmoidal sinus keeps pace with that of the frontal, which is to be expected since both structures develop from the middle meatus. The sinus, its rudimentary structures present in the fourth fetal month, is an anatomical and clinical entity at birth. It develops steadily and reaches adult size in early adolescence, from the twelfth to fourteenth year; extensive pneumatization has been seen as early as the tenth year.

Maxillary Antrum. The maxillary antrum is present as early as the seventieth day of fetal life as a pouching out of the infundibulum ethmoidale (furrow of the middle meatus); the largest sinus at birth, it is seen as a definite slitlike cell, large as a small bean, lying lateral to the nasal cavity; like the ethmoidal sinus, its greatest importance clinically is in infancy and childhood. The adult stage is reached between the fifteenth and eighteenth years, full development being dependent upon the eruption of the molar teeth.

Sphenoidal Sinus. This sinus is present as early as the third month of fetal life as a pouching out of the mucosa into the cartilaginous nasal capsule in the posterior portion of the nose; at birth it is a definite cell structure entirely nasal in position. It enters the sphenoidal bone only after absorption of the intervening nasal cartilage and is completely surrounded by sphenoid bone by the end of the third and beginning of the fourth year of life. It reaches adult size about the fourteenth year of life.

Lining Membrane. The mucous membrane of the nasal cavity extends in to line the accessory sinuses; in these spaces, its stroma is thin and delicate, owing to fewer glands and blood vessels and to the absence of vascular spaces and elastic tissue seen in certain structures of the nose, such as the inferior turbinate.

This continuity of lining membrane accounts for the frequent involvement of the sinuses in acute rhinitis. Fortunately, this involvement is usually slight, amounting only to some congestion, edema and perhaps transudation of small amounts of serum, but it is enough to account for the occasional prolongation of the head infection with its attendant feeling of pressure, tightness, marked nasal occlusion and discharge of mucus. This common clinical picture formerly received the name of catarrhal sinusitis, but its recognition as a distinct entity is not justified, since it is but an early stage in the progressive changes which eventuate in acute suppurative sinusitis. These changes resolve spontaneously in most cases without special treatment; only when some factor predisposing to their continuance is present, such as obstructed nasal drainage, unusually severe infection, poor physical condition of the patient, or nasal allergy, do they eventuate in acute suppurative sinusitis.

ACUTE STAGE OF SUPPURATIVE SINUSITIS

Acute suppurative sinusitis most frequently follows acute head infection and so occurs with greatest frequency in winter but may be seen at any time of year. One particularly severe type involving especially the frontal sinus occurs after swimming and is attributed to the irritating effect of water in a nose already harboring infection. Many causes are considered as contributory in the development of acute and chronic sinusitis. The general physical condition of the patient, the presence of other diseases, avitaminosis, disorders of glands of internal secretion such as hypothyroidism, degree of natural resistance of the respiratory tract to infections, occupation with degree of exposure to cold and dampness, superheated houses with low humidity in winter and public buildings too cold and humid in summer from improper air conditioning, too frequent and too extreme temperature changes, these and other factors all play a part in the development of sinus infections.

The pathologic changes seen are those common to inflammation of soft tissue and are characterized by congestion, edema, infiltration of the mucous membrane with histiocytes, cells of the plasmacytic series (plasma cells), lymphocytes and neutrophils; the surface epithelium may undergo necrosis and disintegration. These changes are uniform throughout the involved sinus, in contradistinction to those of chronic sinusitis in which various stages of the inflammatory process may be seen in one cavity.

The organisms responsible for acute upper respiratory infections are found in acute suppurative sinusitis; the bacterial flora varies from time to time as it does in all respiratory infections but the organisms commonly found are the various streptococci, micrococci (staphylococci) and pneumococci. Fungi are occasionally the cause of sinus infections.

SYMPTOMS

The symptoms are general and local. The general symptoms are those found in any acute infection and may include fever, usually of slight or moderate degree but high in severe infections or complications, malaise, restlessness, lassitude, inability to concentrate, insomnia, depression and dizziness. Symptoms due to involvement of distant structures by absorption, such as iritis, neuritis, or arthritis may be present but are more commonly seen in chronic than in acute sinus infections, in which most symptoms are due to the local inflammatory process.

Headache. Headache is one of the most common local symptoms in acute suppurative sinusitis, its intensity depending upon the severity of the infection and the adequacy of drainage. It may be generalized or localized in the region of the affected sinus; this localization is not always exact enough to offer unfailing indication of the involved sinus. A sphenoidal sinusitis characteristically causes posterior (occipital) headache but may also cause frontal headache; an acute antrum infection may also cause frontal headache. Sinus headache is characterized by its tendency to occur at approximately the same hour daily during the acute stages. This is usually early in the morning and is thought to be due to interference with drainage during the night and to the increased congestion of head membranes in the recumbent position. However, daily headache may come at other hours, occasionally in the afternoon or at night. As convalescence proceeds, the daily headache tends to come at a later hour, be less severe, and of shorter duration until it disappears entirely.

Tenderness or Pain. Tenderness or pain over the sinus is often quite marked and, in contradistinction to headache, is usually a reliable guide to the involved sinus, the cheek in cases of antrum involvement, the mesial portion of the infra-orbital area in frontal and ethmoidal infection, the frontal area in cases of frontal sinusitis.

Neuralgic Pain. This is commonly present in acute sinus infections and is referred to the area of distribution of sensory nerves affected by the inflammatory process within the sinus. In acute maxillary sinusitis, severe pain may be experienced in the teeth underlying the sinus so that the patient consults a dentist; in fronto-ethmoidal involvement, neuralgic pain may occur in the temple, the parietal or the vertex area and in posterior ethmoidal and sphenoidal infections, the pain commonly occurs in the forehead or behind the eye, over the mastoid process, the posterior cervical muscles, or in the ear. There is also, in many cases, a generalized sense of fulness and pressure in the head which is most uncomfortable; this is quite characteristic of ethmoidal infections in which the discomfort is experienced between and behind the eyes.

Anosmia. Owing to intranasal swelling which prevents the air current from reaching the olfactory area, anosmia may be present, and taste, which is usually less affected, may also be involved.

Nasal Occlusion. Unilateral or bilateral occlusion is present in varying degrees and in severe cases may be quite marked.

Nasal Discharge. Discharge is always present in varying degree; in the early stages of acute rhinitis from which the sinusitis develops it is watery, becoming thick and purulent as the condition progresses. The discharge may be in either or both the anterior and posterior portion of the nose; when posterior, it is responsible for the postnasal discharge commonly present and its frequent attendant pharyngitis with sore throat, laryngitis with hoarseness and bronchitis with cough.

Sore Throat. Lateral pharyngitis with thickening of the lateral bands is frequently seen in acute sinusitis with postnasal discharge; cervical glands, especially the posterior group, are often enlarged and tender and the neck is stiff and sore, owing to cervical myositis.

Acute bronchitis, often present with acute sinusitis, may represent the pulmonary involvement of a generalized acute upper respiratory infection; aspiration of purulent postnasal discharge may also cause or accentuate the condition.

DIAGNOSIS

Physical Findings. Acute sinusitis, especially of the posterior series, may be attended by no external signs about the head, other than slight redness and excoriation about the anterior nares. There may be, however, swelling over the cheek in antrum involvement, edema of the lids, especially the upper, and fulness in the mesial portion of the supra-orbital area in ethmoidal and frontal involvement and swelling over the frontal area in cases of frontal sinusitis. Such physical findings indicate a severe infection, often with insufficient drainage.

The nasal membrane is red, thickened, often edematous, and purulent or mucopurulent discharge is present; its location indicates in a general way its source. Secretion coming from the middle meatus has its origin in the anterior series of sinuses, the antrum, anterior ethmoidal cells and frontal sinus. Secretion coming from above the middle turbinate has its origin in the posterior series of sinuses, the posterior ethmoidal cells and the sphenoid sinus. (It is to be remembered that the action of the cilia and mucous blanket of the nose and throat may quickly change the location of or completely remove nasal discharge; repeated examination may be necessary to fix exactly the true source of discharge seen within the nose.)

Smears. Smears of the secretion in acute suppurative sinusitis show it to be composed almost entirely of neutrophils; great numbers of bacteria are often present. In allergic sinusitis, eosinophils are prominent and in mixed reactions both types of cells are found.

Transillumination. When positive, showing a definite shadow over a sinus, the frontal or maxillary, transillumination suggests thickened membrane or fluid; a negative finding does not eliminate these conditions.

X-ray. Always of great value in giving exact anatomic information, x-ray examination is usually not necessary in establishing a diagnosis of acute suppurative sinusitis. It may, however, be very helpful in judging the extent and progress of the infection and in giving information concerning complications such as osteomyelitis or osteitis.

TREATMENT

General. Treatment of acute suppurative sinusitis is both general and local. In the early stages, general treatment is the more important and consists of measures applicable to any acute illness. The sick patient should have complete *bed rest* in a properly ventilated room; an optimum temperature of 21 or 22° C. (70 or 72° F.) and a humidity of 45 or 50 degrees should be maintained if possible. An ordinary steam kettle will provide moisture, but a cold humidifier is more efficient and comfortable. An *anodyne* should be given to control headache and pain; a sedative may be indicated.

The *sulfonamides*, especially *sulfadiazine*, may be tried; they occasionally seem to be of benefit, especially in involvement of soft tissue, such as orbital cellulitis, but have not been uniformly effective.

Penicillin in adequate intramuscular administration seems to be definitely beneficial and should be used, if possible, over a period of days in severe cases.

Local. Local treatment in the early stages of acute suppurative sinusitis is limited. *Heat* in some form is helpful in most cases, although
occasionally cold applications are preferred. *Warm, moist packs* are
excellent and *heat pads,* and *hot water bottles* are also effective. The
ordinary 250 watt carbon filament bulb in a reflector (Fig. 180) provides
considerable infra-red radiation.

Marked nasal obstruction should be relieved by the instillation of a
vasoconstrictor at regular intervals. There are many proprietary prepa-

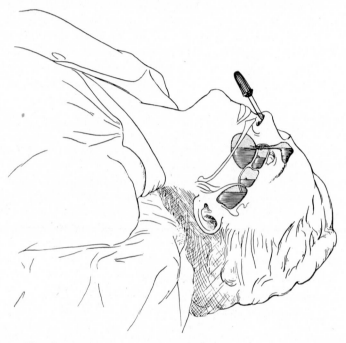

Fig. 83. The "head low" position for the instillation of nose drops. In this procedure, only a small amount of medication is used (usually 5 or 10 drops), which would
not be enough to produce a fluid level in the sinuses to the point shown in this illustration. In fact, the simple instillation of nose drops does not allow medication to enter
the sinuses to any degree. In "displacement irrigation," however, several cubic
centimeters of medication are used to produce a fluid level in the sinuses.

rations which contain ephedrine or a synthetic ephedrine-like substance,
as well as various other constituents, such as chemical bactericidal
agents, sulfonamide drugs, or the newer biotics such as penicillin and
tyrothricin. The important result desired is *vasoconstriction* to promote
sinus ventilation and drainage, and for this purpose, a simple 1 per cent
solution of ephedrine hydrochloride in isotonic saline solution is preferred (Figs. 83, 84).

It is to be remembered that marked and prolonged vasoconstriction
is often followed by undesirable congestion due to vasodilation and

paresis; for this reason, extreme or prolonged vasoconstriction is less desirable than that of moderate degree. The hyperemia and congestion of the nasal membrane is part of its defense mechanism and should not

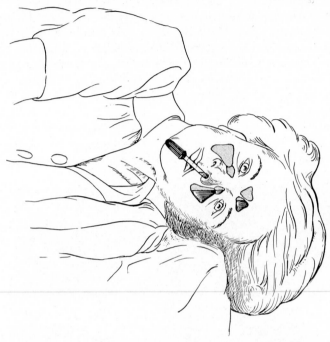

Fig. 84. The Parkinson position for the instillation of nose drops. This represents the most desirable position with the patient on a side and head lower than shoulders. The nose drops are then introduced into the dependent nostril. Again, no medication actually forms this much of a level within the sinuses, but the aim of the procedure is to introduce a medication to produce vasoconstriction of the mucosa of the nasal space including the sinus ostia.

be interfered with to the point of producing ischemia; nasal medication should be dispensed with as soon as possible.

SUBACUTE STAGE

In a patient progressing favorably, the symptoms of the acute stage lessen in severity. The general symptoms, the malaise and fever dis appear and the headache, pain, nasal obstruction and discharge gradually lessen. In the subacute stage, more active intranasal treatment may be used if the progress is retarded. The frontal and sphenoid sinuses may be irrigated by means of proper cannulas; the antra may be washed either through the natural ostium or a needle puncture in the inferior meatus (Fig. 85). Three types of maxillary sinus cannulas are shown in Figure 179. The pointed one is used to pierce the middle meatus membrane. Many drugs and chemicals have been used in these irrigations, none with sustained or outstanding success; good results have followed the instillation of penicillin. The simple cleansing action of any solution is probably its most important effect.

Proetz displacement irrigation (Fig. 86), a method of cleansing a sinus cavity by the exhaustion of its contained air by suction and the subsequent introduction of the irrigating fluid by the resulting negative pressure, is especially applicable to the ethmoidal and sphenoidal sinuses. Here it is effective in ridding the numerous cells of their contained mucoid or mucopurulent secretion and so restoring to normal activity the cilia and mucous blanket; it is less effective in the frontal sinus.

The principal therapeutic action of the medication used (ephedrine $\frac{1}{2}$ to $\frac{1}{4}$ per cent in isotonic saline solution) is obviously one of vasoconstriction. This shrinkage of the membrane of the ostia of the sinuses combined with the actual entrance of some of the medication into the

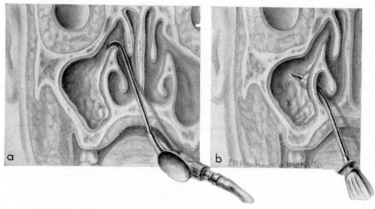

Fig. 85. a, The most commonly used modern method of irrigating a maxillary sinus
b, A method in which a trocar is inserted through the meatal wall.

sinus and the negative pressure of the act which dislodges obstructing secretions, accounts for the value of the procedure. The introduction of medications which might have an antibacterial action has never been considered effective. An antibacterial agent in sufficient strength to be effective would be expected to have a deleterious effect on ciliary activity. Recently, however, the combination of a vasoconstrictor and penicillin has been advocated. This combination may prove to have some value. Two types of suction bulbs for this procedure are shown in Figure 178.

Nasal packs, or pledgets of cotton saturated with a mild silver protein, usually 10 to 25 per cent argyrol, and inserted into the middle meatus, have been extensively used for many years and are considered by many to effect considerable shrinking and decongestion with improvement in sinus drainage. Others consider them not only ineffective but actually harmful, in that they interfere with the action of the cilia and mucous blanket.

The middle turbinate may be infracted mesially if it is closely applied to the middle meatus or swollen so that it impedes frontal and ethmoidal drainage; this procedure is often of definite value.

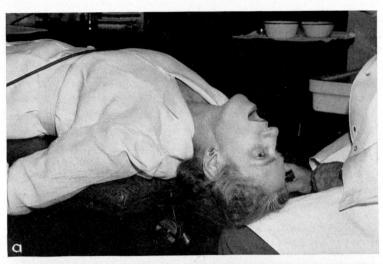

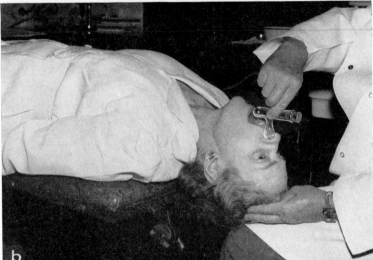

Fig. 86. (a) The position of the patient for displacement irrigation. The patient is requested to breathe entirely by mouth, the medication is instilled into the side to be treated and the tip of the suction bulb is inserted (b), and alternate action and release of negative pressure is produced by holding a finger on and off the vent in the suction bulb.

Short wave diathermy, a method of applying heat a little more deeply in the tissues, may be used in the subacute stage, especially if neuritic pain or deep tenderness persists; it is not used in the presence of marked nasal congestion or of obstruction of sinus ostia because of the increased discomfort which may result under such circumstances. Light doses of x-ray have been reported as lessening the discomfort of acute sinusitis.

In a patient progressing favorably, improvement is steady, though often slow, requiring from two or three to several weeks. The last sign to disappear is the postnasal discharge, which becomes less and less purulent until it is mucopurulent and finally mucoid. The sinus membrane may return completely to normal after an acute infection and the patient may never have another attack, or, depending somewhat on the duration and severity of the infection, there may be left a residual fibrosis and round cell infiltration of the stroma which predisposes the patient to recurrence of the sinusitis with subsequent head infections. If these latter changes are marked and accompanied by persisting deep seated infection in the stroma of the nasal mucosa, a chronic sinusitis is the final result of the acute infection.

SURGERY

Indications for Surgical Treatment. Cases of acute suppurative sinusitis due to unusually virulent infection or occurring in patients with low resistance or with anatomical drainage obstructions or under circumstances in which adequate treatment is not possible occasionally develop indications for surgical treatment. The common surgical indications are the prevention of chronicity in cases failing to respond to medical treatment (although such cases are usually allowed to become chronic before surgery is instituted), excessive, uncontrolled pain from retained secretion, and threatened complications, either intracranial or orbital.

The surgery of acute suppurative sinusitis has but a single purpose and that is to secure adequate drainage of the involved cavities and so meet the indications previously mentioned. In achieving this end, nasal tissue and physiologic function are disturbed as little as possible; the complete anatomical dissections often indicated in chronic infections have no place in the treatment of acute infections.

The approach of choice is external. This is always so in the case of frontal and ethmoidal infections; the sphenoidal sinus is of necessity always approached by the intranasal route. Acute antritis rarely requires surgical treatment. General anesthesia is used because of the inadvisability of infiltrating soft tissue with local anesthetic solutions in the presence of acute infection; also, local anesthesia is not fully effective under such conditions.

Various factors enter into the result of the surgical treatment of acute suppurative sinusitis, among them being the physical condition of the patient, the anatomy of the sinus involved, the virulence of the infection and extent of involvement, the presence of uncontrolled allergy, the proper choice of surgical procedure and its proper execution; these factors are better discussed in connection with each sinus.

Frontal Sinus

Anatomy. The frontal sinus varies in size from a small cell lying at or just above the level of the supra-orbital margin to a relatively large cavity extending up to the hair line, laterally to the malar process of the frontal bone and posteriorly over the orbit almost to its apex. It may be divided into compartments by partial septa and is connected with the nasal cavity through the nasofrontal duct, which may be comparatively short and straight opening directly into the middle meatus or long and narrow reaching the middle meatus only indirectly through the anterior ethmoidal sinus. The duct may end in an anterior ethmoidal cell.

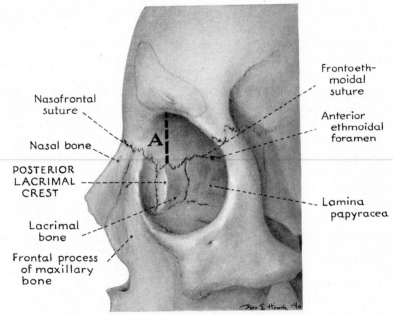

Fig. 87. A frontal sinus trephine should be made entirely through the floor of the sinus. This floor consists of lamellar bone in which there is no marrow.

Upon the development of the frontal sinus depends its relations and therefore the complications which occur during its involvement in infection. It forms the roof of the orbit, and orbital lesions varying in degree from edema and congestion to phlegmon and abscess may occur as the result of frontal sinusitis; when unusually well developed, the orbital extension of the frontal sinus may be in contact with the optic nerve and lesions of the latter structure may result from infections in the former. The posterior wall forms part of the anterior wall of the anterior cranial fossa, and pathologic changes in this wall or infection passing through it may cause localized encephalitis or brain abscess in the frontal lobe of the cerebrum. When the sinus is well developed in the vertical portion of the frontal bone, the veins of the sinus mucosa may be in continuity with the venous spaces of the diploic bone; in such cases, an osteomyelitis of the frontal bone may follow an acute frontal sinus infection.

Indications for Surgery. When frontal sinusitis is attended by severe increasing pain, retained secretions, or threatened complications and is uncontrolled by sulfonamides or antibiotics (penicillin), surgical drainage of the sinus is indicated.

Technic. This drainage is performed by the external approach under general anesthesia, entry into the sinus being gained through the thin, hard bone of the mesial portion of its floor (Fig. 87), every effort being made to avoid cancellous or diploic bone, which might become infected if surgically invaded. Enough of the floor is removed to permit adequate drainage of the cavity, but no attempt is made to remove the acutely inflamed lining; if underlying ethmoidal cells are involved in the process, they are entered through the lamina papyracea, broken down and both cavities drained through a large opening into the nose. The anterior wall of the sinus is not removed unless it is diseased and the posterior wall is removed only in case of suspected involvement of the frontal lobe.

An uncomplicated infection of the frontal sinus usually responds satisfactorily to adequate drainage, as do orbital infections. Frontal lobe abscess responds well if proper drainage can be secured and maintained; often this is difficult, and undrained pockets or secondary abscess cavities result ultimately in death. Osteomyelitis of the frontal bone differs in type. It may be of slow development and self limiting, spontaneous sequestration and healing occurring, or it may be an extremely virulent, rapidly spreading process, the control of which demands extensive resection of the frontal bone. Sulfonamides and antibiotics should be used in all these conditions.

Ethmoidal Sinus

Anatomy. The ethmoidal sinus, like the frontal, is subject to great variation in development and relations. Its cells may extend over the roof of the orbit, almost to the apex, pneumatizing the body and lesser wing of the sphenoid bone and bringing the sinus into direct relation with the optic nerve, the two structures being separated by a layer of bone of tissue paper thickness or by mucous membrane only; in a series of skulls of average development, a layer of bone from 2 to 5 mm. in thickness intervened between these structures. This relationship may account for impaired vision in disease of the posterior ethmoidal cells.

An ethmoid cell may invade the posterior-superior mesial angle of the maxillary sinus, simulating a double antrum; one may invade the middle turbinate to make of it a cystlike structure, or mound into the floor of the frontal sinus to form the so-called frontal bulla, a separate cell in the frontal sinus, which may sometimes confuse the diagnosis and complicate treatment.

Superiorly, the ethmoidal sinus is separated from the middle cranial fossa by thin, dense bone. Disease or fracture of this structure may result in intracranial disease such as meningitis.

Laterally, the lamina papyracea separates the ethmoidal sinus from the orbit; fracture, disease, or dehiscence of this structure may permit the entrance of infection into the orbit with resulting disease of that structure varying from simple edema and congestion to phlegmon and abscess.

Indications for Surgical Intervention. Acute suppurative disease of the ethmoidal sinus without evidence of the complications previously mentioned may, but rarely does, call for surgical intervention to relieve the pain and toxemia of an empyema of the sinus. Surgical intervention in acute suppurative ethmoiditis is most frequently demanded to relieve an impending or already present orbital complication, especially abscess. This is a comparatively frequent complication, especially in children, and while many cases are controlled by medical treatment, especially since the advent of the sulfonamides and antibiotics, surgery is occasionally required.

Technic. Under general anesthesia an external incision is made and the sinus is entered through the lamina papyracea, the cells broken down, drainage into the nose established and the orbital abscess drained; the thin floor of the frontal sinus is removed whenever this cavity is also involved, as it frequently is. The results of this procedure are usually very good, both the orbital and ethmoidal infection clearing with return to normal.

Maxillary Antrum

Anatomy. The antrum of Highmore, the largest of the sinuses at birth, is located in the maxilla lying alongside the nasal cavity; it may be as large as a small bean. As the maxilla develops, the antrum enlarges laterally and downward until in adult life it occupies most of the maxilla. It overlies the bicuspid and molar teeth and its full development downward and posteriorly is conditioned by the eruption of the permanent bicuspid and molar teeth, especially the third molar.

The antrum, the largest of the accessory sinuses, consists usually of a single cell (the ostium of which is near its roof); inadequate drainage is a factor in its frequent involvement in suppurative processes. Its walls may be thick or thin, depending on the extent of pneumatization of the maxilla, but its pneumatization pattern is much simpler than is the case with the ethmoid or sphenoid sinuses; its relations are fewer and simpler and its complications less frequent.

The most important relation of the antrum is with the teeth of the upper jaw; the two bicuspid teeth and the first and second molar usually underlie its floor (Fig. 64). The canine tooth and the third molar may also come into close relationship with the cavity of the sinus when it is unusually well pneumatized. The floor of the antrum overlying the teeth may be several millimeters thick so that the relation between the roots of the teeth and the cavity is not a close one, or the intervening floor may be very thin so that the roots of the teeth protrude into the cavity itself. Under such conditions, apical disease of the underlying teeth frequently causes disease of the antrum; various writers estimate the incidence of such a cause as from 20 per cent to 50 or 60 per cent.

The antrum, when well developed, may hollow out the alveolar process of the maxilla, producing the alveolar recess, into which the roots of the upper teeth may protrude, or it may invade the hard palate, forming the palatal recess; in well developed cases, the palatal recesses may almost meet in the midline beneath the floor of the nose.

The roof of the antrum forms the floor of the orbit and antral disease may cause orbital complications, just as may the ethmoid sinus, but much less frequently. Suppurative antritis may infrequently cause osteitis or osteomyelitis of the superior maxilla, especially in young children.

Indications for Surgery. Acute suppurative disease of the antrum rarely requires surgical treatment. When retained secretions cause excessive pain or threaten neighboring structures, irrigation, preferably through the natural ostium in the middle meatus or by needle puncture through the naso-antral wall in the inferior meatus, may be performed. Very rarely antrotomy in the inferior meatus may be necessary, but surgical procedures involving bony tissue are to be avoided in the presence of acute infection.

In general, it may be said that surgical treatment is necessary in relatively few cases of acute suppurative sinusitis, that its purpose is to control pain and prevent complications and that when adequate drainage is secured the results are good, and a cure may be expected. If complications are present, the result of surgical treatment will depend on the gravity of the complication; chronicity may ensue after an acute suppuration if the infection was unusually virulent, the resistance of the patient low, or the surgical procedure inadequate.

Sphenoidal Sinus

Anatomy. The complex anatomy of the sphenoid bone and its intimate relation with many important structures permit endless variation in the pneumatization pattern of the sphenoidal sinus and in its complex relations; nowhere else in the body are there so many vital structures within such limited space. These relationships are responsible for many clinical conditions not always obviously associated with disease of the sphenoid sinus.

When a recess of the sinus is in close relation with a sensory nerve, only a thin lamella of bone or, at times, mucous membrane separates the structures; disease in the sinus cavity may result in neuralgic pain over the distribution of the sensory nerve. When a recess of the sinus is in close approximation to the optic nerve, various degrees of impaired vision due to scotomas caused by optic neuritis may result. Posteriorly, the sphenoid sinus may be related to the hypophysis cerebri, the optic commissure (in 50 per cent of the patients), or portions of the brain stem. Laterally, it is close to the cavernous sinus, which has within its walls the oculomotor, the trochlear, the ophthalmic and the maxillary nerves and in its cavity the internal carotid artery and abducens nerve. Inferiorly, it is related to the pterygoid (vidian) nerve, the choanae and the nasopharynx. Inferolaterally, it may be related to the optic nerve and ophthalmic artery; it may be related superoposteriorly or inferiorly with the sphenopalatine fossa and its contained sphenopalatine ganglion.

When the sinus pneumatizes the lesser and greater wings of the sphenoid, it comes into close relation with the ophthalmic, the oculomotor, trochlear, abducens, frontal, lacrimal and nasal nerves; when the lesser wing of the sphenoid and the anterior clinoid process are invaded, the optic nerve is in intimate association with the cavity. When the great wing of the sphenoid (pterygoid process) is invaded, the cavity may come into close association with the foramen rotundum and maxillary nerve, the foramen ovale and mandibular nerve and the pterygoid (vidian) nerve. The sinus may also invade the orbital process of the palate bone, the palatine recess, on the superomedian aspect of the orbit, or the ethmoid bone, the ethmoidal recess; the latter may contact the posterior extension of the supra-orbital portion of the frontal sinus.

Consideration of the infinite variation in the anatomy of the sphenoid sinus as outlined above and realization that its recesses may bring the diseased lining of the sinus into contact with the related nerves, vessels and ganglia will explain the varied and often puzzling clinical pictures of neuralgias, cephalalgias, meningitis, osteitis or osteomyelitis of the base of the skull, and disturbed vision encountered in diseases of these cavities.

Technic. The surgical approach to the sphenoid is entirely intranasal and is much better performed under local than under general anesthesia. The ostium may be enlarged or the entire anterior wall, including the basisphenoid, may be resected; in this latter procedure, care must be taken not to injure the sphenopalatine artery which courses across the lower part of the anterior wall of the sinus.

The result of these procedures is usually good, the diseased mucosa returning to normal if adequate ventilation and drainage is secured. The presence of deep recesses, especially in the pyterygoid process, may modify the result obtained.

CHRONIC SUPPURATIVE SINUSITIS

Chronic suppurative sinusitis may result from one attack of severe acute suppurative sinusitis, but it more frequently ensues as the result of repeated attacks of mild acute sinusitis. The factors which increase the severity and duration of an acute infection are naturally those conducive to the development of chronicity, such as unusually virulent infection, lack of resistance or poor physical condition in the patient, improper treatment, or lack of treatment through neglect or economic necessity. Anatomical variations, as pointed out previously, have much to do with the development of chronicity. A frontal sinus with deep lateral recesses or a tortuous nasofrontal duct, a sphenoid sinus with marked pneumatization of the root of the pterygoid process or the basisphenoid or poorly drained ethmoid cells are more apt to develop chronic infections than sinuses in which these conditions do not exist. Any obstruction to sinus ventilation and drainage, such as that offered by a deviated septum, an enlarged middle turbinate or bulla ethmoidalis, or a hypertrophied processus uncinatus, definitely increases the possibility of a chronic infection developing from an acute one. Apical disease of the teeth underlying the antrum plays a very definite role in the development of chronic antritis. Allergic rhinitis, with its attending edema, is a factor in many cases of chronic sinusitis.

PATHOLOGY

In chronic suppurative sinusitis, the pathologic changes have become permanent, spontaneous healing being no longer possible, yet the tissue reactions represent nature's attempt to effect a cure. These reactions are found principally in the stroma, which becomes the seat of proliferative changes involving cells having to do with repair, such as histiocytes, cells of the plasmacytic and lymphocytic series (plasma cells and lymphocytes) and fibroblasts; neutrophils are also found. The end result may be fibrosis with sclerosis, often especially marked about blood vessels, impairing the blood supply, or about the glands, resulting in either atrophy or cystic dilatation; minute encapsulated abscesses may be present throughout the stroma.

The epithelium may remain intact with functioning cilia and mucous blanket over a markedly inflamed stroma, or it may show various stages of desquamation with loss of cilia, even to frank ulceration. Occasionally, the long-continued inflammatory reaction leads to metaplasia of the pseudostratified ciliated columnar epithelium and the formation of stratified squamous epithelium, or to hyperplasia, resulting in the so-called hyperplastic sinusitis with villi and polyps.

In contrast to acute suppurative sinusitis, in which the pathologic changes are uniform throughout the involved sinus, in chronic suppurative sinusitis, various stages of the inflammatory process may be found in the same cavity; an area of intact epithelium overlying a stroma, the seat of slight or moderate inflammatory reaction, may adjoin an area of ulcerated epithelium overlying an intensely inflamed stroma, the seat of numerous small abscesses. Logical therapy attempts to reinforce nature's reparative processes; therefore, extensive removal of the diseased mucosa is not warranted unless restoration to normal is obviously impossible. Frequently, adequate ventilation and drainage will enable the reparative processes to achieve such restoration.

Diseased mucosa surgically removed is replaced, not by normal mucosa, as was formerly believed, but by mucosa the stroma of which is less vascular and more fibrotic than normal; this mucosa is less able to resist infection. The regenerated epithelium may be normal with normal cilia and normal mucous blanket.

Chronic suppurative sinusitis has been exhaustively studied bacteriologically; the results vary depending on the year and locality in which they are made. In general, the organisms found in acute sinusitis are found also in the chronic infections—hemolytic and nonhemolytic streptococci, pneumococci and hemolytic and nonhemolytic micrococci (staphylococci). In addition, saprophytes and fungi are occasionally found.

Chronic sinusitis is a common disease; the absence of urgent symptoms encourages many of its victims to ignore it until some secondary effect or acute exacerbation forces it upon their attention.

Many disorders have been reported to be the result of chronic suppurative sinusitis; occasionally the relationship has been established by the cure of the complication when the sinus infection cleared. Fortunately, the majority of chronic sinus infections run their course without such complications, but the possibility of their occurrence should always be borne in mind.

SYMPTOMS

General symptoms indicative of absorption which have been reported are fatigue, lassitude, aprosexia, anorexia and vertigo. Mental disturbances, sleeplessness and depression are occasionally seen, especially in infection of the frontal, ethmoidal and sphenoidal sinuses; sphenoiditis, in particular, has been reported to be the cause of psychic disturbances, presumably because of its close association with the base of the skull and the attendant dural congestion. Arthritis, neuritis and iritis are occasionally the result of sinus infection.

Local symptoms of chronic sinusitis are not as frequent or severe as those seen in acute sinusitis.

Pain and Tenderness. Localized pain and tenderness are not usually present unless associated with an acute exacerbation of the chronic inflammatory process, in which case they have much the same character and location as that seen in acute infection.

Eye Disorders. Suppuration within posterior ethmoidal cells or the sphenoid sinus may cause visual disturbance by involvement of the optic nerve where it is in close relationship with these cells; obstruction of the lacrimal duct causes various types of conjunctivitis. Reflex irritation of chronic sinusitis has been credited with causing blepharitis, phlyctenular keratitis, asthenopia, blepharospasm and ptosis.

Headache. The severe headache so characteristic of acute sinus infections is not seen in the chronic type of disease, except in acute exacerbations. Headache, when present, is dull, persistent, less definitely localized or related to any special sinus, and is usually indicative of some obstruction to drainage or ventilation.

Nasal Occlusion. Nasal occlusion is a common symptom and may be due to hypertrophy of intranasal structures such as turbinates, processus uncinatus or bulla ethmoidalis, or to polyps, the result of infection; deviation of the nasal septum is frequently present and may be responsible for much obstruction.

Discharge. Discharge, either anterior into the handkerchief or posteriorly into the pharynx, not always pathognomonic of sinus disease, is a very common symptom, usually present in some degree; it varies considerably, but in general is purulent in character, as is the drainage from any infected area.

The point of appearance of the discharge in the nasal cavity is indicative of its source and hence of the sinus involved. Careful repeated study may be necessary to determine this point; the statements made in this connection in the discussion of acute sinusitis apply equally to the location of discharge in chronic sinusitis.

The postnasal drainage may cause chronic sore throat, laryngitis, or bronchitis with nocturnal cough, especially in childhood.

Anosmia. Anosmia may be caused by intranasal swelling or local inflammatory reaction in the olfactory area preventing the air currents from reaching the terminals of the olfactory nerve. Sneezing may be caused by the local irritation of polypoid hypertrophies or polyps, although it always suggests the possibility of an allergenic factor in the process.

Pulmonary Infection. Special mention should be made of the association of chronic bronchitis and bronchiectasis with chronic suppurative sinusitis, although the relationship between these conditions is not clear. The sinusitis may cause the pulmonary complication, either by direct aspiration or through descending lymph channels or both lesions may represent simultaneous involvement of different portions of the respiratory tract. In any case, it is considered good treatment to make every effort to clear up sinusitis coexisting with pulmonary infection, although cure of the latter by such procedure cannot be promised.

The intranasal examination reveals varying degrees of hypertrophy or atrophy of soft tissue, chronic passive congestion of the mucosa and purulent or mucopurulent discharge.

Throat. The throat often presents chronic pharyngitis; the posterior wall is covered with purulent discharge or glazed with a thin layer of dried secretion. The lateral margins of the posterior wall, the so-called lateral bands, are often inflamed and thickened. Cervical glands, especially the posterior group, may be enlarged and the cervical muscles tender and tense, owing to chronic myositis from absorption.

DIAGNOSIS

X-ray studies are of great value, not only in giving exact knowledge of the anatomy of the sinuses, but also in depicting the extent and severity of the disease. Good films will demonstrate the thickness of the sinus

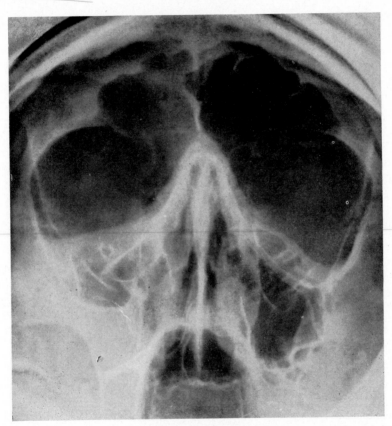

Fig. 88. An x-ray view in the Waldron-Waters position of a chronic sinusitis involving the right maxillary, ethmoid, and frontal sinuses. There is a fluid level visible in the involved maxillary sinus.

mucosa, the presence or absence of fluid, polyps, cysts, or osteitis or necrosis of the bony walls of the cavity (Fig. 88). Such studies, made after the instillation into the sinus of an opaque medium such as iodized oil (lipiodol), may delimit more clearly the pathologic processes; it also gives us information about the function of the cilia, the mucous blanket and the sinus ostia by the speed of elimination of the opaque medium.

The nasopharyngoscope is useful in studying the postnasal area, especially the spheno-ethmoidal recess; the antroscope often gives valuable information about the interior of the antrum. Transillumination is not conclusive; clear sinuses may contain fluid and shadows may be due either to thickened membrane or to variation in the thickness of bone.

Smears of the nasal secretions should always be made; a persistent appreciable eosinophilia is always indicative of an allergenic factor in the pathologic process, provided parasitic infestation can be ruled out.

Bacteriologic studies are helpful as a guide to the use of sulfonamide drugs and the antibiotics.

MEDICAL TREATMENT

The treatment of chronic suppurative sinusitis is essentially surgical, but certain general and local measures should always be tried before resorting to surgery.

General. The general physical condition and the hygiene of the patient should be carefully checked and abnormalities and errors corrected so far as possible. Climatic treatment may be tried if the patient can afford it. Patients with sinusitis characterized by boggy membranes and much discharge usually do better in a dry, warm climate, such as is found in the far southwestern United States; patients with scanty, sticky discharge attended by much crusting are often more comfortable in a warm, moist climate, such as is found in Florida and the West Indies. Any such change of climate must be maintained for a considerable period of time, at least a year, preferably two, in order to derive full benefit from it and permit conclusions as to its effectiveness.

Local. Local treatment as used in acute suppurative sinusitis is usually of little help in chronic conditions. However, it should be tried; the result is occasionally surprisingly good and indicates that the pathologic process was not irreversible. Occasionally, cannula irrigation of the sphenoid or maxillary antrum, or Proetz displacement of the ethmoid will clear up a case which had all the earmarks of chronicity; such results are, however, not frequent.

X-ray therapy has been advocated, mostly by roentgenologists, in the treatment of hyperplastic sinusitis; results have not been notable.

The *sulfonamide* drugs used locally in the nose are usually ineffective; used by mouth, they have been disappointing, although the occasional case, especially that complicated by involvement of soft tissue, such as orbital abscess, may be definitely benefited.

Penicillin, used locally in the nose or parenterally, has proved disappointing in most cases of chronic suppurative sinusitis; acute complications, such as osteomyelitis of the frontal bone and thrombosis of the cavernous sinus and acute exacerbations of chronic sinusitis are often greatly benefited or completely controlled.

It may be said, in summary, that the general and local measures effective in acute sinusitis are much less useful in chronic conditions and in most instances are quite ineffectual; surgical treatment is almost always indicated.

SURGICAL TREATMENT

Indications. Surgical treatment of chronic suppurative sinusitis is indicated to relieve the local discomfort due to nasal obstruction or discharge, to prevent impending complications or to control already present complications such as optic neuritis, osteomyelitis of the frontal bone or maxilla, orbital abscess, or cavernous sinus thrombosis, and to eliminate the sinus disease when it may possibly act as a focus of infection in such systemic disorders as arthritis.

To accomplish this, three criteria, originally formulated by Küster, should be met as far as possible. The diseased cavity must be opened as completely as possible to inspection, diseased tissue must be removed as completely as possible, and a permanent opening large enough to insure adequate drainage and ventilation must be installed. All surgical procedures are planned to conserve nasal tissue so far as possible and interfere with nasal physiology as little as possible.

In acute suppuration, surgical treatment, when necessary, is carried out under general anesthesia and by the external approach. In chronic suppuration, either type of anesthesia and either type of approach may be used, as conditions indicate; these will be discussed in more detail in connection with each sinus.

Maxillary Antrum

The maxillary antrum is the sinus most often involved in chronic suppuration because of its low position with the head erect, which permits seepage into it from infected overlying sinuses, ethmoid and frontal, and because its ostium is placed high in the nasal wall, which predisposes to stagnation of secretion, although the cilia and mucous blanket are remarkably effective mechanisms in keeping the cavity clean.

Partial septa may form pockets which interfere with drainage, and occasionally a large posterior ethmoid cell may invade the upper posterior mesial angle of the antrum, forming, in reality, a second antrum or so-called double antrum, which may be missed entirely unless careful diagnostic studies are made; failure would attend any operation on a maxillary sinus in which such an infected second antrum was overlooked.

The teeth underlying the antrum, the bicuspid teeth and first two molars, rarely the canine or third molar, must always be carefully examined and all diseased teeth removed; infected teeth are a frequent cause of chronic antritis, called dental antritis because of its origin, and characterized by a peculiarly foul discharge.

Chronic suppurative antritis rarely causes pain or discomfort but is attended by nasal obstruction and discharge, often foul; cacosmia may be present. Complications are not frequent; the most common one is a localized osteitis of the alveolar process, often starting in and localized about a diseased tooth root.

Examination will show inflammatory reaction of varying degree in the middle meatus; antrum irrigation will usually be returned with the fine flakes, shreds and granular detritus of a chronic sinusitis; x-ray will reveal thickened membrane, polyps, cysts, or, occasionally, fluid.

Technic. Antrotomy, or "window resection," made in the inferior meatus (Fig. 89), with the installation of as big an opening as possible, will cure a very large percentage, estimated as high as 85 per cent,

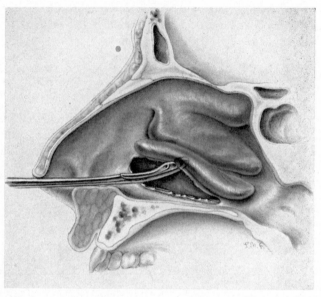

Fig. 89. The purpose in making an antrum window is to produce a large opening in the naso-antral wall of the inferior meatus which will allow ventilation of the sinus and gravity drainage.

of patients with chronic suppuration of the antrum. This is almost always performed under local anesthesia and is attended by little reaction or discomfort. Some time, often a period of months, is required before the effect of the improved ventilation and drainage on the pathologic process in the antrum is noted, but a surprising amount of hyperplasia and even polyposis will clear up after antrotomy.

The so-called radical antrum operation, or Caldwell-Luc, is reserved for cases which have not responded to antrotomy or for those cases with extreme polyposis or in which tumor, especially malignant tumor, foreign body, fracture, or disease of the bony walls is present. The approach is through the canine fossa (Fig. 90), which is resected to permit inspection of the antrum cavity and removal of the diseased tissue; antrotomy is made under the inferior turbinate and the incision over the canine fossa closed. Local anesthesia is preferred, although general anesthesia may be used. Its results are usually excellent unless suppuration in an overlying sinus has been neglected, in which case the disease of the antrum will probably continue.

Ethmoidal Sinus

Chronic suppurative disease of the ethmoid sinus is a common disorder but is usually attended by little discomfort; the principal symptoms are nasal congestion and discharge. Anosmia may occur. Examination shows inflammatory hypertrophy, perhaps with polyps, of the structures of the middle meatus, especially the processus uncinatus

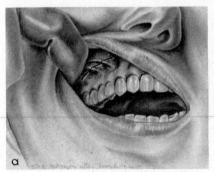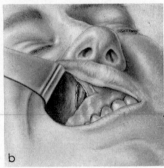

Fig. 90. The purpose of the Caldwell-Luc ("radical antrum") operation is to clean out under direct vision the diseased tissue in the sinus. A horizontal incision (a) is made in the canine fossa, the soft tissue is elevated, the sinus is entered through its anterior wall and enough of the wall is removed to provide adequate exposure. Then the diseased membrane in the sinus is removed and a large window made under the inferior turbinate (b). The incision in the canine fossa is then sutured.

and the middle turbinate. Purulent secretion will be seen in the middle meatus in involvement of the anterior group and above the middle turbinate in disease of the posterior group.

Technic. Surgical interference is indicated for relief of the nasal congestion and discharge and to prevent and control complications such as orbital infection, impaired vision (in disease of the posterior cells) and meningitis; as in the case of the frontal sinus, anatomy is a factor in the selection of the operation. If the sinus is small and does not have extensive cell systems outside the capsule proper (such as extensive cell development in the roof of the orbit), the intranasal approach may be used. Local anesthesia is used because it produces hemostasis and permits much better examination and demarcation of the operative field than does general anesthesia, in which bleeding is apt to obscure the landmarks. The intranasal approach (Fig. 91) is followed by less reaction than the external approach but is fraught with more danger than is the external operation (Fig. 92) because the operative field is not so easily delimited. If the sinus is large with extensive development, especially in the roof of the orbit, the external approach is indicated.

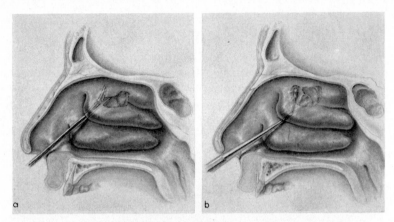

Fig. 91. The purpose of an ethmoid operation is to reduce the many-celled ethmoid labyrinth into one cavity or one large cell. When this is done intranasally, the operative field is visualized entirely by light reflected through the naris and the cells are removed with biting forceps (a) and curette (b) working under the middle turbinate.

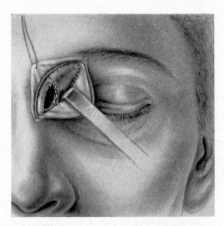

Fig. 92. An external ethmoidectomy can be done under better visualization as cell by cell can be carefully removed. The external scar is negligible.

This may be performed under either local or general anesthesia; local anesthesia is preferable in properly selected cases; general anesthesia may be used, but bleeding is a complicating factor. The approach is through a curvilinear incision about the inner canthus. The ethmoid capsule is entered through the lamina papyracea and the cells exenterated; the frontal and sphenoidal sinuses may be included in the operation.

The results of surgical treatment of chronic ethmoiditis are usually good if allergenic factors are controlled and if a complete exenteration of the cells has been accomplished; cells inaccessible by any surgical approach may continue to suppurate and prevent complete cure of the process.

Frontal Sinus

Fortunately, acute suppuration of the frontal sinus heals spontaneously or with proper treatment in a high percentage of cases. When the infection becomes chronic, local or medical treatment is usually of no avail. The patient rarely has pain or headache except with acute exacerbations, when he may have dull frontal headache. Examination shows inflammatory hypertrophy of the tissues in the anterior part of the middle meatus and pus in the same area, appearing first in the area of the nasofrontal duct.

Technic. When a chronic suppuration is present, the anatomy of the sinus (see discussion under Acute Suppurative Sinusitis) has much to do with the type of surgical procedure indicated. When the sinus is small or medium in size, without dependent lateral recesses or septa dividing it into pockets, with but limited development of its horizontal portion (cells in the roof of the orbit) and with a short, straight nasofrontal duct connecting it with the middle meatus of the nose, an intranasal approach under local anesthesia is the procedure of choice. Removal of the anterior third of the middle turbinate and exenteration of the anterior ethmoidal cells, especially those of the frontal recess, will frequently so improve ventilation and drainage that cure is effected. Such a procedure is not an operation upon the frontal sinus but upon the ethmoid sinus; its effectiveness is due to the fact that the frontal sinus often drains through the anterior ethmoidal area and the exenteration of the latter gives the necessary improvement in ventilation and drainage of the former.

If the above procedure has been tried and has failed, or if the sinus is a large one with dependent lateral recesses, septa interfering with drainage, marked development of its horizontal portion in the roof of the orbit, or a narrow, long tortuous nasofrontal duct, an external approach is indicated; this is the approach necessary in fracture of the posterior wall of the sinus, tumor, foreign body, or impending complication. The incision is made under the inner end of the supra-orbital margin and extended as far as necessary around the inner canthus.

Entry into the sinus is effected through the thin, hard bone of the mesial portion of the floor. Enough of the floor is removed to permit satisfactory inspection of the interior of the sinus and removal of diseased tissue; every effort is made in this procedure to avoid entering cancellous or diploic bone. If the anterior wall of the sinus is diseased or if adequate inspection and treatment of the interior of the sinus cannot be accomplished through the floor of the sinus, the anterior wall must be removed. If the orbital portion of the sinus is well developed, as it frequently is in sinuses requiring the external approach, these cells are completely exenterated and their intercellular walls removed. If the ethmoid cells, especially the anterior group, are involved in the suppurative process, they are exenterated and a large opening installed into the nose. In this surgical treatment, adequate exposure is necessary in order to permit as complete removal as possible of all diseased tissue.

The most difficult problem in frontal sinus surgery is the maintenance of a permanent nasofrontal communication, once it has been installed. Recent work with inlays of metals such as tantalum or with acrylic resins have given promising results. A tube made of one of these substances is allowed to remain in the nasofrontal duct until epithelization is completed.

Complications. The most common complications of frontal sinus disease and surgery are those mentioned in the discussion of acute suppurative frontal sinusitis, osteomyelitis of the frontal bone and abscess of the frontal lobe of the brain. Penicillin has proven effective in some cases of osteomyelitis and gives hope of more effective control of this dreaded complication. A proliferative osteitis following surgery may render impossible the maintenance of a permanently open nasofrontal duct.

The results of frontal sinus surgery depend on the thoroughness with which diseased tissue is removed from the sinus and from the underlying ethmoid cells, and the maintenance of a patent nasofrontal duct. If these objectives can be secured, the surgery will be successful; if not, it will fail.

Sphenoidal Sinus

The anatomic variations of the sphenoidal sinus and the complications encountered in its disease are described in the section devoted to acute suppurative sphenoiditis.

Chronic suppurative disease of the sphenoid sinus, frequently associated with chronic ethmoiditis, is often overlooked because it is not carefully searched for; postmortem studies of large groups of patients have shown that unsuspected suppuration may be present in the sphenoid sinus and be the cause of fatal complications, such as osteomyelitis of the base of the skull or of meningitis.

Chronic suppurative sphenoiditis may exist with few or no symptoms, or the patient may complain of dull suboccipital headache (occasionally frontal), neuralgias in the distribution of the pterygoid nerve and sphenopalatine ganglion, and of postnasal discharge. Repeated examination with postnasal mirror and nasopharyngoscope will demonstrate chronic inflammatory reaction and pus in the spheno-ethmoidal recess; irrigation will show the fine granular detritus of a chronic sinus infection, and x-ray may reveal increased density due to thickened membrane.

Technic. The only surgical approach to the sphenoid (when infection is limited to this sinus) is intranasal under local anesthesia and involves enlargement of its ostium in mild cases or, in more severe infections, resection of the entire anterior wall formed by the upper part of the basisphenoid. Some rhinologists deprecate any interference with the natural ostium, preferring to leave it undisturbed and to make an accessory ostium lower down in the face of the sphenoid; they believe that the natural ostium never functions well once it has been interfered with.

Sphenoid sinus suppuration is usually well controlled, provided adequate drainage and ventilation can be maintained. Dependent recesses with poor natural drainage are often slow to clear up although the cilia and the mucous blanket are remarkably effective in promoting healing.

HYPERPLASTIC SINUSITIS

Hyperplasia of the sinus mucosa associated with scanty mucoid or mucopurulent discharge is characteristic of a common form of chronic sinusitis. It is caused by long continued, low grade infection or by repeated attacks of acute infection and results in marked hyperplasia of the sinus membrane, especially in the ethmoidal and maxillary sinuses, with polyposis in the middle meatus. The sinus membrane is pale and thick and often associated with the same changes in the nasal mucosa.

The hyperplasia involves the epithelium, being greater in this condition than in allergic hyperplasia and with more marked squamous characteristics. Many of the ciliated columnar cells are replaced by goblet cells secreting mucus. The basement membrane is thickened and the stroma thickened and edematous but not so markedly as in allergic reaction. Eosinophils are not found; contraction of fibrous tissue elements may give the mucosa a papillary appearance. The periostium may be thickened; the underlying bone may or may not show absorption.

Two theories have been advanced to explain these changes in the sinus mucosa; one is that of long continued or often repeated attacks of acute inflammation, the whole process being on an infectious basis; the other, that of allergic origin with chronic infection superimposed. The pathologic changes are very similar to those of allergic sinusitis except that tissue eosinophilia is not present and edema is not so marked. The theory of allergic origin finds support in the fact that hyperplastic sinusitis is often associated with allergic conditions such as asthma.

SYMPTOMS

The patient may have no symptoms except a chronic mucoid or mucopurulent discharge and an increased susceptibility to what he believes to be "colds in the head," but which are exacerbations of the chronic sinus infection. Local pain and tenderness of the severity of acute suppurative processes are not seen. The patient may have diffuse dull headache of the pressure type caused by obstruction to ventilation and drainage. Hyperplastic ethmoiditis, especially, is apt to cause deep pressure discomfort between and behind the eyes; the patient may have no discomfort at all.

DIAGNOSIS

Examination of the nose shows the pale hyperplastic mucosa, perhaps with polyps or polypoid hypertrophy of the mucous membrane, especially of the middle meatus. Strings of mucoid or mucopurulent secretion are seen in the nose and postnasal space. Smears of this secretion do not usually show eosinophils.

X-rays demonstrate the thickening of the mucosa and the presence of polyps or cysts; contrast media often increase the definition of the film. A shadow on transillumination suggests thickening of the sinus membrane but is not conclusive; antroscopic examination of the cavity will show thickened membrane and polyps, but is usually not necessary.

TREATMENT

Treatment of this type of sinusitis is almost entirely surgical. Roentgen therapy has been advocated, principally by roentgenologists, in the lesser degrees of hyperplasia, but the results have not been sufficiently satisfactory or certain to win an assured place for this type of therapy.

Indications for Surgery. Surgical treatment is indicated to relieve the patient of the local discomfort, the nasal occlusion, postnasal discharge and pressure headache, especially in ethmoidal disease, or to clear up frequent exacerbations of the sinus infection, the so-called colds from which the patient suffers; occasionally disease of other organs may be due to absorption from the sinus focus. The relation of this type of sinusitis to asthma is of special interest. If the lung condition is due to sensitization to chronic infection in the sinuses, treatment of the latter is definitely indicated; in asthma which is definitely the result of sensitivity to extrinsic factors, surgical treatment is not indicated because it will surely be of no avail. Although much study has been given to this subject, great diversity of opinion still exists, owing largely to the difficulty of uniform classification of the sinus and chest diseases. In general, when the hyperplasia is primarily infectious in origin, good results may be expected from surgical treatment; when the hyperplasia is fundamentally allergic or contains an allergenic factor, the results of surgical treatment will be disappointing.

Surgical Technic. Surgical procedures, such as removal of nasal polyps or submucous resection of the nasal septum, are often indicated and may be performed in allergic patients, with considerable relief of the nasal obstruction but without effect on the hyperplasia of the sinus membrane. When treatment of the hyperplastic sinusitis is indicated, usually on account of the local symptoms, less frequently because of absorption, surgical removal of the diseased membrane is called for. The Caldwell-Luc operation on the maxillary sinus or the intranasal or external operation on the ethmoid sinus, depending partly on its anatomy, is indicated; the membrane should be removed as completely as possible; incomplete operations compromise the result of the surgical treatment. An unrecognized and untreated allergenic factor in the hyperplastic process will almost certainly result in failure of surgical treatment.

ALLERGIC SINUSITIS

Allergic sinusitis, always associated with allergic rhinitis, is a common disease, resembling in many respects chronic hyperplastic sinusitis of infectious origin, and frequently confused with it. One opinion, indeed, holds that all hyperplastic processes within the nose and sinuses and all polyps are primarily allergic in origin; when infection is present, it is a secondary superimposed process. This opinion is not universally accepted.

The pathologic changes of infectious and allergic sinusitis are similar in many respects; the latter condition usually presents a paler membrane, a more marked edema of the stroma and a frequent blood, tissue and nasal smear eosinophilia.

DIAGNOSIS

The diagnosis in typical cases is not difficult. There is usually a history of allergy, either familial or personal; nasal examination shows the pale diffuse hyperplasia of the mucosa, perhaps with polyps, and a watery mucoid secretion, smears of which show a definite eosinophilia. X-ray studies show a thickening of the membrane in all sinuses, in contradistinction to that seen in infectious hyperplasia, in which it may be limited to one or more of the sinuses; the shadow is said to have a diffused cloudy white appearance characteristic of allergic thickening.

Nasal obstruction and discharge are present in varying degree, often associated with itching in the nose, postnasal space or palate. Perhaps the most frequent and characteristic symptom is the frequent attack of nasal stuffiness, watery discharge, sneezing and itching of sudden onset, brief duration and rapid disappearance. The patient thinks it is a "cold in the head" and is surprised by its abortive course. Such upsets are usually caused by increased exposure to the offending allergen.

TREATMENT

Identification and elimination of the offending allergen is of prime importance; where this cannot be accomplished, desensitization with agents such as histamine or house dust frequently are of definite and considerable help.

Removal of polyps and submucous resection are indicated to control obstruction; sinus infection severe enough to call for treatment in the nonallergic patient, especially when it is causing systemic symptoms, may be treated by acceptable surgical methods only after every effort has been made to eliminate all allergenic factors and with the realization that any uncontrolled allergy will probably compromise the result to greater or less degree. The success of treatment is measured largely by the completeness of control of allergic causes.

SINUSITIS IN CHILDREN

Most of the discussion on sinusitis in adults applies with equal force to that condition in children, but there are certain features peculiar to and characteristic of sinusitis in childhood that should be emphasized.

First is the undoubted fact that sinusitis in infants and children is very frequently overlooked or is considered an ordinary cold which will clear spontaneously or which the child will outgrow. Then, too, infants and small children ordinarily do not have pain or headache with sinusitis and when it is present, they do not complain of it. Symptoms, especially in chronic cases, are not always too obvious and the examination necessary to uncover them, while usually simple, occasionally calls for time and patience on the part of the examining physician. One of the most important reasons for the disregard of sinusitis in infancy and childhood is the failure to realize that both the maxillary and ethmoidal sinuses are present at birth and large enough to be of clinical importance; many of the persistent or recurring colds of children are due to infection in these cavities.

Another important factor in this disregard of childhood sinusitis is the undue attention focused on adenoids and tonsils and the universal tendency to attribute all children's ailments of infectious origin to disease of these structures; certainly they are many times at fault, but it is equally certain that in many cases the sinuses and not the tonsils and adenoids are responsible for a clinical situation.

Postmortem studies of large groups of infants and young children have demonstrated the presence of suppurative sinusitis in a surprisingly large percentage of cases, in some groups as high as 30 per cent.

There are certain predisposing causes of sinusitis in infancy and childhood, not present in adult life, which must be reckoned with. First of all, the acute exanthemas in childhood, especially scarlet fever and measles, cause much sinusitis; mouth breathing and nasal obstruction due to large adenoids, while not causing the sinusitis, serve to prolong its course and prevent complete convalescence. The sinus ostia are relatively large, permitting access of infected secretion from the nasal passages and the patient, in his earlier years, has not yet acquired the resistance to infection present in later life.

SYMPTOMS

General symptoms may be any of those experienced by adult patients. Children show pallor, lassitude, weight loss, anorexia and secondary anemia due to sinus infection more frequently and more promptly than do adults with comparable infections.

Nasal obstruction and discharge are present in varying degree; discharge may be almost entirely postnasal and so escape casual observation. It is, however, responsible for persistent sniffling and for nonproductive nocturnal cough, so characteristic of childhood sinusitis. Mouth breathing, due to recurrent adenoid or to lymphoid hyperplasias in the postnasal space, is frequent; pain, headache, and local tenderness are not usually present in the uncomplicated case.

Nasal examination, both with mirror and nasopharyngoscope, is possible, even in quite young children, if time and patience are exercised; if necessary, the child may be immobilized in blankets or given a light anesthesia. Rhinoscopic findings are comparable with those of adults and have the same significance. Examination of the pharynx often reveals a heavy mucoid or mucopurulent postnasal discharge; this may not be evident until the child gags when the secretion is brought down from the postnasal space by the wiping action of the soft palate. This discharge may be indicative of sinusitis or an infected adenoid. Cervical adenitis is almost always present. General physical examination should always be performed and will frequently show underweight and anemia as above mentioned. A low basal metabolic rate accounts for hyperplastic changes in some cases.

TREATMENT

The treatment of sinusitis in infants and children is almost always medical: rarely is surgery necessary. *Vasoconstriction* with $\frac{1}{2}$ per cent ephedrine sulfate solution, the instillation performed with the head in either the Proetz or Parkinson lateral position, and sinus irrigation with Proetz displacement or, in maxillary sinusitis, with needle or cannula, are important and useful procedures. In chronic sinusitis, especially of the maxillary antrum, *antrotomy* performed in the inferior meatus may be necessary; radical surgical procedures are rarely, if ever, justified in the sinusitis of childhood.

The complications of sinusitis in infancy and childhood are those seen in adult life: probably the most common one is orbital infection, cellulitis, phlegmon, or abscess, caused by acute ethmoiditis. Most of these infections yield to medical treatment, hot moist packs, treatment of the causal sinusitis and use of the sulfonamides and antibiotics; penicillin, especially, has been effective. In the exceptional case, surgical treatment is necessary; this consists in drainage through an external incision, not only of the orbital abscess but also of the underlying acute ethmoiditis.

Another complication seen in young children is osteitis or osteomyelitis of the maxilla, originating either in the antrum or around the buds of deciduous teeth; redness, swelling and fistula formation with sequestration may result. Incision and drainage with removal of sequestra may be necessary.

The recognition and control, as far as possible, of the nasal allergy so frequently present in infancy and childhood is extremely important and at times difficult. Inhalants are the common cause of allergic rhinitis in both children and adults; the occurrence of eczema and hives in sinus patients calls for a thorough allergic investigation.

The general health and hygiene of children suffering from sinusitis is of great importance; proper food, rest, fresh air and vitamin dosage are essential. Iron and liver are indicated for the secondary anemia frequently present.

ROLE OF TONSILLITIS AND ADENOIDITIS

The role of chronic tonsillitis and adenoiditis in the causation and prolongation of sinusitis is important and frequently misunderstood. Marked hypertrophy of the adenoid causes nasal obstruction and mouth breathing, factors which make for chronicity in any nasal or sinus infection present; such adenoids should be removed. Chronic tonsillitis is often present in sinusitis and should be treated on its own merits and on the usual indications, not in the belief that it causes, or that tonsillectomy will cure, the sinusitis; the removal of the tonsils when definitely infected is indicated for the improvement in the health of the patient, which should follow. This procedure is performed upon proper indication, not for any direct effect on the sinuses.

REFERENCES

Barach, A. L., et al.: Penicillin Aerosol and Negative Pressure in the Treatment of Sinusitis. Am. J. Med., *1*:268, 1946.

Campbell, P. A.: Aerosinusitis—A Résumé. Ann. Otol., Rhin. & Laryng., *54*:69, 1945.

Cardwell, E. P.: Penicillin Administered Locally in Treatment of Disease of Nasal Accessory Sinus: Evaluation of Bacterial Sensitivity. Arch. Otolaryng., *44*:287, 1946.

Crowe, S. J., and Lett, J. E.: The Etiology, Treatment and Prevention of Chronic Sinus Infection. Ann. Otol., Rhin. & Laryng., *57*:364, 1948.

Dunn, R. E.: Penicillin in Treatment of Infections in the Nasal Passages and Sinuses. Australian & New Zealand J. Surg., *16*:163, 1947.

Goodyear, H. M.: Surgery of the Frontal Sinus. Laryngoscope, *57*:340, 1947.

Hunnicutt, L. G.: Modern Treatment of Chronic Sinusitis. J.A.M.A., *133*:84, 1947.

McMahon, B. J.: Treatment of Sinusitis in Children. Ann. Otol., Rhin. & Laryng., *53*:644, 1944.

Rawlins, A. G.: Chronic Allergic Sinusitis. Laryngoscope, *57*:381, 1947.

Rekling, E., and Worning, B.: Sinusitis in Childhood. Mod. Med., *34*:1381, 1947.

Schenck, H. P.: Antibiotics in the Treatment of Sinus Infections. Ann. Otol., Rhin. & Laryng., *56*:39, 1947.

Schenck, H. P.: Indications for Surgery in the Light of the Use of Antibiotics. Surg., Gynec. & Obst., *84*:850, 1947.

Shea, J. J.: Intranasal Surgery. *Ibid.*, *84*:859, 1947.

Smith, A. T., and Spencer, J. T.: Orbital Complications Resulting from Lesions of the Sinuses. Ann. Otol., Rhin. & Laryng., *57*:5, 1948.

Symposium on Diseases of the Paranasal Sinuses. Proc. Staff Meet., Mayo Clin., *19*:465, 1944.

Van Alyea, O. E.: Nasal Sinuses. Baltimore, Williams & Wilkins Co., 1942.

Van Alyea, O. E.: Management of Chronic Sinus Disease. Ann. Otol., Rhin. & Laryng., *54*:443, 1945.

Van Alyea, O. E.: Treatment of the Acute Nasal and Sinus Infection. North Carolina M. J., *8*:63, 1947.

Weille, F. L.: External Sinus Surgery. Surg., Gynec. & Obst., *84*:853, 1947.

Weille, F. L.: Problems of Secondary Frontal Sinus Surgery. Ann. Otol., Rhin. & Laryng., *55*:372, 1946.

Williams, H. L.: Fundamental Conceptual Changes in Regard to Chronic Suppurative Sinusitis. *Ibid.*, *57*:541, 1948.

Wishart, D. E. S.: Diagnosis and Treatment of Sinusitis in Children. Laryngoscope, *54*:97, 1944.

CHAPTER XVII

COMPLICATIONS OF SINUSITIS

JEROME A. HILGER, M.D.

Extension from infection of the sinuses to neighboring or distant structures may be divided into: cranial complications, lower respiratory complications, focal infection (extension to tissues remote to the sinuses), and oro-antral fistula.

CRANIAL COMPLICATIONS

Anatomy. *Structures in Proximity to the Sinuses.* Anatomically, the structures of importance which are contiguous to the paranasal sinuses are the orbit and its contents, the diploic frontal bone, the meninges and the cranial contents, including the brain and the venous sinuses.

Communicating Channels. There is an intervening bony plate or fibrous tissue septum between all of the paranasal sinuses and the neighboring tissues. It is inconceivable in the light of fundamental pathological changes that direct extension ever occurs in the spread of infection from a sinus cavity. Fundamentally and microscopically it is necessary that some communicating channel be used to convey the infection. The lymphatic and venous systems are the principal routes of extension.

Communicating lymphatic pathways have not been demonstrated between extracranial and intracranial structures, except in the demonstrations by Rouviere and others of cranioneurolymphatics in the region of the olfactory nerve. Since the existence and function of the latter are controversial at best, it is probable that in few instances are they an important factor in communication of infection from the paranasal sinuses to the intracranial cavity. There is, however, an intercommunicating venous network between the cranial cavity, the orbit and the paranasal sinuses. It is by means of the venous network that the vast majority of infections extend from the paranasal sinus spaces. The perforating vessels in the fibrous tissue of the fronto-ethmoid suture line which has not been obliterated by bony union in children are a ready means of extension of sinus infection from the ethmoid sinuses to the orbit in the younger age group. In adults, the thin, bony floor of the frontal sinus is perforated by numerous venules and gives similar route of extension in the older age groups from the frontal sinus to the orbit. The ease of communication between small veins of the mucoperiosteal lining of the frontal sinus and the anterior temporal and frontal diploic veins admits ready extension from the frontal sinus mucosa to the venous system of frontal diploic bone. From this involvement, the thrombophlebitis may readily extend to the epidural, subdural and subarachnoid spaces, and to the cortex of the brain by venules which communicate freely between the vessels of the diploic venous system and the intracranial venous system.

The venous network in the mucoperiosteum of the maxillary sinus is in continuity with the marrow spaces of the maxillary bone and with the pterygoid venous plexus. In the posterior ethmoid and sphenoid sinuses, similar relationship exists with the cavernous sinus.

PATHOLOGY AND BACTERIOLOGY

The mucoperiosteal lining of the paranasal sinuses has tremendous power of resistance and healing. Fundamental local factors in healing are drainage and ventilation of the infected mucosa. Systemic factors are grouped immunologically as general resistance of the host to the invading organism. When resistance is low, infection develops and certain anatomic and physiologic factors may make for impaired ventilation and drainage of a paranasal sinus. Extreme edema and closure of the ostium may result. This is particularly prone to occur in the frontal sinus because of the frequently tortuous course of the longer nasofrontal duct. In such circumstances, a favorable medium exists for the further growth of certain micro-aerophilic and anaerobic cocci, and the vicious circle of further edema and obstruction results. The inflammatory process involves the veins of the mucoperiosteal lining and thrombophlebitis with intravenous infection then exists. Laboratory demonstration of bacteremia is often possible. Extension through larger and deeper veins of the mucoperiosteum and eventually to the communicating venules mentioned previously can readily occur. By this process it is possible, therefore, for infections of the paranasal sinuses to extend throughout the communicating venous system to the frontal diploic bone, to the epidural and subdural spaces, the subarachnoid space, the cortex of the brain, or into the large venous sinuses of the head. It is also possible for extension to occur to the periorbita and hence into the venous channels of the orbital contents, and from the maxillary sinus to the marrow spaces of the maxilla and to the pterygoid venous plexus and the internal jugular vein.

GENERAL TREATMENT

In very acute upper respiratory infections, *physiologic rest* for the nasal mucosa is important. Patients should be kept at rest in an atmosphere of comfortable temperature and adequate humidity. The addition of *simple nasal decongestants* in physiologic solution for use locally in the nose every three to four hours is a slight help. Pain can be minimized with *elevation of the head, local application of heat; analgesics* and *opiates* as necessary. Local manipulative procedures within the nose are unwise. There is little that can be accomplished by local manipulation except the destruction of valuable cilia.

When systemic reaction of fever and malaise are in evidence, chemo-therapeutic or antibiotic agents should be used early in adequate dosage. Because of the rapid rate of progress of many infections, it is not always possible to obtain bacteriologic evidence of the nature of the infecting organism and its sensitivity to a particular agent. In the early stages, therefore, the use of these agents is necessarily empirical.

Extension of an infectious process from a sinus is usually heralded by marked pain and tenderness over the involved sinus and evidence of

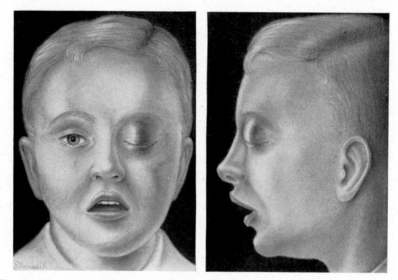

Fig. 93. The characteristic appearance of orbital cellulitis developing from acute ethmoiditis.

early edema. When these signs are combined with severe systemic reaction, rising temperature and chill, venous extension is developing and more definitive measures are necessary.

ORBITAL CELLULITIS AND ABSCESS

Symptoms. When manifest acute nasal suppuration is present as a primary acute infection or as an acute exacerbation of a pre-existing chronic suppuration of the frontal, ethmoid, or sphenoid sinuses, the first sign of extension into the orbit is edema in the region of the inner canthus, which is usually accompanied by marked local pain over the involved sinuses and by a febrile reaction. Since the venous system is the route of extension, the invasion of the blood stream is usually signaled by an initial sharp rise in temperature and frequently by a chill. If the process of extension is not checked by appropriate measures at this point, edema of the lid increases and the periorbita and orbital contents are displaced outward and downward (Fig. 93). As the cellulitis advances,

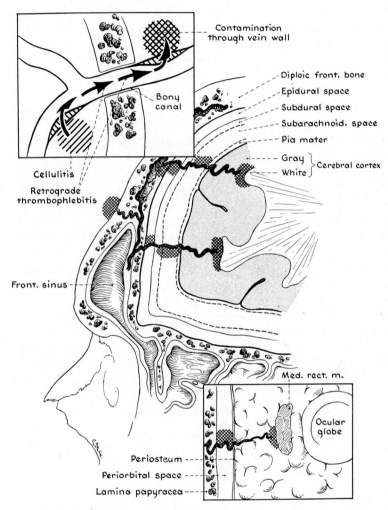

Fig. 94. Diagrammatic representation of the venous system as the highway of extension of suppuration from the sinus mucosa to adjoining structures. Note the depth at which brain abscess develops because of the venous anatomy of the cerebral cortex.

fixation of the extra-ocular muscles, chemosis of the bulbar conjunctiva and proptosis signal the invasion of the orbit deep to the periorbita.

Treatment. *Drainage* of the involved area by inner canthus incision and *elevation of the periorbita* from the lamina of the ethmoid bone are necessary.

RETROBULBAR NEURITIS

Retrobulbar neuritis is no longer considered a disease resulting from extension from infected paranasal sinuses. It must be mentioned to be depreciated. In the search for a cause for retrobulbar neuritis, it is apparent that there is no justification for exploration of an ethmoid abyrinth which does not show advanced changes of chronic suppuration.

BRAIN ABSCESS

Once the venous system is infected in the mucoperiosteum of a sinus, it is conceivable that hematogenous metastatic extension may occur anywhere in the brain. However, brain abscess usually develops by directly extending thrombophlebitis. Hence, the usual site of formation is at the termination of the involved perforating veins which extend through the dura and arachnoid mesh to the juncture between the gray and white substance of the cerebral cortex (Fig. 94). It is at this point that the terminals of the venous drainage to the surface of the brain approximate the terminals draining centrally into the cerebral veins.

The contamination of the brain substance may occur at the peak of a severe suppurative sinusitis and the process of brain abscess formation may continue as the sinus involvement progresses satisfactorily through the stages of normal resolution. The possibility of encephalitis, therefore, must be considered in all cases of severe acute suppurative frontal, ethmoidal, or sphenoidal sinusitis attended in the acute phase by the sharp rise in temperature and chill characteristic of intravenous infection. A case of this type must be observed in subsequent months. Lack of appetite, loss in weight, moderate cachexia, low grade afternoon fever, recurring headache and occasional unexplained nausea and vomiting may be the only sign of an encephalitis which is localizing in cerebral abscess and extending into new cortical areas. A neurosurgeon should have the opportunity of following the course from its inception.

FRONTAL OSTEOMYELITIS

The anterior temporal and the frontal diploic veins are the principal channels in the wide-open mesh of the diploic venous system of the frontal bone. Innumerable small vessels perforate the cortical plates to the external periosteum and to the internal periosteum (dura). Within the frontal bone there is no natural barrier to limit the process of extending thrombophlebitis once it enters the diploic venous system.

Symptoms. Localized pain and tenderness are extreme. Systemic fever and chill are usual. External frontal edema and abscess may be presumed to be paralleled by epidural edema and abscess and to presage further intracranial extension (Fig. 95).

Treatment. Coincident with the appearance of external edema, the extending process may be halted by a small trephine opening through the thin bony plate of the floor of the frontal sinus (Fig. 87). Surgical drainage through the diploic anterior wall will encourage further extension and should never be considered. Free ingress of air through the trephine immediately creates an atmosphere unfavorable to the further growth of the micro-aerophilic infecting organism.

When indicated by the disease process, early and radical *removal of all infected frontal bone*, allowing a margin of healthy bone, may interrupt the continuing process of venous extension before intracranial contamination has occurred. In deciding the need for and extent of bone removal, x-ray examination is a relatively valueless procedure since one is combating primarily an infection of the venous system and only secondarily a resultant and lagging bony involvement.

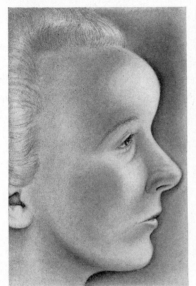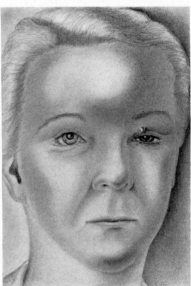

Fig. 95. External manifestation of osteomyelitis of the frontal bone. At this stage it may be presumed that extensive infection of the internal periosteal (dural) veins as well as deeper veins is present. Drainage at the inner canthus cannot check this already extensive venous involvement. Wide removal of the involved diploic bone is indicated.

MENINGITIS

Thrombophlebitis extending directly from the mucoperiosteum of the frontal, ethmoidal, or sphenoidal sinus or from the infected diploic venous system of the frontal bone may open into the epidural, subdural, or subarachnoid spaces.

Symptoms. External periosteal edema is convincing clinical evidence that the meninges have also been approached by the extending infection. To the preceding sharp febrile reaction and chill will be added evidences of meningeal irritation with generalized headache, nuchal rigidity and increased spinal fluid pressure and cell count. Epidural and subdural involvement may be attended by a state of meningismus closely simulating the true leptomeningitis of subarachnoid involvement in which organisms can be found in the spinal fluid by direct smear of the centrifuged specimen or by culture.

Treatment. *Chemotherapeutic* and *antibiotic drugs* given systemically and intraspinally and combined with supportive measures have improved the prognosis in meningitis immeasurably. *Surgical drainage* of the involved sinus or *removal of the osteomyelitic bone* may be necessary to prevent additional venous involvement and extension.

CAVERNOUS SINUS THROMBOSIS

It is anatomically possible that a thrombophlebitis developing in the mucoperiosteal lining of any sinus can by extension reach the large venous sinuses of the dura and from thence the cavernous sinus.

Symptoms. This process is attended by signs of sepsis with sharp rise in temperature, chill and laboratory evidence of bacteremia. Bulbar chemosis and bilateral proptosis develop rapidly and to a remarkable degree, owing to venous obstruction. The patient is very ill and the usual termination is death.

Treatment. The use of *heparin* to retard thrombus formation during aggressive antibiotic and chemotherapy has resulted in some recoveries.

LOWER RESPIRATORY COMPLICATIONS

Upper respiratory infections can extend to the lower respiratory tract by airborne contaminated droplets during inspiration. There are no lymphatic or venous channels to carry the invading organism from the upper respiratory tract to the lower. Infected secretions which are swept by ciliary action from the paranasal sinuses and nasal spaces into the pharynx do not contaminate the lower respiratory tract by direct surface extension. The seemingly important influence of gravity in this connection is fallacious. The alert laryngeal cough reflex and the powerful upward ciliary streaming from the tracheobronchial tree into the hypopharynx completely precludes extension by gravity.

Airborne droplet extension probably occurs commonly in the acute and subacute phase of upper respiratory infection. It is of doubtful importance in the production of lower respiratory infection from chronic suppurative sinusitis. The viscosity of the mucopurulent secretions tends to hold them to the mucous membrane surface. The systemic resistance engendered in the host by the local chronic suppurative process in the sinus mucosa helps further to protect against pulmonary extension.

Symptoms. Chronic productive cough and chronic postnasal discharge are symptoms commonly associated in respiratory allergy. The nasal phenomena of edema and hypersecretion are frequently misinterpreted as chronic suppurative sinusitis. The cough of allergic bronchitis does not result from postnasal drainage. The nasal mucosal and bronchial mucosal changes have no cause and effect relationship upon each other. They are the parallel result of respiratory allergic involvement. There is submucosal edema, goblet cell degeneration of the surface epithelium and, of most importance, there is loss of cilia over large areas. The latter completely disorganizes normal drainage, either nasal, bronchial, or both. This physiologic obstruction may be virtually complete despite a patent sinus ostium or bronchial lumen. It cannot be corrected by local treatment. When secondary infection is superimposed, the stage is set for persistent suppuration in the sinuses and bronchi. Chronicity is due to the nature of allergic change. Therapy as for a primary infection is unsatisfactory. Recurrent exacerbations both nasal and pulmonary are the rule.

It is the physiologic block of this fundamental allergic change which sets the stage for most multilobar bronchiectasis. Therapy misdirected to concomitant sinusitis can have no primary influence on the bronchial change. Secondary infection in the paranasal spaces does not by drainage affect the bronchi, though secondary bronchial infection is recurrently projected into the postnasal space by cough and can recurrently infect the nose and sinuses.

Recognition of basic allergic change is important in treatment of chronic respiratory disease. Ignorance of it lends to infection a primary importance which is frequently not justified.

FOCAL INFECTION

The Mechanism of Distant Involvement. The infectious process of sinusitis can conceivably involve distant tissues in the body in only one of two manners: by metastatic extension, or by sensitization of distant tissues to exotoxins produced locally in the infected sinus mucosa.

Metastatic Extension. Metastatic extension of infection necessarily involves a transient bacteremia. It is uncommon. It occurs in extremely virulent inflammatory involvement of the sinuses in which the resistance of the host is low and permits true bacteremia to occur with all of its attendant systemic symptoms, with high fever, chill and positive blood culture if taken at the time of blood stream invasion. It is obviously true that bacteremia can result in focal lodgment in any tissue. There is particular predilection for the highly vascular beds of the kidneys and lungs, and for the end vessels of brain and synovial membrane and endocardium. Localization in these tissues produces more striking clinical symptoms than would occur in gross tissue like muscle where inflammation would not interfere with vital function.

Exotoxins. The usual hypothesis of focal infection does not imply true bacteremia and metastatic extension. It states that tissue changes distantly are the result of sensitization of the tissues to an exotoxin produced in the infected sinus mucosa and absorbed into the general

circulation. This theory circumvents many of the rational objections to
the entire focal theory. However, distant symptoms frequently have a
chronicity and recurrent nature which do not correlate well with manifestations of infection in the sinus mucosa. Actually, many of the
diseases which in the past several decades have been regarded as focal
diseases have since been removed from this general classification of
medical ignorance and have been given their proper interpretation as
disorders resulting from chronic circulatory change unrelated to infection of any sort. It is for this reason that disease still thought of as
focal in origin must be examined extremely critically.

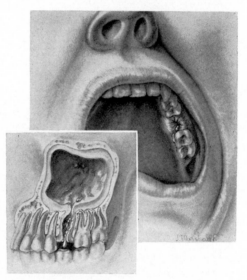

Fig. 96. Oro-antral fistula and chronic suppurative maxillary sinusitis. Infection
in the maxillary sinus must be resolved before closure of the fistula is feasible. Note
the high position of the maxillary ostium.

ORO-ANTRAL FISTULA

Anatomically, the last four upper teeth on each side are in intimate
contact with the floor of the maxillary sinus. The sinus cavity is normally
separated from the apices of these teeth by a thin layer of bone. This is
particularly thin and sometimes absent over the first molar tooth.
Dental cyst formation or apical abscess involving one or more of these
molar and second premolar teeth may open beneath the mucoperiosteum
of the sinus cavity. Furthermore, extraction of a molar or second premolar tooth may remove the intervening thin bony plate (Fig. 96).

When communication is established between the oral cavity and the
maxillary sinus through a tooth space, a severe suppurative maxillary
sinusitis may result. It tends to persist as long as the communication
remains patent, and may persist after it spontaneously closes. It is

characteristically a foul suppuration due to a mixed infection including spirilliform and fusiform organisms.

The communication or dental fistula through the alveolar process impairs the healing of the maxillary sinusitis, and the suppurative sinus involvement usually encourages persistence of the fistula. Extension of the suppurative process to the ethmoidal and frontal sinuses is not uncommon.

Treatment. Early care with parenteral administration of *penicillin* and insufflation of a combined *sulfonamide* and *penicillin powder* into the sinus cavity through the fistula can control the infection and permit the normal healing process to close the fistula.

Involvement of the sinus mucosa in the advanced chronic stage may still be amenable to similar care through the fistulous opening or intra-nasally through the natural ostium of the maxillary sinus.

Where sequestration in the floor of the sinus or advanced granulo-matous change in the mucosa exists, the sinus is best entered through the canine fossa and the focal areas removed under direct vision.

At the same time or at a later procedure, as judgment dictates, the fistulous opening in the alveolus may be closed by a pedicled flap carried across it from the palatal mucosa or from the mucosa of the buccal gutter.

REFERENCES

Anderson, F. M.: Subdural Empyema Secondary to Frontal Sinusitis. Ann. Otol., Rhin. & Laryng., *56*:5, 1947.

Brunner, H.: Chronic Osteomyelitis of the Skull. Ann. Otol., Rhin. & Laryng., *52*:850, 1943.

Brown, L.: Osteomyelitis of the Frontal Bone. Arch. Otolaryng., *39*:485, 1944.

Bucy, P. C., and Haberfield, W. T.: Cranial and Intracranial Complications of Acute Frontal Sinusitis. J.A.M.A., *115*:983, 1940.

Davis, E. D. D., Mygind, S. H., Howells, G. H., and Capps, F. C. W.: Orbital Cellulitis Due to Sinus Infection and Its Treatment. J. Laryng. & Otol., *52*:834, 1937.

Davison, F.: Does Chronic Sinusitis Cause Bronchiectasis? Ann. Otol., Rhin. & Laryng., *53*:849, 1944.

Furstenberg, A. C.: Osteomyelitis of the Skull: The Osteogenetic Processes in the Repair of Cranial Defects. Ann. Otol., Rhin. & Laryng., *40*:996, 1931.

Hubert, L.: Orbital Infections Due to Nasal Sinusitis. New York State J. Med. *37*:1559, 1937.

Lillie, H. I.: Osteomyelitis of Maxilla Secondary to Suppurative Maxillary Sinusitis. Ann. Otol., Rhin. & Laryng., *55*:495, 1946.

McQuiston, R.: Maxillary Sinusitis of Dental Origin and Management of Antral Fistula. Ann. Otol., Rhin. & Laryng., *54*:373, 1945.

Maxwell, J.: Chronic Proliferative Osteomyelitis of Skull. Ann. Otol., Rhin. & Laryng., *55*:719, 1946.

Mellinger, W. J.: The Venous Circulation as a Factor in Osteomyelitis of the Skull. Ann. Otol., Rhin. & Laryng., *49*:438, 1940.

Mosher, H. P.: Osteomyelitis of the Frontal Bone. J.A.M.A., *115*:1179, 1940.

Mosher, H. P., and Judd, K. D.: An Analysis of Seven Cases of Osteomyelitis of the Frontal Bone Complicating Frontal Sinusitis. Laryngoscope, *43*:153, 1933.

Pate, W., and Courville, C. B.: Intracranial Complications of Infections of the Nasal Air Passages and Accessory Sinuses. Bull. Los Angeles Neurol. Soc., *10:*114, 1945.

Ray, B. S., and Parson, H.: Subdural Abscess Complicating Frontal Sinusitis. Arch. Otolaryng., *37:*536, 1943.

Skillern, S. R.: Osteomyelitic Invasion of the Frontal Bone Following Frontal Sinus Disease. Ann. Otol., Rhin. & Laryng., *48:*392, 1939.

Schultz, E. C.: Subdural Empyema of Frontal Sinus Origin. Ann. Otol., Rhin. & Laryng., *55:*882, 1946.

Williams, H. L.: Acute Infections of the Upper Respiratory Tract. Journal Lancet, *60:*95, 1940.

Woodward, F. D.: Osteomyelitis of the Skull: Report of Cases Occurring as a Result of Frontal Sinus Infection with Staphylococcus Pyogenes Aureus. J.A.M.A., *95:*927, 1930.

CHAPTER XVIII

HEADACHE AND NEURALGIA OF NASAL ORIGIN

The nasal space and in particular the accessory sinuses are often blamed for chronic head pain when the cause of this symptom cannot otherwise be easily explained. This fact apparently accounts for the frequency with which various surgical procedures have been performed within the nose and sinuses to relieve victims of chronic head pain. However, the rhinologist has not made all of the mistakes. Moench remarked, "The person with a headache often finds himself a medical orphan. He is fortunate indeed if the headache is transient, for otherwise he may find himself on an excursion to ophthalmologist, otolaryngologist, neurologist, dentist, psychiatrist, osteopath and chiropractor. Thereupon he is x-rayed, massaged, analyzed, fitted with glasses, relieved of his turbinates and teeth, and too often emerges with his headache intact."

Probably the reason why the rhinologist has been led astray, has been his limited knowledge of the cause and the character of the various patterns of headache, and the ease with which that which looks like significant disease is found within the nasal space. This indicates how important it is for any physician who treats persons with headache to know something about the mechanism giving rise to this disorder and its many causes.

THE MECHANISM OF HEADACHE

In recent years considerable information on the mechanism of headache has accumulated. The research publications of the Association for Research in Nervous and Mental Disease assembled in a volume entitled "Pain," reveal some of the pain pathways and mechanism.

These studies determined that:

1. Of the tissues covering the cranium, all were more or less sensitive to pain, the arteries being especially so.

2. Of the intracranial structures, the great venous sinuses and their venous tributaries from the surface of the brain, parts of the dura at the base, the dural arteries and the cerebral arteries at the base of the brain, the fifth, ninth and tenth cranial nerves, and the upper cervical nerves were sensitive to pain.

3. The cranium (including the diploic and emissary veins), the parenchyma of the brain, most of the dura, most of the pia arachnoid, the ependymal lining of the ventricles, and the choroid plexuses were not sensitive to pain.

CAUSES OF HEADACHE

From the data available, six basic mechanisms of headache from intracranial sources have been formulated. Headache may result from:

1. Traction on the veins that pass to the venous sinuses from the surface of the brain and displacement of the great venous sinuses.

2. Traction on the middle meningeal arteries.

3. Traction on the large arteries at the base of the brain and their main branches.

4. Distention and dilatation of intracranial arteries.

5. Inflammation in or about any of the pain-sensitive structures of the head.

6. Direct pressure by tumors on the cranial and cervical nerves containing many pain-afferent fibers from the head.

Traction displacement, distention and inflammation of cranial vascular structures are chiefly responsible for headache.

Pain referred to the head from disease of tissue not in the head does not occur, with the rare exception of pain in the jaw or neck with angina pectoris. Sepsis or fever of any organ may be associated with headache, but this is not referred pain.

The inference is that the mechanism of headache as a symptom of disease outside of the head is dependent upon a vasomotor phenomenon. With this understanding, a study of headaches associated with changes in intracranial pressure, brain tumor, the presence of fever, migraine and hypertension revealed that:

The headache associated with either decreased or increased intracranial pressure results from traction upon or displacement of pain-sensitive intracranial structures and is independent of generalized intracranial pressure changes per se.

Brain tumor headache is produced by traction upon intracranial pain-sensitive structures, chiefly the large arteries, veins and venous sinuses and certain cranial nerves.

Observations of the amplitude of pulsations of the cranial arteries during headache associated with experimentally induced fever showed that the spontaneous increase and decrease of intensity of the headache paralleled the changes in amplitude of pulsations in these arteries. The observation was made that increasing the cerebrospinal fluid pressure in the subarachnoid space relieved fever headache (Pickering).

The headache of migraine seems to be due to dilatation and distention of the extracranial and possibly the dural branches of the external carotid artery.

The headache associated with hypertension arises from dilatation and distention of certain branches of the external carotid artery. It bears no direct relationship to the level of blood pressure or pulse pressure.

CLASSIFICATION OF HEADACHE

Most of the classifications of headache have been unsatisfactory because they have been too complicated. I have modified an old one of Auerbach. It is simple, rather complete and calls attention to the basic condition of which the headache is a symptom. This classification lists three main groups: the headaches from systemic disorders or general diseases; those headaches which are more or less independent of a disorder within any particular organ or dependent on any systemic disorder; and those associated with disorders localized within the head.

Headache from systemic disorders or general disease:
1. Infectious diseases.
2. Circulatory disturbances; hypertension, hypotension.
3. Abnormal blood states; anemia, alkalosis, uremia, hypoglycemia, polycythemia, etc.
4. Gastro-intestinal disorders.
5. Miscellaneous: relaxation states, caffeine withdrawal, cerebrovascular syphilis, etc.

Independent forms of headache:
1. Migraine.
2. Histamine headache.
3. Headache of emotional origin.
4. Headache from disorders in the neck.

Headache from disorder localized within the head:
1. Intracranial disease.
2. Ocular disorders.
3. Nasal space disease.

HEADACHE FROM SYSTEMIC DISORDERS OR GENERAL DISEASE

Infectious disease as a cause of headache is common during the acute phase of the disease. In the common disorder rather loosely diagnosed as the "flu" or "grippe," the headache is toxic in origin with an alteration in the brain blood volume. Often these headaches are erroneously diagnosed as "sinus" headaches, particularly if the upper respiratory tract is congested as part of the disorder.

The exact mechanism by which headache is produced in many systemic disorders is not clear, but it is believed that a disturbance in the hydrodynamic mechanism within the head plays a prominent role. This hydrodynamic alteration may be caused in part by emotional states often associated with the systemic disorder. Thus more than one factor plays an important role. Moench has provided a graphic representation (Fig. 97) which helps to visualize the mechanical effect of the alteration of blood volume on pain-sensitive structures. With the understanding of the basic mechanisms in the production of headache, it is not difficult to understand how the various disorders listed can produce this disturbance.

INDEPENDENT FORMS OF HEADACHE

Migraine Headache. Migraine, more commonly known as a "sick headache" has been defined by Grinker as a headache characterized by

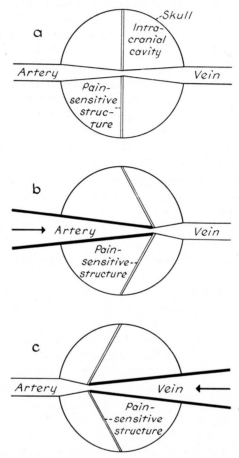

Fig. 97. (a) Normal intracranial vascular relations. (b) Distortion of pain-sensitive structures by alteration of normal arteriovenous relationship in hypertension, vasodilatation, increased blood volume or arteritis. (c) Distortion of pain-sensitive structures by increased venous pressure (increased blood volume, congestive heart failure, orthostatic hypotension). (Drawn from Moench.)

periodic paroxysms of intense pain preceded or accompanied by characteristic sensory or motor disturbances or a combination of these, with general vasomotor or psychic phenomena. The most frequent beginning site is in the neighborhood of an eye; the sensation may be either above the eye, lateral to it, or deep within it. There is a tendency for the pain to become diffused and involve the whole side of the head, or it may become generalized. The patient may describe the pain as dull, boring, pressing, throbbing, hammering, viselike, or shooting. The pain tends gradually to increase to an intense degree.

Duration. The duration of the headache is variable. It usually lasts more than a day, often for several days. Abortive attacks may last two or three hours. An attack may appear at any time of day and even awaken the patient at night.

Symptoms and Signs. The patient may have a foreboding—an aura of impending headache; this is really part of the attack.

Gastro-intestinal symptoms usually present are nausea and vomiting. Complete anorexia during the headache and abdominal pains are not infrequent, and the patient is usually constipated.

Throughout an attack, the patient often exhibits a general hypersensitiveness. He is irritable, though mentally slow, complains of photophobia and abhors noise.

Certain signs referable to the cervical sympathetic function may be noted, such as pallor and hyperidrosis of one side of the face and one pupil smaller than the other with absence of normal reaction.

There may also be evidence of general sympathetic dysfunction, such as bradycardia, generalized perspiration, urinary frequency and pyrexia in children.

Cause. The cause of migraine is unknown. Among the theories advanced are that it is a reflex phenomenon, a toxic metabolic disorder, that it results from mechanical obstructions to the central ventricular system, or that it is a vasomotor disturbance. The last mentioned theory seems to have the most support. Vaughan has reported a high percentage of cases in which an allergenic factor was the cause. There is doubt, however, that allergenic substances such as foreign proteins etc., are ever the cause of the classical migraine with its periodic attacks.

A variety of conditions seems to have a role in precipitating attacks, such as mental and emotional excitement, fatigue, dietary indiscretions and in women, the menstrual relationship.

There seems to be a hereditary factor, over 50 per cent of the patients giving a history indicating a direct homologous heredity.

Incidence. The incidence of migraine is difficult to estimate. Puberty is the most frequent time of onset. Relatively few people develop migraine after 40 years of age. The condition is more than twice as common in females as in males.

The patient is symptomless between attacks. The course is lengthy and may continue in the same form for years, although the character of the attack may change. The frequency and severity of an attack may be altered in either direction. Natural menopause may be accompanied by a cessation of the attacks.

Treatment. The treatment consists of avoiding the factors which seem to precipitate attacks. The most effective medication is *ergotamine tartrate* (gynergen). This comes in 1 cc. ampules. From ½ to 1 ampule (0.25 to 0.5 gm.) is given hypodermically (intramuscularly) and repeated once if symptoms are not abated or if they return.

Ophthalmic Form. A localized form of migraine referred to as the ophthalmic form occurs in which the prodromata and early symptoms are referable to the visual system. Scotomas and homonymous hemianopsia characterize this form. A rare ophthalmoplegic migraine has been described in which the function of the oculomotor nerve is impaired.

Histamine Headache. A new clinical picture representing more or less of an entity in headache has been described in recent years. First this was given the name of "erythromelalgia of the head," then "histaminic cephalgia" and is now referred to as "histamine headache." These terms were supplied by Horton and his investigators. Williams has referred to the picture as a "vasodilating head pain."

In the typical picture of a histamine headache, the following characteristics are noted:

1. The occurrence is usually in later age decades.

2. The attack is hemicranial and of short duration (under one hour) and tends to occur at night and awaken the patient from sleep.

3. Pain is confined to the distribution of the external carotid artery and tenderness is felt along the branches of the temporal artery.

4. The pain may be excruciating, constant, boring, and involves the eye, the temple, neck and face.

5. The skin over the involved area may become reddened with increased surface temperature and swelling of the temporal vessels.

6. There is tearing and conjunctival injection on the involved side, associated with rhinorrhea and nasal stuffiness.

7. The headache can be reproduced by injecting 0.1 to 1.2 mg. of histamine subcutaneously or intravenously.

Treatment. Temporary relief can often be obtained by *compressing the carotid artery* with the patient in an erect posture. An intravenous injection of 0.1 cc. of 1:100,000 *epinephrine* if there are no contraindications, may afford relief. *Desensitization to histamine* is more effective treatment. One method advocated is to give *histamine diphosphate* subcutaneously twice daily and increase from an initial dose of 0.01 to 0.05 mg. according to the patient's tolerance up to 0.4 mg. This is continued for one month and then the frequency of the dose is gradually decreased. Others recommend smaller initial doses.

Headaches of Emotional Origin. The incidence of headache in emotional states particularly in the pathologic type of person is apparently very great. Stresses of all types, often a combination of worry, fatigue and excitement, contribute to a physiological disturbance which initiates the headache. This type in many instances could rightly be classed under systemic disorders.

In the majority of cases of this form of headache, there is no actual pain, but an oppression, constriction, or heaviness of the head; or the patient may complain of a sensation of pulling or drawing in the occipital region. The sensations are often complained of as situated in or behind the forehead and extending down into the eyes and the root of the nose. Less frequently, the temples are involved. The sensation may also be likened to an elastic band encircling the head. Sometimes the patient

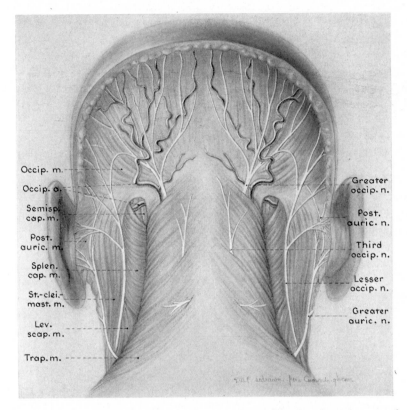

Fig. 98. The superficial structures in the posterior neck and occiput that may be involved in headache or neuralgia originating in this area.

refers to a sensation of the head feeling hollow or empty. Some describe paresthesia of the temples and forehead. Occasionally, the pain may assume a neuralgic character. This form of headache has no periodicity. It tends to be more or less constant. Many patients have vague general complaints which, in their analysis and from the fact that a physical study of the person shows no sign of disease, suggest hypochondria.

A diagnosis is made primarily on a careful history and the absence of physical findings suggesting an organic cause.

Headache from Disorders in the Neck. A number of causes for headache and neuralgia have been found in the posterior part of the neck (Fig. 98). Auerbach described what he believed to be a clinical entity under the title of nodular or induration headache. Small palpable, tender, nodular, or indurated areas occurred in the occipital muscles or fascia of the neck. These caused an occipital ache which remained localized or spread up over the temples. Exposure to cold and chilling precipitated the pain. The nodular or indurated area consisted of a localized muscle spasm causing irritation of sensory nerve endings in the area involved. Treatment with local application of heat, the use of antineuralgics, and supplementary massage invariably brought relief.

Occipital headache originating in the posterior part of the neck has been described as due to myalgia, fibrositis, hypertonic neck muscles and arthritis of the cervical spine. There is a marked similarity in the cause, age group, manifestations and treatment.

The chief precipitating factor seems to be exposure to the cold. The symptoms are aggravated by fatigue and tight-fitting apparel such as a hat, cap, or collar. The discomfort is usually unilateral and consists of a dull but definite ache which is aggravated by movements of the head and neck. When sought for, tender spots may be found on careful palpation over the superior nuchal line, the trapezius, the splenius and scalenus muscles, or the sternocleidomastoid and its fibrous attachment to the mastoid tip. If areas of myositis or localized muscle spasm exist, these will be definitely palpable as thickening or nodules. The fibrositic areas may be palpable, but in an arthritis of the cervical spine, objective evidence is usually lacking except by x-ray examination.

Treatment. The treatment has in part been referred to in the use of *heat, antineuralgics* and *massage.* Obviously, massage would not be expected to aid a cervical arthritis. The search for and *eradication of toxic foci, avoidance of chilling and fatigue,* and the *administration of foreign proteins* are recommended.

These conditions are uncommon in children and are usually found in the middle age group.

Williams believes that headache localized in the muscles of the posterior part of the neck and elsewhere about the head may be a myalgia which is an expression of physical allergy due to a local release of histamine. He has found that treatment with *nicotinic acid* (100 mg. daily) gives more uniform results than desensitization with histamine.

HEADACHE FROM DISORDERS LOCALIZED WITHIN THE HEAD

Intracranial Disease. The victim of chronic headache usually suspects a disorder localized within the head and the physician should always have in mind the possibility of intracranial disease as a source of head pain which becomes a chronic problem. The possibilities are numerous and the cause may be found among the following:

1. Vascular conditions: arteriosclerosis, hemorrhage, thrombosis, emboli, aneurysms, syphilitic arteritis.

2. Inflammations: encephalitis from a virus such as is found in the epidemic form, from mumps, influenza, etc.; meningeal inflammations from bacteria, viruses, or parasites, abscesses which usually originate from middle ear and mastoid disease, frontal sinusitis, or may be embolic.

3. Tumors: primary or metastatic.

4. Head injury.

Ocular Disease. Headache from ocular disturbance is due to one or more of four conditions: refractive errors, muscular imbalance, intra-ocular inflammation and pathological tension. Invariably attention is directed to the eyes by a history of the discomfort coming on after use of the eyes in the acts of accommodation, or the fact that the discomfort is actually within the eye. Usually this discomfort is not a unilateral one except in cases of localized disease as in an inflammatory process or in a pathological tension of one eye. The headache from refractive error is usually frontal; that from muscle imbalance may be occipital.

Nasal Space Disease. This source of headache from a disorder localized within the head is discussed in detail in the concluding paragraphs of this chapter.

FACIAL NEURALGIAS

Any discussion of head pain if it is to be complete must include a consideration of the facial neuralgias.

The facial neuralgias are not encountered in clinical practice as commonly as is some form of headache. Many of the classifications of facial neuralgia are complicated. I have found it useful to list these neuralgias in six groups:

1. Trigeminal neuralgia, primary and secondary.
2. Glossopharyngeal neuralgia, primary and secondary.
3. Vidian and sphenopalatine neuralgia.
4. Neuralgia from disturbances of the temporomandibular joint.
5. Atypical facial neuralgias.
6. Some rare affections such as:
   (a) Geniculate ganglion neuralgia.
   (b) Tympanic plexus neuralgia.
   (c) Great superficial petrosal neuralgia.

TRIGEMINAL NEURALGIA

The diagnosis of primary trigeminal neuralgia (tic douloureux) is never difficult to make because of its character. The pain is one of sudden onset, is sharp, lancinating and knife-like, brought on from trigger zones about the face which react to light contacts or draughts of air. It usually occurs in persons beyond middle age and is confined mainly to the ophthalmic and maxillary divisions. Attacks may occur every few seconds with intervals of freedom, and periods of repeated attacks may last from a few days to a few weeks. Remissions of months to years occur. The disease is always unilateral. The cause is unknown.

In the secondary type, the pain as a rule is of a more chronic type and the attacks are longer and less severe. Trigger zones are rare. The cause is found in some lesion irritating one of the nerve roots. Dental and nasal disease are the more common factors.

GLOSSOPHARYNGEAL NEURALGIA

Primary glossopharyngeal neuralgia, a tic douloureux of this nerve is relatively rare. The paroxysms of stabbing pain in the ear with trigger zones in the tonsillar area of the involved side accompanied by salivation provide a picture in which the disgnosis is not difficult. A secondary form is common. This picture is seen in the earache following tonsillectomy in the absence of evidence of middle ear disease. It can be caused by any inflammatory process involving the tonsillar area and the adjacent area of the tongue. One must not forget, however, that pain in the ear in the absence of middle ear disease is produced by lesions involving the trigeminal nerve (teeth and temporomandibular joint) and the vagus nerve (a lesion in the pharynx, on the rim of the larynx, or in cervical glands).

VIDIAN AND SPHENOPALATINE GANGLION NEURALGIA

The vidian nerve, which is the posterior root of the sphenopalatine ganglion, or the ganglion itself is occasionally found to be involved in neuralgic pain on one side of the face. This pain may have a sudden onset, is severe, localized around or back of the eyeball, radiates to the temple, back of the ear to the occiput and down into the neck and even into the shoulder. This description was made by Vail who believed it represented an irritation of the vidian nerve in its course below the floor of the sphenoid sinus. The picture for the most part fits the previously described sphenopalatine ganglion neuralgia of Sluder. The latter described two syndromes from involvement of the ganglion. One was neuralgic and the other "sympathetic," in which the painful picture is supplemented by vasomotor and secretory phenomena.

Since the passing of Sluder and of Vail we have heard relatively little about these conditions. Many neurologists have seemed unwilling to accept Sluder's explanation of these pictures which are occasionally encountered. With the newer knowledge regarding vasomotor disturbances, it seems likely that this explanation rather than one of sinus inflammatory change may account for some of the painful and probably all of the vasomotor phenomena. Williams explains the picture of sphenopalatine neuralgia, particularly the sympathetic syndrome, on the basis of a physical allergy. There are no doubt cases of vidian neuralgia caused by an irritation of the vidian nerve in the floor of the sphenoid sinus. Introducing cocaine into the sphenoid sinus will control

the pain and clinch the diagnosis. Also there are instances of suspected
sphenopalatine neuralgia in which cocaine placed over the site of the
sphenopalatine foramen relieves pain, indicative of neuralgic disturbance
of the adjacent nerve structures.

In some instances in which the sympathetic phenomena are prominent,
strong silver nitrate used as irritant or caustic in the area of the sphenopalatine foramen wi'l relieve the nasal symptoms. It seems probable,
therefore, that vidian or sphenopalatine neuralgia is produced from
inflammatory changes within a sinus but that much of that which has
been called sphenopalatine neuralgia was a vasomotor phenomenon
and could fit into the picture of physical allergy described by Williams.

NEURALGIA FROM DISTURBANCE IN THE TEMPOROMANDIBULAR JOINT

Neuralgia from disturbance in the temporomandibular joint may
result from a change in the bite, most often caused by a loss of molar
support. Costen has reported numerous cases. In my experience, the
neuralgia is usually located in front of the ear of the involved side.
Costen has described headache from this disturbance as vertex, occipital,
or supra-orbital in location.

ATYPICAL NEURALGIAS

The atypical facial neuralgias comprise a group of ill defined heag
pains, which have been described as deep-seated pains of an achind,
burning, or throbbing type which often cannot be accurately described
by the patient. The distribution of the pain is within a circular area
within the vascular supply of the head. Sympathetic phenomena, such
as lacrimation, edema, corneal injection, unequal pupils, blurred vision
and photophobia, are present in about half of the cases. The writings on
this subject suggest many possible causative factors. A diagnosis of
atypical neuralgia is apparently made when the disorder does not fit
to a considerable degree one of the well defined neuralgias. Many of these
could be vasomotor disturbances on the basis of a physical allergy.

RARE NEURALGIAS

A geniculate ganglion affection is diagnosed by finding the zoster
zones involving the external canal and often the concha. Tympanic
plexus neuralgia is a rare type of partial tic involving the tympanic
branch of the glossopharyngeal nerve (Reichert). Great superficial
petrosal neuralgia is the pain accompanying some cases of petrositis.
It is retro-ocular in location on the involved side.

THE NASAL SPACE AS A SOURCE OF HEADACHE OR NEURALGIA

The layman and many physicians are prone to attribute the symptoms
of headache and often of neuralgia to the sinuses when some obvious

cause is lacking. The widely prevalent symptoms of transient nasal congestion and the common postnasal discharge have centered attention on the nose. More objectively, the irregularities of the nasal septum and x-ray evidence of sinus disease have suggested the possibilities of this apparent close anatomical relationship.

It is probable that our mistakes in evaluating the role of the nasal space in the symptom of head pain, particularly a chronic pain, are due, first to an inadequate history, and, second, to a lack of information on the problem of headache and neuralgia in general.

INTERPRETATION OF THE LOCAL FINDINGS IN THE NASAL SPACE

If one had to make a diagnosis as to the cause of a case of headache in which a nasal origin was suspected, and either the history or the local findings were available, the history would certainly be found to be the more valuable. Every observing clinician sees frequent cases of marked irregularity of the nasal septum, hypertrophied turbinates, and x-ray shadows indicating extensive changes within the sinus linings, but in which the patients' complaints do not include headache as a symptom. In numerous cases of chronic bilateral suppurative pansinusitis with polyps, I have made a point of questioning the patient in regard to the symptom of headache. More often than not the patient will remark that headache is not one of his problems. But, in contrast, instances of contact or congestive headache are frequently encountered in which the nasal interior showed only a very moderate abnormality but in which prompt relief of the discomfort was obtained by simple shrinkage with ephedrine or some similarly acting substance, or by cocainization of the contact.

Because of the unreliability of attempting to correlate the findings in the nasal space with the symptom of headache, accurate diagnosis in many cases must rest on certain tests, which often are a form of treatment and thus may be termed therapeutic tests.

Therapeutic Tests. It is generally accepted that in acute rhinitis and sinusitis with suppuration, the most important item of treatment is the matter of adequate *drainage* of any accumulation of pus and ventilation of the sinus involved. If pain is present, the usual experience is that when drainage is established the pain promptly subsides and disappears. This supports the idea that the actual cause for pain in the majority of cases is the factor of tension. In chronic suppurative sinusitis, pain is usually present only at times of acute exacerbation when drainage is blocked. The therapeutic tests, then, on which the otolaryngologist can rely, are (1) simple *shrinkage* or *cocainization* in cases of congestive or contact headaches and (2) the effect of *drainage* and *ventilation* in cases of suppuration within any of the several sinuses.

In cases of suspected vidian neuralgia, the instillation of cocaine (4 per cent) into the sphenoidal sinus will relieve the pain; cocainization of the area over the sphenopalatine ganglion will relieve a neuralgia of that nerve structure.

It has been my experience that when these tests are applied when the pain is present in cases of headache or neuralgia of a chronic type, the tests are reliable in establishing whether or not the nasal space is a causative factor in the pain.

REFERENCES

Alvarez, W.: Migraine. M. Clin. North America, 24:1171, 1940.

Auerbach, S.: Headache. London, Oxford University Press, 1913.

Boies, L. R.: The Symptom of Headache. Journal Lancet, 64:400, 1944.

Brenner, C., et al: Post-traumatic Headache. J. Neurosurg., 1:379, 1944.

Brickner, R., and Riley, H.: Autonomic Facio-cephalgia. Bull. Neurol. Inst. New York, 4:422, 1935.

Costen, J. B.: A Syndrome of Ear and Sinus Symptoms Dependent on Disturbed Function of the Temporomandibular Joint. Ann. Otol., Rhin. & Laryng., 43:1, 1943.

Dandy, W. E.: Glossopharyngeal Neuralgia (Tic Douloreux). Arch. Surg., 15:198, 1927.

Dreisbach, R., and Pfeiffer, C.: Caffeine-Withdrawal Headache. J. Lab. & Clin. Med., 28:1212, 1943.

Eckardt, L., McLean, J., and Goodell, H.: Experimental Studies on Headache: The Genesis of Pain from the Eye. Research Nerv. & Ment. Dis. Proc., 23:209, 1943.

Fay, T.: Atypical Facial Neuralgia: A Syndrome of Vascular Pain. Ann. Otol., Rhin. & Laryng., 41:1030, 1932.

Glaser, M. A.: Atypical Facial Neuralgia; Diagnosis, Cause and Treatment. Arch. Int. Med., 65:340, 1940.

Gray, P., and Burtness, H.: Hypoglycemic Headache. Endocrinology, 19:549, 1935.

Grinker, R. G.: Neurology. Springfield, Ill., Charles C Thomas, 1943.

Hartsock, C.: Headache from Arthritis of the Cervical Spine. M. Clin. North America, 24:329, 1940.

Hartsock, C.: Headache of Gastrointestinal Origin. Ibid., 24:341, 1940.

Hartsock, C., and McGurl, F.: Allergy as a Factor in Headache. Ibid., 22:325, 1938.

Horton, B. T.: Use of Histamine in the Treatment of Specific Types of Headaches. Collect. Papers Mayo Clin. & Mayo Found., 32:1028, 1940; and J.A.M.A., 116:377, 1941.

Horton, B. T., McLean, A. R., and Craig, N. W.: A New Syndrome of Vascular Headache. Proc. Staff Meet., Mayo Clin., 14:257, 1939.

Hunt, J. R.: Geniculate Neuralgia. Arch. Neurol. & Psychiat., 37:253, 1937.

Kamman, G.: Some Painful Conditions about the Head and Face. Journal Lancet, 60:111, 1940.

McAuliffe, G., Goodell, H., and Wolff, H.: Experimental Studies on Headache: Pain from the Nasal and Paranasal Structures. A. Research Nerv. & Mental Dis. Proc., 23:185, 1943.

McDonald, R.: Headache of Renal Origin. M. Clin. North America, 24:365, 1940.

McLaurin, J. G.: Headache of Otorhinologic Origin and Certain Reflexes caused by Fifth Nerve Irritation. Ann. Otol., Rhin. & Laryng., 50:469, 1941.

Mithoefer, W.: Hypertonic Neck Muscles as a Cause of Headache. Ibid., 43:67, 1934.

Moench, L. G.: Headache. Chicago, Year Book Publishers, Inc., 1947.

Moore, P. M., Jr.: Headaches of Nasal Origin. M. Clin. North America, 24:311, 1940.

O'Sullivan, M. E.: Termination of 1000 Attacks of Migraine with Ergotamine Tartrate. J.A.M.A., *107*:1208, 1936.

Penfield, W., and Norcross, N.: Subdural Traction and Post-traumatic Headache: A Study of Pathology and Therapeusis. Arch. Neurol. & Psychiat., *36*:75, 1936.

Pfeiffer, C., et al.: Etiology of Migraine Syndrome: The Physiologic Approach. J. Lab. & Clin. Med., *28*:1219, 1943.

Pickering, G. W., and Hess, W.: Observations on the Mechanism of Headache Produced by Histamine. Clin. Sc., *1*:77, 1933.

Profant, H.: Temporal Arteritis. Ann. Otol., Rhin. & Laryng., *53*:308, 1944.

Ray, B., and Wolff, H.: Experimental Studies on Headache: Pain-sensitive Structures of the Head and Their Significance in Headache. Arch. Surg., *41*:813, 1940.

Reichert, F.: Compression of the Brachial Plexus: The Scalenus Anticus Syndrome. J.A.M.A., *118*:294, 1942.

Seydell, E.: Indurative or Myalgic Headache. Arch. Otolaryng., *32*:860, 1940.

Schumacher, G., and Wolff, H.: Experimental Studies on Headache: A Contrast of Histamine Headache with Headache of Migraine and that Associated with Hypertension; A Contrast of Vascular Mechanisms in Pre-headache and in Headache Phenomena of Migraine. Arch. Neurol. & Psychiat., *45*:199, 1941.

Sluder, G.: Headaches and Eye Disorders of Nasal Origin. St. Louis, C. V. Mosby Co., 1920.

Spriggs, E.: A Clinical Study of Headaches (Croonian Lecture). Lancet, *2*:1, 1935.

von Storch, T.: The Migraine Syndrome. M. Clin. North America, *22*:689, 1938.

Studies on Headache: The Mechanisms and Significance of the Headache Associated with Brain Tumor. Bull. New York Acad. Med., *18*:400, 1942.

Sutherland, A., and Wolff, H.: Experimental Studies on Headache. A Further Analysis of the Mechanism of Headache in Migraine, Hypertension and Fever. Arch. Neurol. & Psychiat., *44*:929, 1940.

Thomas, J., and Johnston, C.: Headaches of Allergic Origin. M. Clin. North America, *24*:285, 1940.

Tucker, J.: Headache in Cardiovascular Disease. *Ibid.*, *24*:321, 1940.

Vail, H. H.: Vidian Neuralgia from Disease of the Sphenoid Sinus. Arch. Surg., *18*:212, 1927.

Vail, H. H.: Vidian Neuralgia. Ann. Otol., Rhin. & Laryng., *41*:837, 1932.

Vaughan, W. T.: An Analysis of the Allergic Factor in Recurrent Paroxysmal Headaches. J. Allergy, *6*:365, 1935.

Williams, H. L.: Intrinsic Allergy as it Affects the Ear, Nose and Throat: The Intrinsic Allergy Syndrome. Tr. Am. Acad. Ophth., July–Aug., p. 379, 1944; and Ann. Otol., Rhin. & Laryng., *53*:397, 1944.

Williams, H. L.: The Syndrome of Physical or Intrinsic Allergy of the Head: Myalgia of the Head (Sinus Headache). Proc. Staff Meet., Mayo Clin., *20*:177, 1945.

Wilson, H.: Psychogenic Headache. Lancet, *1*:367, 1938.

Wolff, H. G., Gasser, H. S., and Hinsey, J. C.: Pain. Baltimore, Williams and Wilkins, 1943.

Woltman, H. W.: Headache: A Consideration of Some of the More Common Types. M. Clin. North America, *24*:1159, 1940.

CHAPTER XIX

EPISTAXIS

Conrad J. Holmberg, M.D.

Epistaxis means hemorrhage from the nose. The source of a severe nose-bleed may be obscure. Fortunately, the majority of nasal hemorrhages are not serious and are due to spontaneous rupture of minute vessels in a small area in the anterior part of the cartilaginous nasal septum. This area is commonly known as Kiesselbach's plexus. Control of bleeding from this area is usually a simple matter.

BLOOD VESSELS

The blood vessels from which expistaxis may come include the following:

1. Sphenopalatine branches of the internal maxillary artery, located high and posteriorly in the nose and running forward on the septum and laterally to the turbinate.

2. Anterior and posterior ethmoidal branches of the ophthalmic artery, supplying the roof of the nasal fossae. (The ophthalmic artery is a terminal branch of the internal carotid.)

3. Descending palatine branch of the internal maxillary artery; at its termination it passes upward through the incisive canal to anastomose with terminals of the sphenopalatine artery.

4. Septal branch of the superior labial artery, a branch of the external maxillary. (It is also called the superior coronary artery.) This vessel ascends from the upper lip into the anterior naris and onto the septum. The junction of these vessels often forms a prominent network of dilated vessels (Fig. 99). The bleeding may be arterial or venous. Some of the veins of the anterior septal region open into the sphenopalatine vein; others join the anterior facial vein or accompany the ethmoidal arteries to enter the ophthalmic veins. Usually a large dilated vein running across the floor of the nose is visible when recurrent bleeding occurs from this anterior plexus.

ETIOLOGY

The causes of nosebleed can be roughly divided into local or primary vascular conditions and general or secondary systemic conditions.

Local causes:

1. Trauma: from nose picking, a blow on the nose, the irritation of foreign bodies, instrumental, or operative injury.

2. Acute infections: acute rhinitis, inflammatory or allergic, causing local capillary or venous congestion.

3. Chronic infections or trophic changes as occur in anterior rhinitis sicca, atrophic rhinitis, membranous rhinitis, tuberculosis and syphilis, from lupus, mercurial and phosphorus poisoning, etc. A perforation of the septal cartilage usually leaves raw bleeding margins.

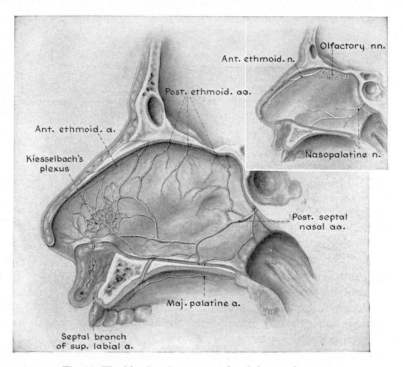

Fig. 99. The blood and nerve supply of the nasal septum.

4. Violent sneezing or blowing nose, causing capillary congestion.

5. Congestion from inhalation of irritating dusts or chemical fumes.

6. New growths in the nasal cavity, nasopharynx and sinuses.

7. A rare local cause is hereditary hemorrhagic telangiectasia (Osler's disease).

General and systemic causes:

1. Hypertension and arterial vessel changes, as in arteriosclerosis, chronic nephritis, hepatic cirrhosis, syphilis, diabetes, climacteric changes, chronic alcoholism.

2. High venous tension, as in emphysema, bronchitis, whooping cough, mitral stenosis, pneumonia, tumors of the neck, thoracic aneurysms.

3. Blood diseases: hemophilia, purpura, leukemia, some anemias, chlorosis, scurvy, malaria.

4. Cardiac conditions and rheumatic fever.

5. Early stages of some acute infectious fevers, such as typhoid fever, influenza, measles, varicella, scarlatina, typhus, erysipelas, diphtheria.

6. Vicarious menstruation.

7. High altitudes.

Nosebleed is more common in males than in females; it is rare in infancy and most frequent between early childhood and puberty. In advanced life, the disorder has a more serious import.

PATHOLOGY

In the majority of cases of nosebleed there is an erosion of a superficial vessel and nothing more than a bleeding point is visible. Certain parts of the nose are more exposed and subject to greater trauma than others. The vascularity of the mucosa varies in different regions of the nose and is greatest over the anterior septum and anterior ends of the turbinates. A curvature of the cartilaginous septum exposes the convexity to increased trauma. Repeated exposure and irritation with subsequent bleeding reduces tissue vitality, invites secondary inflammatory reactions and finally trophic changes. This results in scabbing and crusting, loss of mucosal tissue and ultimate ulceration with perforation of the cartilage. The margins of the perforation accumulate crusts which separate to leave a bleeding surface underneath.

SYMPTOMS AND DIAGNOSIS

The symptoms are usually limited to those of an outflow of blood from the anterior or posterior nares, or both. The patient may be seen with a large oozing blood clot protruding from the anterior naris, after some efforts have been made in plugging the nose to control the bleeding. The blood may all pass backward if the patient has assumed a reclining position, being largely swallowed and later appearing in vomitus or sometimes coughed up. When blood is vomited or coughed up, a source of bleeding in the lower respiratory tract and gastro-intestinal tract must, of course, be considered. Following severe loss of blood, the patient may be seen in varying degrees of shock, with lowered blood pressure, rapid pulse and other evidence of circulatory depression. In robust persons, however, the majority of cases of epistaxis are comparatively void of hazard to the general health. Under careful examination with a speculum and adequate illumination, the bleeding site can be seen in the average case after obstructing clots are removed.

Obviously, a general study of the patient is indicated in all but the very simple cases. Routine study of the blood along with special tests where indicated will reveal blood dyscrasias as an underlying cause when this factor is present.

TREATMENT

In a majority of cases, the treatment is local and self limiting; that is, it is recovered from without any special treatment or with the very simplest of maneuvers such as compressing the nares, insertion of a simple cotton plug, and so on. In cases which are not readily controlled by simple measures, the following considerations are valuable: have the patient in an erect sitting position or not lower than a semirecumbent position, and preferably with head tilted forward. This facilitates clot formation by back pressure against the bleeding vessel rather than a trickling of blood into the pharynx; sedation, in the form of morphine hypodermically, may be indicated to promote quiet and physical relaxation.

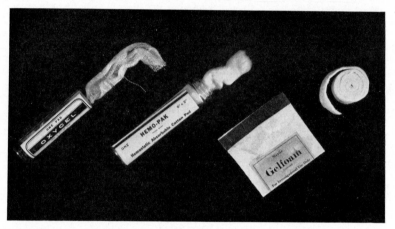

Fig. 100. Three materials in modern use for the control of nasal hemorrhage by topical packing.

The armamentarium for dealing with a persistent nosebleed should be at hand on a prepared tray. The following items are important:

1. Cotton for pledgets or packs.
2. Epinephrine (adrenalin) 1:1000 solution.
3. 10 per cent cocaine solution.
4. Gauze strip for packing.
5. Electric cautery.
6. Instruments for visualization and packing: head mirror, nasal speculum, bayonet forceps and suction tube.
7. Material for making a postnasal pack or plug: gauze squares, strong cord, string or silk, small rubber catheter.
8. An additional item of recently proven value is material used as a hemostatic agent in the form of gauze or cotton oxidized cellulose and known as "oxycel," "hemo-pak," or "gelfoam" (Fig. 100). Many persistent cases of bleeding can be controlled by *insertion of a pack* which is left

in for a day or two until the edema or thrombosis seals the bleeding point (Figs. 101, 102). In some instances when the bleeding point is seen, a red hot cautery point will seal the point permanently. Chemical cauterizing

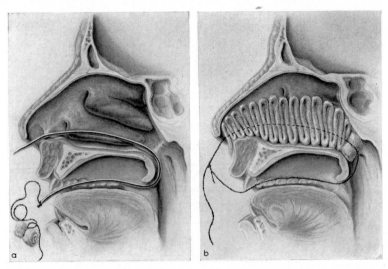

Fig. 101. Posterior choanal packing combined with an anterior nasal pack. (a) Rubber catheter directed posteriorly through the nose and drawn into the mouth; packing attached to catheter which is drawn back through the nose pulling the pack securely into the post-nasal position. (b) Post-choanae pack in position secured with one string through the nose and the other through the mouth; anterior nasal packing filling the entire nasal cavity and placed in orderly fashion against the posterior pack.

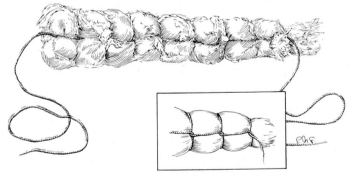

Fig. 102. The Mackenty choanal plug is made out of cotton bound with twine. It is pulled into the choana from the nasopharynx.

agents such as silver nitrate, chromic acid, and trichloracetic acid are of little value in an active case of bleeding.

When the newer oxidized cellulose packs are used, this material is usually left in position until it dissolves out in approximately four days.

Occasionally a patient is encountered with a septal deflection which exposes the venous plexus to irritation. A *submucous resection* may be needed to correct this condition.

Intramucosal injection of a sclerosing agent has been advocated to destroy a bleeding site. There is risk that this may contribute further to the trophic changes already present. General measures include the treatment of blood dyscrasias, cardiac conditions, and acute infections when these diseases are associated with epistaxis.

For severe uncontrolled arterial hemorrhage, *ligation* of the external carotid artery or the internal maxillary artery (by an antral approach) or the internal carotid artery for bleeding from the ethmoidal vessels may be necessary when all other efforts have failed.

Blood transfusions are indicated in the presence of severe blood loss.

REFERENCES

Fox, S.: Treatment of Epistaxis by Sclerosing Solutions. Laryngoscope, *54:*398, 1944.
Hollender, A. R.: Office Treatment of the Nose, Throat and Ear. Chicago, Year Book Publishers, Inc., 1943.
Houser, K.: Oxidized Cellulose Gauze Packing for Nasal Bleeding. J.A.M.A., *132:*143, 1946.

CHAPTER XX

ATROPHIC RHINITIS

CONRAD J. HOLMBERG, M.D.

A high percentage of infections involving the nasal mucosa cause hypertrophy of this structure. Not uncommonly, however, an atrophy is encountered in a condition which represents a clinical entity, atrophic rhinitis.

Atrophic rhinitis is characterized by an atrophy of the structures in the nasal fossae (Fig. 103), resulting in abnormal patency, dryness, and

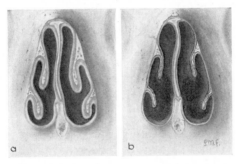

Fig. 103. The atrophied nasal fossa can be compared to a tree which has lost its leaves as compared to one in full bloom.

crusting and often accompanied by infection with organisms (*Klebsiella ozaenae* and *Bacillus foetidus*) which produce a fetid odor. The presence of this odor has resulted in the use of the term "ozena" as a name for the condition. This comes from the Greek word "ozein" meaning "to smell."

ETIOLOGY

The cause of this disease has not been definitely established; it is resistant to treatment, and thus presents one of the perplexing problems of the rhinologist. Numerous theories as to cause of the disease have been advanced; these include endocrine, metabolic, inflammatory, anatomic and constitutional derangements. Several factors have been suggested as important in the development of the disease. These are:

Heredity. The disease is more prevalent in some families, and in some races, than in others. It has been traced through several generations. The Negro race is relatively free from the disease; it is prevalent in the yellow race and common in the white race. It is more frequently found in women by a ratio of 3:1 and usually appears at or before puberty.

It is occasionally seen in persons with abnormalities in shape of the skull and malformation of nasal fossae, palate and adjoining structures. An arrested development of the turbinate bones and a congenital inhibition of the development of the nasal mucosa are considered predisposing inherited factors. It is occasionally associated with atrophic vaginitis in girls.

Disease. Secondary changes of hyperplastic rhinitis or suppurative disease of the nasal accessory sinuses may cause atrophic rhinitis; the atrophic process results from proliferation and pressure of newly formed connective tissue stimulated by chronic sinus secretion. The contraction of these tissue cells decreases the blood supply and reduces nourishment to the mucous membrane, thus interfering with glandular function and ultimately resulting in atrophy. Some investigators consider this form a purely secondary atrophic condition with changes only in the mucous membrane, as contrasted with a primary form involving bony structure as well. The latter condition may result without pre-existing rhinitis or sinusitis.

Sequelae of acute exanthems are a causative factor, since the condition often appears early in life.

Removal of Turbinal Structures. Secondary changes may result from injury or excessive drying of the mucosa incident to extensive removal of turbinal structures.

Microorganisms. Bacterial infection is commonly found in association with the disease, but not generally accepted as the cause. The organisms considered to be responsible for the fetid odor and the crusting are the *Klebsiella ozaenae* and the *Bacillus foetidus* (of Perez and Hofer). Other organisms isolated from the nasal secretions are: *Proteus vulgaris, Escherichia coli, Klebsiella pneumoniae,* pseudodiphtheritic bacillus, micrococcus (staphylococcus) and streptococcus. Klebsiella organisms have been isolated in nasal cultures in a group of cases studied at the Mayo Clinic. The bacterial flora is largely saprophytic.

PATHOLOGY

There is marked atrophy of the nasal mucosa and a decrease in the connective tissue of the submucosa, with thickening, fibrosis and then obliteration of blood vessels, together with a diminution or complete destruction of glandular elements. In the early stages, the changes are comparable to those of a chronic inflammatory process. In later stages, there is a desquamation and loss of the normal columnar epithelial cells and their cilia, which are eventually replaced by squamous, stratified nonciliated epithelium. The blood vessels undergo fibrosis and eventually an obliterating endarteritis. In the late stage, the epithelium is largely of squamous cell type with subepithelial fibrosis and the underlying bone undergoes atrophic or degenerative changes. With atrophy of the mucous glands, the character of the secretion changes, becomes tenacious, crusted and often mucopurulent. As a rule, there is no ulceration except that due to trauma in the mechanical removal of crusts.

The changes in circulation of the nasal mucosa and finally retrogression of the epithelium and underlying structures have been attributed by some investigators to a degeneration of the sphenopalatine ganglion.

There has been an attempt to separate atrophic rhinitis from ozena on a histologic basis, on the contention that atrophic rhinitis is a result of chronic infection with lymphocytic infiltration and not a disease of blood vessels or a fibrotic process, whereas ozena presents fibrosis without evidence of lymphocytic infiltration, thus suggesting a primary disease.

SYMPTOMS

Dryness and crusting with an offensive odor to the altered nasal secretion are the most common complaints of the patient. The dirty greenish colored crusts are usually retained and may extend to the posterior pharyngeal wall. The discharge and crusts may entirely occlude the nostril. They are tenacious and difficult to expel except by mechanical means. The offensive stench is due to the presence of the bacilli mentioned, to the decomposition of the secretion and action of other saprophytic bacteria. Mucopurulent secretion is usually present beneath crusts.

Partial or complete loss of smell (anosmia) often prevents the odor being detected by the patient.

Nasal obstruction is common and is due to the extensive crusting, which frequently forms a cast of the nasal chambers.

Inspection after removal of crusts reveals roomy nasal cavities with thinned-out turbinates, covered by pale, atrophic and shiny mucous membrane. When crusts are firmly adherent, slight bleeding may occur following their removal. Ulceration of the mucosa of the anterior part of the septum (anterior rhinitis sicca) may be caused by constant picking of the nose, terminating in ulceration or a gray plaque of fibrous tissue replacing the mucosa when healed.

The nasopharynx is commonly involved and hearing impairment may result from catarrhal changes in the eustachian tube.

The pharynx is also frequently affected, presenting a dry, glazed mucosa often covered with adherent crusts (pharyngitis sicca).

Laryngeal extension may cause cough and voice changes (laryngitis sicca).

Pain is not usually present, although a dull headache above the root of the nose together with mental depression and lassitude are frequent complaints.

Secondary infection in the paranasal sinuses may result from extension of the diseased mucosa and mechanical blockage of the sinus ostia.

DIAGNOSIS

The diagnosis of a fully developed atrophic rhinitis is easily made. The examiner finds abnormal patency of the nasal cavity which is filled or partly filled with the characteristic dirty, tenacious secretion and crusts. The atrophic mucosa covering the shrunken turbinates is present in variable degree. The foul odor is unmistakable, but this finding must be differentiated from other disease of the nose producing necrosis of mucous membrane and bone, namely, tertiary syphilis, rhinolith, or foreign body in the nose with suppuration and crusting, chronic suppurative sinusitis, malignant disease of the paranasal sinuses or of the nose, postradiation changes and lupus or tuberculosis of the nose. In marked primary or secondary anemias, the erectile tissue overlying the turbinate bones may be pale and atrophic (in state of collapse) but the tenacious stagnant secretion is most always absent in this condition.

In syphilis, there is a history of other symptoms as a rule; the condition is most often unilateral and localized to one area of deep ulceration involving the septum or hard palate. Serologic examination will, of course, aid in ruling out this disease. Foreign bodies in the nose are most commonly found in children. They produce suppuration and sometimes ulceration from pressure necrosis. In suppuration of the nasal accessory sinuses, there is free discharge of mucopurulent secretion from the middle meatus rather than tenacious crusting.

TREATMENT

The aim of the treatment is to remove crusted secretions and to stimulate normal secretion, but because of the resistance of this disease to treatment, several procedures and numerous medications have been advocated. Among these, the most effective procedures are in the form of (1) irrigation, (2) medicated tampons and (3) sprays of oily medications, particularly the estrogenic substances.

Irrigation. Once or twice a day, nasal irrigation, or douching is performed from an irrigating reservoir such as a fountain syringe, douche bag (Fig. 173), nasal syphon, or the small glass nasal irrigation instrument. The irrigating fluid should be comfortably warm when tested on the back of the hand. The can or douche bag should be about two feet above the patient's head, which is held face down over a basin. The irrigating tip is inserted into one nostril and the solution allowed to flow gently into the nose and out the other nostril. This will occur if the mouth is held open and the breathing is carried on through it. After half of the fluid has been used in irrigating through one nostril, the direction of flow is reversed by changing to the opposite one. If the patient has to cough, sneeze or gag, he closes the tube temporarily by clamping or pinching it off. At the finish of the irrigation, the patient is instructed to allow all of the fluid to run out before he attempts to blow his nose, so as to avoid forcing any solution into his eustachian tubes.

A fairly efficient method of washing the nasal cavities may be carried out by snuffing a warm solution from the palm of the hand. Isotonic saline solution is commonly used.

The solution is drawn into one nostril from the palm with a strong snuff. It enters the nasopharynx, from which it is hawked out and then expectorated into a basin. The snuffing is done through alternate sides until a water glass full of the solution has been used. Nose blowing is avoided until all of the fluid has run out.

Another method of douching may be accomplished with the use of a specially constructed glass bulb, the Bermingham nasal douche (Fig. 173b). This bulb can be filled with the solution and the flow controlled by a finger held on or off the vent on the top of the bulb.

A warm alkaline solution made by dissolving a teaspoonful of the following mixture:

		Gm.
Sodium bicarbonate		30
Sodium chloride		30
Sodium biborate		30

to the pint of water is effective. This treatment is, of course, carried out by the patient. The effectiveness of the treatment is usually in direct proportion to the faithfulness with which it is performed. An isotonic saline solution may be used, which is made by dissolving one teaspoonful of salt in two glasses of water that has been boiled and cooled. Following each irrigation, a nasal spray is used to stimulate secretion (see below).

Tampons. Removal of crusts in many cases can only be done effectively by the physician. In some cases, however, the patient may successfully use self introduced tampons or applicators. One of the following medications on these tampons or applicators are effective in loosening crusts and all but the peroxide stimulates secretion:

> Half strength hydrogen perox de
> Lugol's solution
> Ichthyoldine

For local application to stimulate secretion, the following iodine preparation is useful:

		Gm. or cc.
1. Iodine		0.3
Creosote		0.3
Potassium iodide		2.0
Glycerin		30.0

Some physicians prefer to omit the creosote.

Nasal Spray. In recent years, the use of estrogenic substance by local application in the form of a nasal spray has been advocated. The treatment is based on the estrogenic hormone properties of producing hypertrophy of normal mucous membranes in the nose. The estrogenic substances have also been given parenterally. Histologic studies are reported to show increased hyperemia and hypertrophy of the sub-epithelial glandular system of the nasal mucosa. Experiments on the effect of estrogenic substances on ciliary motion of the bucco-esophageal mucosa of frogs show that crystalline estrone, estriol, and estradiol dissolved in isotonic saline solution stimulate ciliary activity when given in minute doses, and depress the action when given in large doses. Some investigators believe, however, that the initial improvement noted in patients during the first two or three weeks of treatment is due to the increased attention given the condition, such as cleansing and douching, rather than the direct effect of the estrogenic substance. The following procedure of intranasal application of the estrogenic substance is suggested:

(1) Remove crusts as thoroughly as possible by saline douche or by mechanical means.

(2) Spray the nasal cavity with estrogenic substance in olive or corn oil two or three times daily. The dosage is variable with the particular commercial form of estrogenic substance. Convenient preparations of 20,000 units per 30 cc. are put up in suitable nasal atomizers. The treatment is first demonstrated to the patient who then carries it out on himself.

Miscellaneous Forms of Therapy. Many other forms of therapy or particular medications have been advocated. Among these are the following:

Insufflation of powders containing iodine or iodides in various forms combined with potassium iodide taken internally.

The use of a bland oil or mild astringents to soften crusts. (As a rule, in the late stages, the crusts must be detached and removed mechanically by forceful blowing, by forceps, or by cotton tipped applicator.)

Irrigation with a solution of potassium permanganate (2 grains to 500 cc. of warm water) to reduce the offensive odor.

The local use of prostigmine methyl sulfate or acetylcholine has been advocated for their vasodilating action in an effort to produce reactivity of the mucous glands.

Diathermy followed by ultraviolet radiation to improve the circulation in the mucosa.

A vaccine made from the strains of the Perez and Hofer bacillus.

Surgical procedures designed to narrow the abnormally patent nasal space by moving in the lateral nasal wall or implanting ivory, or autogenous material beneath the mucoperichondrium of the floor of the nose and the septum. The latest of these which shows promise is an acrylic resin which produces little local reaction. The fact that so many therapeutic procedures have been advocated is indicative of the ineffectiveness of any method of therapy in the cure of this disease.

REFERENCES

Fitzhugh, W. M., Jr.: Atrophic Rhinitis and Ozena. Arch. Otolaryng., *42*:404, 1945.

Henner, R., and Busby, W.: Prostigmine Therapy of Atrophic Rhinitis. *Ibid.*, *38*:426, 1943.

Mortimer, H., Wright, R., and Collip, J.: Atrophic Rhinitis, The Constitutional Factor and the Treatment with Oestrogenic Hormones, Canad. M.A.J., *37*:445, 1937.

Pollock, H. L.: A New Conception of the Etiology of Atrophic Rhinitis. Am. Laryng., Rhinol. & Otol. Soc., p. 375, 1931.

Ruskin, S. L.: A Differential Diagnosis and Therapy of Atrophic Rhinitis and Ozena. Arch. Otolaryng., *15*:222, 1932.

Thornell, W. C.: Ozena—Bacteriologic and Pathologic Studies. Proc. Staff Meet., Mayo Clin., *21*:90, 1946.

CHAPTER XXI

INJURIES TO THE NOSE

John J. Hochfilzer, M.D.

One of the most common injuries received in this age of automotive transportation is that to the nasal structure. The external nose is the most protruding and least protected structure of the human body and is commonly traumatized sufficiently to cause a serious impairment of function.

Fractures and dislocations of the nasal structures are often overlooked. There is a tendency to consider these injuries as rather trivial; they are rarely associated with constitutional symptoms. For that reason, the advantage of early treatment is often lost.

The nasal framework consists of the nasal bones, the upper and lower lateral cartilages, the bony and cartilaginous nasal septum, and the frontal process of the maxilla. The nasal bones articulate at the sides with the maxilla from whose level they rise, at the root with the frontal bone, and on a median line with each other (Fig. 57). They are in contact beneath with the bony and cartilaginous elements of the septum again on their median line and with the cartilaginous septum and upper lateral cartilages at their distal ends. For full discussion of external nose anatomy, see Chapter XI.

Nasal fractures are usually the result of a direct blow to the external nose. The nasal structures of infants and small children are soft, an arrangement on the part of nature to offer maximum safety at an age when nasal trauma is likely to be most frequent.

Nasal injury occurs at all ages, but is most common in children and in youth.

FRACTURES

Types of Fracture. Several types or combinations of nasal fracture are possible (Fig. 104). Classifications as to types have been suggested. From a practical standpoint, the following considerations are important:

1. The nasal bridge may be thickened, broadened, and flattened, or definitely dislocated to one side or the other.

2. The septum may be dislocated generally or at the columnella.

3. Compound fractures are infrequent in comparison with ordinary fractures. Involvement of the bones comprising the nasal bridge in a

compound fracture is more important than the elements of the septum but compound fracture involving the bones of the nasal bridge or the septum should receive consideration as to the possibilities of infection. Next in importance would be the restoration of the displaced fragments so as to insure the maximum of nasal function.

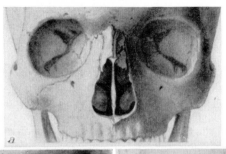

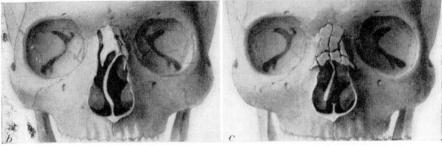

Fig. 104. Types of nasal fractures. (a) Simple depression of one nasal bone, usually with more or less comminution. (b) Lateral displacement of the bony nasal bridge with separation of the articulation on each side between the nasal bone and the maxillary bone. The septum is usually bent or deviated in this type of fracture and dislocation. (c) Flattening of the nasal bridge with comminution. The septum is bent, fractured, and dislocated. (Boies, L. R. In: Allen, E. V. (ed.): Specialties in Medical Practice. Vol. 1. New York, Thomas Nelson & Sons.)

Symptoms and Signs. The common indications of a nasal fracture are:

1. Swelling and deformity.
2. Ecchymosis.
3. Bony crepitus.

Pain is not severe in the ordinary nasal fracture, although palpation of the swollen and deformed nose may produce considerable tenderness.

Diagnosis. The symptoms and signs mentioned above may leave little doubt concerning the probability of fracture of the nasal bridge. X-ray studies are of relatively little value in diagnosis or as a guide to treatment. There are cases in which a fracture exists but in which little can be determined from the x-ray plate. In other cases, little external deformity may be present but a fracture is indicated by the x-ray study.

Treatment. The nasal bones serve only as contour supports. They are thin and flat and are in between two layers of soft tissue, a muco-periosteum internally and periosteum and skin externally. There is no important muscular pull on them. When a fracture of the bony bridge with dislocation and deformity is reduced early, the *soft tissue splinting* as a rule maintains the reduction in good position.

Reduction is usually performed under cocaine anesthesia except in infants and small children in whom it is better to administer a light, brief, general anesthesia of sufficient duration to provide unconsciousness for

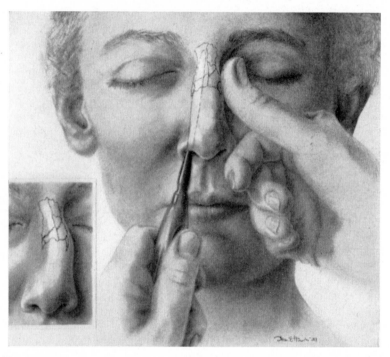

Fig. 105. Reduction of a depressed or dislocated nasal bridge. This reduction is accomplished by raising with an elevator inserted under the nasal bone to be lifted or reset. The thumb of the free hand of the operator is used to press against the convex side of the deformity. (Boies, L. R. In: Allen, E. V. (ed.): Specialties in Medical Practice. Vol. 1. New York, Thomas Nelson & Sons.)

two or three minutes while the elevation of a depressed nasal bone or the repositioning of a dislocated nasal bridge is accomplished.

Technic. An adequate technic for the ordinary case is illustrated in Fig. 105. A blunt elevator of a special design (Fig. 106) or any strong thin blade with rounded margins may be introduced on the depressed side. With a lifting motion, the depressed bone is elevated into position. If there has been a dislocation of the nasal bridge to one side, pressure from the thumb of the free hand is used to push on the convexity caused by the bone not being lifted. The force of the lift is upward and toward the side from which the bone was displaced. The force of thumb pressure on the other nasal bone is also toward the side from which the bridge was displaced. Usually in fresh cases this simple manuever is all that is necessary for a satisfactory reduction.

A deflection of the nasal bridge is usually accompanied by some deflection of the nasal septum. When the deformity of the bridge is corrected, the septum usually goes back into position, although some thickening may have occurred as a result of the trauma.

When the septum is badly traumatized and the fracture is compound with a protrusion of bone or cartilage through the mucosa, it is difficult to reposition the parts and maintain this position. The treatment requires the skill and judgment of an experienced rhinologist. Packing to produce sufficient pressure to maintain alignment of displaced fragments is difficult for the patient to tolerate.

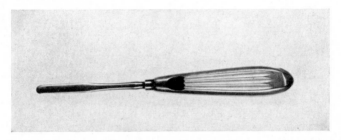

Fig. 106. An instrument for elevation of a depressed nasal fracture. The blade is moderately thin, rounded and sturdy enough so it will not bend when considerable force is exerted. This model was designed by Boies (Storz Instrument Co., St. Louis)

Severe comminution of the nasal bridge particularly if seen several days after the injury may require traction from a specially constructed head gear to maintain the position of corrected contours. Compound fractures of the nasal bridge may produce lacerations and scar formation which will later require plastic surgery of soft tissue and bony support to provide a good cosmetic appearance.

DEFORMITIES

The modern developments in plastic surgery offer the victims of nasal deformity an opportunity for a marked improvement in appearance (Fig. 107). The common deformities are:

1. Depression of the nasal bridge (saddle nose) from inadequately or untreated nasal fracture, or the effects of infection or disease resulting in a sagging of the nasal bridge.

2. A nasal hump usually associated with too long a nose. This is often the result of factors of growth and race, but may be the result wholly or in part from injury.

3. Lateral dislocation of the nasal bridge. This is entirely due to

trauma and usually is the result of a blow on the side of the nose, which is inadequately treated or not treated at all.

There are, of course, various types of combinations of these deformities. There are also noses with too broad a bridge, which can be narrowed; there are noses with too large a tip, which can be reduced by skilful plastic reshaping of the alar cartilages; there are nostrils which are misshapen or too small, which can be improved as to function and appearance. There are instances of loss of nasal substance or the entire nose from trauma, such as gunshot wounds, or from infection or other disease, in which the plastic surgeon can rebuild the external nose wholly or in part.

Plastic Repair. Most plastic procedures on the nose are performed under local anesthesia. The incisions are made through the nasal vestibules except for some approaches through the columnella. Where there

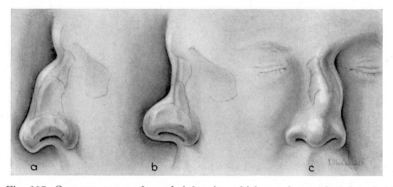

Fig. 107. Common types of nasal deformity which can be repaired by plastic surgery: (a) the humped nose, (b) the saddle nose, and (c) lateral displacement of the nasal bridge.

is a hump to remove, this is done with a saw or chisel. A narrowing of the nasal bridge is then necessary and this is accomplished by loosening the nasal bones by saw or chisel and moving them inward.

The elevation and narrowing of the nasal tip requires shortening of the proper cartilages and the septum.

A graft of cartilage (preserved cartilage is now widely used) or ivory is used to repair a saddle nose. Paraffin injections are now considered obsolete because the paraffin rarely remains permanently in position and also causes more foreign body reaction than other substances.

The laterally dislocated nasal bridge can be repaired by separating the nasal bones and resetting them in proper midline position.

Modern results in plastic surgery of the nose are excellent in the hands of well trained and skilful surgeons. The ideal background for this is a thorough training in rhinology combined with adequate training and experience in the principles and maneuvers of plastic nasal surgery.

REFERENCES

Fomon, S.: The Surgery of Injury and Plastic Repair. Baltimore, Williams & Wilkins Co., 1939.

Hersh, J.: Management of Fractures of the Bony Nasal Vault. Ann. Otol., Rhin. & Laryng., *54*:534, 1945.

Maliniac, J.: Fracture-Dislocations of the Cartilaginous Nose: Anatomico-pathologic Considerations and Treatment. Arch. Otolaryng., *42*:131, 1945.

New, G. B.: Fracture of the Nasal and Malar Bones. S. Clin. North America, *15*:1241, 1935.

Part III

The Throat

CHAPTER XXII

APPLIED ANATOMY AND PHYSIOLOGY
OF THE THROAT

The word throat is broadly used to cover an area containing several distinctly separate structures which differ as to anatomy and function.

PHARYNX

The pharynx is in a sense a musculocutaneous bag which is funnel-shaped, wide above and narrow below (Fig. 108). The upper one-third, the *nasopharynx*, is the respiratory portion and is immobile except for its floor, the soft palate. The middle and lower thirds are mobile; they can be obliterated. The middle portion of the pharynx is termed the *oropharynx* and extends from the inferior border of the soft palate to the lingual surface of the epiglottis. The lower portion of the pharynx is the *laryngopharynx* which leads into the larynx and trachea anteriorly and the esophagus posteriorly.

The posterior wall of the pharynx extends from the base of the skull to the level of the inferior border of the sixth cervical vertebra. It is at this level that the esophagus begins. The introitus of the esophagus is formed by the cricopharyngeus muscle (the inferior constrictor), which is often referred to as the "upper pinchcock" of the esophagus. The length of the posterior wall of the pharynx approximates 5.5 inches (14 cm.). The anteroposterior diameter of the adult nasopharynx varies but little from that at birth, but the nasopharynx doubles in length in the first six months of life.

THE NASOPHARYNX

Chapter XXIV is a detailed discussion of the nasopharynx.

The relatively small nasopharyngeal space contains or is in close relationship to a number of structures which have clinical importance (Figs. 109, 110). These anatomical structures are:

1. Adenoids.

2. Lymphoid tissue on the lateral pharyngeal wall and in the recessus pharyngeus, known as Rosenmüller's fossa.

3. Rathke's pouch (site of evagination of embryonic structures which form the hypophysis cerebri).

4. Torus tubarius—the reflection of the pharyngeal mucosa over the rounded protrusions of the cartilaginous portions of the eustachian tubes.

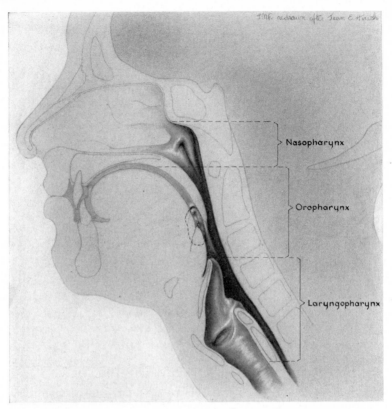

Fig. 108. The throat includes the nasopharynx, tonsils and oropharynx, and extends into the larynx to the upper end of the trachea anteriorly and to the upper end of the esophagus posteriorly. With the exception of the larynx, this area is included in what we technically refer to as the pharynx. (Boies, L. R. In: Allen, E. V. (Ed.): Specialties in Medical Practice. Vol. 1. New York, Thomas Nelson & Sons.)

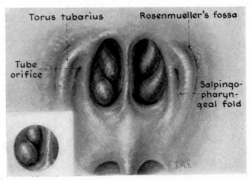

Fig. 109. Nasopharynx as viewed through nasopharyngeal mirror inserted into the throat through the mouth. Mirror shows amount of nasopharynx indicated in small insert at each position, but by moving mirror the entire nasopharynx can be examined, and information on all parts of nasopharynx shown in larger figure can be obtained.

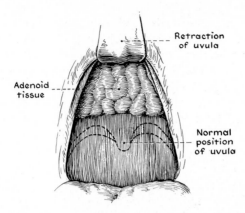

Fig. 110. Adenoid mass as seen at operation and drawn directly from life. A retractor is shown pulling the soft palate and uvula upward to expose the lower portion of the adenoid vegetations. Note the sharp inferior margin of the adenoid mass.

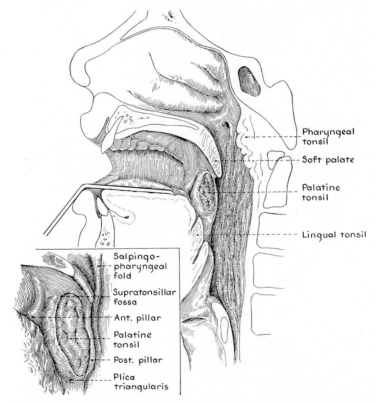

Fig. 111. The relationships of the structures included in the oropharynx. The details of the structures surrounding the tonsils. (Redrawn from Hirsch.)

5. Choanae.

6. Jugular foramina through which pass the glossopharyngeal, vagus and accessory cranial nerves, the inferior petrosal sinus, internal jugular vein and some meningeal branches from the occipital and ascending pharyngeal arteries. The hypoglossal foramen, through which passes the hypoglossal nerve, is adjacent.

7. Petrous portion of the temporal bone and foramen lacerum in proximity to the lateral portion of the roof of the nasopharynx.

THE OROPHARYNX

This area is also referred to as the mesopharynx (Fig. 111). Its boundaries have already been mentioned. The structures within it which are of clinical importance are the:

1. Posterior pharyngeal wall.

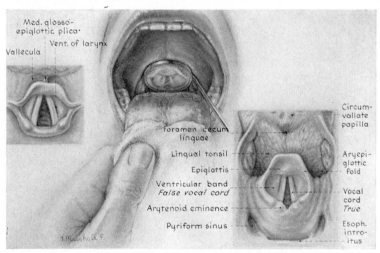

Fig. 112A. The important structures to visualize in an examination of the laryngopharynx are the valleculae, the epiglottis, the ary-epiglottic folds, the ventricular bands ("false" cords), the vocal cords ("true" cords), the openings of the ventricles of the larynx, the anterior commissure, the arytenoid eminences, the pyriform sinuses, and the posterior pharyngeal wall down to the esophageal introitus.

2. Faucial or palatine tonsils and the pillars of these tonsils.
3. Uvula.
4. Lingual tonsils.
5. Foramen caecum.

The posterior pharyngeal wall is important clinically because of its involvement in acute and chronic inflammations, abscesses in the retropharyngeal space and the disturbances in the action of the musculature which is part of it.

Acute and chronic inflammations and abscesses in the retropharyngeal space are considered in detail in Chapter XXV. Disturbances in the action of the muscles of the posterior pharyngeal wall and the soft palate are encountered in several neurological disorders in which the action of the vagus nerve is affected.

THE LARYNGOPHARYNX

When the laryngopharynx is examined with the mirror or by direct laryngoscopy, the first structures noted below the base of the tongue are the valleculae (Fig. 112A). These are two shallow depressions formed by a

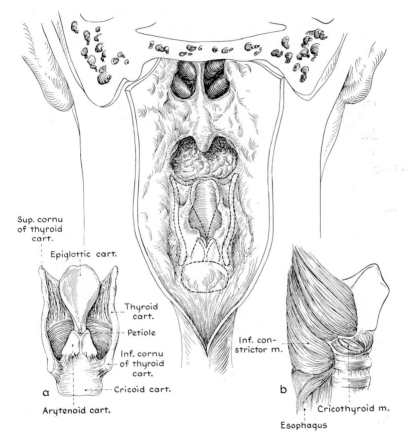

Sup. cornu
of thyroid
cart.

Epiglottic cart.

Thyroid
cart.

Petiole

Inf. cornu
of thyroid
cart.

Inf. con-
strictor m.

Cricoid cart.

a

Arytenoid cart.

b

Cricothyroid m.

Esophagus

Fig. 112B. A diagram of the pharynx as seen from behind. The position of the cartilaginous framework of the larynx (a) is shown by the dotted line in the central figure. The position and direction of the inferior constrictor muscle (cricopharyngeus) as it forms the "upper pinchcock" of the esophagus is illustrated in (b).

median glosso-epiglottic ligament and a lateral glosso-epiglottic fold on each side. The valleculae have been called "pill pockets" because of the tendency in some persons for a pill taken by mouth to lodge at this site.

The epiglottis is the next important structure below the valleculae. In infants, it is shaped like the Greek symbol for omega; as it develops, it opens out, although the infantile form may persist. It may be excessively developed and thin so that it becomes dependent, making examination of the glottis difficult without pressing the epiglottis forward. Its function is probably a protective one to the entrance of the glottis, deflecting fluid or a bolus of food laterally on each side. As fluid or food is deflected laterally, it goes around to the side of the larynx into a pyriform sinus. There is one on each side. Each is a sort of trough which is obliterated as the larynx raises in the act of swallowing. The protective function of the epiglottis is, however, not the most important factor against fluid or food entering the glottis. It is the constrictor or valve-like action of the ventricular bands (false cords) which really protects the glottis (Fig. 112B).

The superior laryngeal nerve passes beneath the floor of the pyriform sinus on each side of the laryngopharynx. This fact is used in applying anesthesia to the pharynx and the laryngeal aperture for endoscopic procedures. A curved metal applicator is used to hold a pledget moistened with cocaine against the sinus floor. Some of the cocaine will be absorbed through the mucosa of the pyriform sinus floor to reach the nerve.

MUCOSA

The structure of the mucosa of the pharynx varies according to its functions. In the nasopharynx, the function is respiratory and the mucosa is a ciliated, stratified columnar epithelium which contains mucous or goblet cells. A basement membrane of a colloid nature lies between the epithelial and submucous layers. Lower down, the function is gustatory and here a nonciliated, stratified squamous epithelium is found. Elastic fibers replace the mucous membrane.

Throughout the entire length of the pharynx are found many cells of the lymphocytic series (lymphocytes) which lie in a fibrous network of the reticulo-endothelial system. That is why the pharynx has been regarded as nature's first line of defense.

MUSCLES

There are three pairs of constrictor muscles and two pairs of elevator muscles in the pharynx. The elevators are the inner muscles and are longitudinal; the constrictors are the outer muscles and are circular. The constrictors are known as the superior, middle and inferior pharyngeal constrictors (Fig. 113). These are fan-shaped. Each lower pair partly covers the next upper pair from behind. The muscles of both sides interdigitate and are partly joined together posteriorly in the median plane of a band of connective tissue. The connecting band is known as the raphe pharyngis.

The superior constrictors are suspended from a median point at the base of the skull instead of from a broad attachment. This leaves an area of variable size laterally on each side. This space is known as the sinus morgagni. It is semilunar in shape and is traversed by the cartilaginous portion of the eustachian tube and the levator and tensor veli palatini muscles.

There are four bellies of origin of the superior constrictor and two bellies of origin of each of the middle and inferior constrictors.

The action of these constrictors is to narrow and obliterate the pharyngeal lumen. The vagus nerve innervates the muscles.

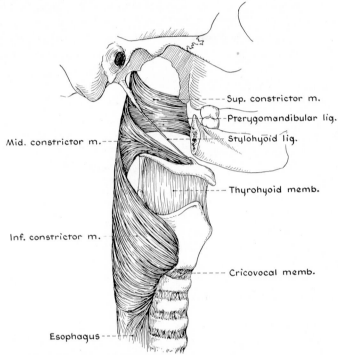

Fig. 113. The relative size, the position, and attachments of the three constrictor muscles of the pharynx. (Adapted from Grant.)

The elevator muscles, which are longitudinal, are the stylopharyngeus and the pharyngopalatinus muscles. The former widens the pharynx and raises the larynx. The latter approximates the pharyngopalatine arch and elevates the inferior part of the larynx and pharynx. The action of both muscles is important in deglutition. Both are supplied by the vagus nerve.

Soft Palate. The soft palate is made up of five pairs of muscles enclosed in a fascial and mucous membrane sheath. The importance of a normal action of these muscles is often overlooked. Some are important in speech and others in the normal function of the eustachian tube. These muscles and their functions are:

1. The levator veli palatinus forms the muscle bulk of the soft palate and acts to narrow the isthmus of the pharynx and widen the ostium of the eustachian tube. Its nerve supply is from the vagus.

2. The tensor veli palatinus forms the tendinous portion of the soft palate and acts to tense the anterior portion of the soft palate and open the eustachian tube. Its nerve supply is from the mandibular branch of the trigeminal.

3. The azygos uvulae is the small muscle which shortens and draws the uvula backward and upward. Its nerve supply is from the vagus.

4. The glossopalatinus muscle forms the anterior pillar of the tonsil and acts to narrow the isthmus of the fauces. It is supplied by the vagus.

5. The pharyngopalatinus muscle forms the posterior pillar of the tonsil and in action both approximates the pharyngopalatine arches and elevates the inferior part of the pharynx and larynx. Fibers from the vagus also innervate this muscle.

Tonsil Fossa. Each faucial (palatine) tonsil fossa is bounded by the anterior pillar (glossopalatinus muscle) and the posterior pillar (pharyngopalatinus muscle) (Fig. 111). The external or lateral boundary is the superior constrictor muscle. The superior margin is known as the upper pole where there is a small space known as the supratonsillar fossa. This contains loose areolar connective tissue. It is the usual site for pus to rupture through when an abscess forms in this area.

The tonsil fossa is lined by a fascia which is part of the buccopharyngeal fascia. This forms its so-called "capsule," which is not a true capsule, since it only lines the fossa. Some of the fibers of the posterior pillar extend under the tonsil and are attached to this fascial sheath. In some instances, this muscle seems to divide the tonsil so that it presents a smaller lower lobe.

TONSILS

The tonsil is a mass of lymphoid tissue supported by a connective tissue framework and tunneled by a complex system of crypts which attain full development late in childhood.

The lingual tonsil is a mass of lymphoid tissue situated at the base of the tongue; it is bisected by the glosso-epiglottic ligament. In the midline just anterior to this mass is the foramen caecum at the apex of the angle formed by the circumvallate papillae. It marks the lingual end of the remains of the thyroglossal duct and may be clinically important if a thyroid mass (lingual thyroid), or a cyst from the thyroglossal duct remains, develop at this site.

PHYSIOLOGY OF THE PHARYNX

The pharynx functions chiefly in respiration, deglutition, voice resonance and articulation. Three of these functions would seem obvious. The function of deglutition merits detailed description.

Deglutition. The mechanism of deglutition functions in three ways.

The first stage is a voluntary one in which the bolus of food is forced past the arches of the fauces. The second stage is involuntary, in which the bolus passes from the mouth through the pharynx. The third stage is also involuntary, in which the food passes down the esophagus into the stomach. The actual steps in the act of deglutition are as follows: Following mastication, the bolus is brought to the base of the tongue and the cheeks are compressed. Then the tongue, hyoid bone and thyroid cartilage are successively raised upward by the muscles which close the mouth and elevate the hyoid bone. The pillars of the fauces (glosso-palatine and pharyngopalatine muscles) contract to narrow the arch. The soft palate then contracts to bring it back to the pharynx and close the nasopharynx. With the elevation of the tongue, hyoid bone and larynx, there occurs simultaneously an elevation of the epiglottis and a closure of the superior aperture of the larynx. The food then passing into the pharynx, is pressed downward to the mouth of the pharynx by contraction of the pharyngeal constrictors. The esophagus is attached anteriorly by a heavy fascial sheath to the plate of the cricoid cartilage in the median line. As a result, when the larynx is elevated, the hypopharynx and pyriform sinuses are opened. Food passage in the esophagus is aided by positive pressure and a peristaltic wave of the esophagus and also by the creation of a negative pressure within the lumen. This negative pressure also acts in the manner of a vacuum or suction to draw down additional food which presents itself at the mouth of the esophagus.

During this act of swallowing, the auditory tube is opened by contraction of the tensor veli palatinus muscle which arises from the tube.

THE PHARYNGEAL SPACES

There are two spaces in relation to the pharynx which are of clinical importance (Fig. 114). One is the retropharyngeal space, which is a potential space. Its anterior wall is the posterior wall of the pharynx. This wall consists (ventrally to dorsally) of pharyngeal mucosa, pharyngobasilar fascia and pharyngeal muscles. The potential space is occupied by a loose areolar tissue of the prevertebral fascia. It extends from the base of the skull above to the farthest point of the cervical fascia below, down to the posterior mediastinum below. Connective tissue fibers in the median line bind it to the spine. Laterally it is bounded by the pharyngomaxillary fossa.

Retropharyngeal abscess is not uncommon in infancy and childhood. Its occurrence results from the fact that a number of lymph nodes occupy the retropharyngeal space. Lymphadenitis may result in suppuration and a breakdown of these nodes. Most of the nodes disappear during early childhood.

The other space is the pharyngomaxillary fossa. This is funnel-shaped, with its base located at the base of the skull close to the jugular foramen and its apex at the great horn of the hyoid bone. The inner boundary of the fossa is the superior constrictor muscle; the outer boundary is the ascending ramus of the mandible and its attached internal pterygoid muscle and the posterior portion of the parotid gland. The dorsal boundary consists of the prevertebral muscles. The fossa is divided into two unequal compartments by the styloid process and its attached muscles. The anterior (prestyloid) compartment is the larger. It may become involved in a suppurative process as a result of infected tonsils, in some

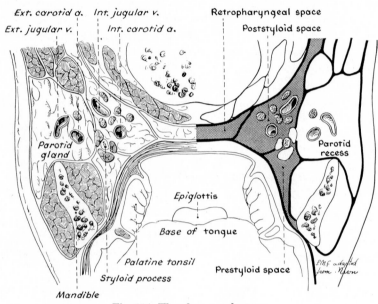

Fig. 114. The pharyngeal spaces.

forms of mastoiditis or petrositis, from dental caries, following surgery and so on. The smaller posterior department contains the internal carotid artery, jugular vein, vagus and sympathetic nerves. Only a thin layer of fascia separates this compartment from the retropharyngeal space.

THE LARYNX

The larynx has the structural form of an inverted triangular pyramidal tube, the framework of which is the large thyroid cartilage atop the sturdy cricoid ring which anchors the upper end of the trachea (Fig. 115). From a practical standpoint, one should have a general knowledge of laryngeal structure in regard to the following:

1. The cartilages united by membranes and ligaments.
2. The histologic structure of the laryngeal mucosa.
3. The functions of the larynx.
4. The five muscles which perform the important laryngeal functions.
5. Innervation.
6. Certain variations of clinical importance in the male, female and infant larynx.

CARTILAGES

On the posterior superior aspect of the sturdy cricoid ring are the two arytenoid cartilages, hitching posts for the vocal cords, which stretch across the laryngeal lumen. The two arytenoids and the unpaired thyroid and cricoid cartilages make up the four major cartilages of the

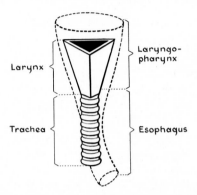

Fig. 115. A diagrammatic representation of the shape and relationships of the cartilaginous larynx ("voice box"). (Redrawn from Turner.)

larynx. The epiglottis and the two paired corniculate and cuneiform make up the five accessory cartilages. The cuneiform cartilages are mounted on the arytenoids (Fig. 116).

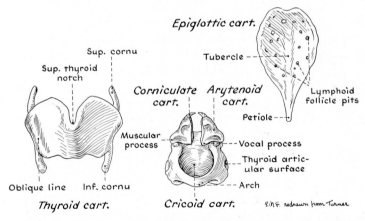

Fig. 116. The cartilages of the larynx. (Redrawn from Turner.)

The cricoid cartilage is the one complete circular cartilage, and maintenance of this complete ring is necessary to an adequate laryngeal lumen. It is shaped like a signet ring with the plate posteriorly. On this plate are the articular facets for the arytenoids and also another pair of facets for the articulation with the thyroid cartilage.

The large thyroid cartilage, incomplete posteriorly, is formed by two quadrangular plates which converge in front and below. In the male, they meet at an acute angle. The uppermost anterior point causes a projection of the skin, the prominentia laryngea, or Adam's apple. In the female, these two quadrangular plates form a wide arch as they converge in front so that the prominentia laryngea is scarcely noticeable.

LARYNGEAL MUCOSA

The conus elasticus is the most important among the various membranes and ligaments uniting the cartilages of the laryngeal structure. This is a connective tissue membrane made up of an especially thick layer of elastic fibrous tissue. It is incorporated with the submucous, or propria, layer of the mucous membrane of the larynx. It extends from the upper margin of the arch of the cricoid to the posterior surface of the angle of the thyroid cartilage anteriorly and to the vocal process of each arytenoid posteriorly. The mucosa is separated in its extension upward to line the laryngeal lumen by a number of muscles from proximity to the perichondrium. It reaches the most medial position at the level of the true cords because of the interposition of the vocal muscles.

At the level of the vocal cords, the conus elasticus is further reinforced by a greater accumulation of elastic tissue fibers in the form of the vocal ligament. This ligament stretches across the laryngeal lumen from the posterior surface of the midportion of the thyroid cartilage to the vocal process of each arytenoid. As the mucosa is reflected up over the vocal ligaments, it is reflected laterally to the thyroid cartilage to form a niche which is known as the ventricle of the larynx. This ventricle, a cul-de-sac, is considered to be a vestigial remains of an appendix which possibly has the function of an accessory air sac in lower vertebrates. From this reflection in the ventricle, the membrane extends upwards to cover the ventricular bands (false cords). The true cord is made up of a muscle, the thyreo-arytenoid, and is covered by this mucous membrane with its conus elasticus reinforced by a special accumulation of elastic tissue fibers. The ventricular band (false cord) is made up of muscle, glandular, lymphoid and adipose tissue.

The mucous membrane of the larynx is a reddish wine color except over the vocal cords where it is an ivory white. Except at certain points such as the laryngeal surface of the epiglottis and vocal ligaments, the mucous membrane of the larynx is not firmly bound down. This accounts for edematous changes in the loose areolar submucous tissue, which cause marked respiratory obstruction and asphyxia. The entire mucous membrane is a ciliated pseudostratified columnar epithelium, except over the vocal cords where it is stratified and squamous in nature. It contains many mucous glands and lymph nodules, except over the vocal cords.

MUSCLES

There are two sets of muscles which function in relation to the larynx. One is a set of muscles attached to the hyoid bone, which are not important in the major functions of the larynx. The other set consists of the intrinsic muscles, which are clinically important chiefly in relation to disturbances in motor function (Fig. 117). The detailed structure of these muscles and their rather complicated function requires special

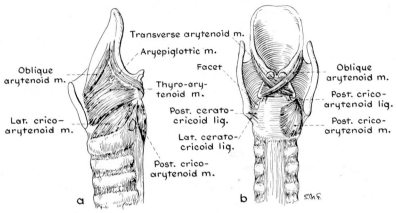

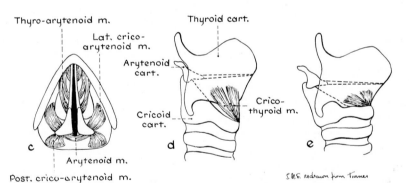

Fig. 117. The appearance of the larynx and attached trachea after removal of all but the muscular and ligamentous structure. (a) side view. (b) posterior view. (c) a diagrammatic representation of the arrangement of the intrinsic muscles. (d) and (e) position, attachments and action of the cricothyroid muscle. (Redrawn from Turner.)

study for one concerned with the numerous disorders associated with them. However, the physician who is not a specialist in laryngology should have a general idea of the muscular structure important to the functions of the larynx and the types of paralysis which may occur. The latter will be discussed in Chapter XXVII.

These intrinsic muscles may be grouped according to function as follows:

(1) The closers of the larynx, which protect the airway on swallowing from fluid, food or other foreign bodies, and (2) the openers of the larynx, which maintain a vital airway.

Closing Muscles. The closing muscles are called adductors. These are the:

1. Lateral crico-arytenoid muscles. There is one on each side. Their action produces a forward pull which brings the cords parallel.

2. Interarytenoid muscle. This muscle, which is unpaired, pulls the arytenoid processes together. It is innervated by the inferior laryngeal nerve, the fibers of which cross the midline. This means that there cannot be a complete unilateral paralysis of the larynx.

3. Internal thyro-arytenoid muscles. The fibers of these muscles are in the substance of the vocal cord. Contraction of these muscles together with the action of the interarytenoid muscles closes the cartilaginous glottis.

There are bands of muscular fibers in the aryepiglottic folds, which aid in closing the lumen of the larynx above the vocal cords.

A fourth pair of muscles which, though not one which closes the larynx, produces tension of the vocal cords and aids in phonation, is the crico-thyroid muscles. These are on the external surface of the cartilages and on contraction pull the thyroid cartilage forward on the arytenoid, increasing the distance from the anterior commissure to the posterior commissure, thus elongating the glottis and tensing the cords. This elongation and tensing enables the thyro-arytenoid muscles in the body of the vocal cord on each side to harden the edges of each cord, which is necessary to raise the pitch on phonation. The cricothyroid muscle receives innervation from the superior laryngeal nerve alone. The inter-arytenoid muscle may receive some of its nerve supply from the superior laryngeal nerve in addition to its innervation by the inferior laryngeal nerve. It is innervated from both sides; thus a unilateral paralysis of this muscle is impossible. All the other muscles are innervated by the inferior nerve.

Opening Muscles. There is only one opener muscle of the larynx among the five muscles that are strictly laryngeal. This is the posterior crico-arytenoid, the most powerful of the laryngeal muscles. There is one on each side. Their action is to slide the arytenoid cartilages outward while tilting the vocal processes of these cartilages backward.

FUNCTION

The larynx has been thought of chiefly in relation to speech. However, Jackson has pointed out nine physiological functions which seem logical as one reflects on the physiology of this structure. These are:

1. Protective function. The larynx closes the airway against intrusion of foreign substances and helps to expel any intruding substance with the cough reflex.

2. Respiratory function.

3. Circulatory function. The effect of changing pressures in the tracheobronchial tree and pulmonary parenchyma exerts a pumping action on circulating blood.

4. Fixative function. The fixation of air in the thorax occurs when the larynx is closed, which is an aid to the act of lifting, straining, and so on.

5. Deglutitory function. The rising action of the larynx participates in getting the bolus of food downward and the closure of the larynx and the function of the epiglottis in guiding the food laterally are aids to deglutition.

6. Tussive function.

7. Expectorative and tussive functions are a second line of defense in case foreign substances get beyond the glottis, and these functions aid in expelling secretions or other endogenous accumulations from the larynx.

8. Phonatory function. This is dependent on a highly developed mechanism but yet it is not nearly of as much importance as some of the protective functions.

9. Emotional function.

NERVES OF THE LARYNX

There are two nerves on each side of the larynx, the superior and inferior laryngeal; both are branches of the vagus.

Superior Laryngeal. This nerve has both sensory and motor functions. It leaves the vagus just above the larynx and divides into two branches. The external branch passes downward to innervate the cricothyroid muscle. The internal branch passes through the thyrohyoid membrane to supply the mucosa of the larynx and epiglottis. Its afferent neurons transmit centrally the sensation of irritation and pain in laryngeal disease. These impulses that are transmitted centrally come back as bilateral motor impulses to the laryngeal and thoracic muscles, thus completing the arc known as the cough reflex, which is the "watchdog" of the lungs (Jackson).

Inferior Laryngeal. These nerves, which are the motor nerves, are given off at different levels on each side. The right one comes off the vagus at the right subclavian artery, passes under the artery and ascends in the groove between the trachea and esophagus to the level of the cricoid cartilage. It then divides into two branches. The anterior branch supplies the lateral crico-arytenoid, the thyro-arytenoid and the arytenoid muscles. The posterior branch is distributed to the right posterior crico-arytenoid muscle and the arytenoid muscle. Its distribution in the latter is to both sides of the median line.

The left inferior laryngeal leaves the vagus as it crosses the arch of the aorta, passes under it and thence upward to the larynx. This longer course of the left inferior nerve and its relationship to the aorta makes it more vulnerable to injury as compared to the right nerve.

The distribution of these nerves is indicative of their complex character. Certain fibers in the same nerve carry impulses to groups of muscles which are directly antagonistic in action. For example, the

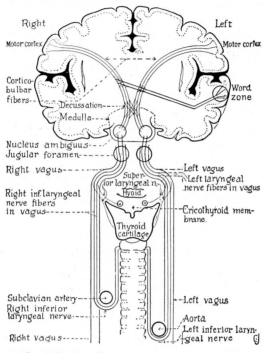

Fig. 118. A pen sketch by Dr. Chevalier Jackson "schematically illustrating in a simplified way the fundamentals of innervation of the larynx for performing its nine functions. For clearness, intervening central structures have been omitted. The laryngeal nerves originate in the nuclei ambigui of which there are two, one on each side of the medulla. Here are activated the autonomic functions of respiration and reflex laryngeal movements. For volitional movements the nuclei ambigui are activated and dominated by impulses, 'orders' received from the cortical executive centers. These bilateral executive centers in turn receive their 'orders,' as to words, from the unilateral language (or word) area located on the left side of the brain (in right handed individuals), represented diagrammatically as distributing its impulses bilaterally. To avoid impairing simplicity, only efferent pathways are indicated in this schema. It must be understood that all these pathways have their complementary afferent pathways." (From Jackson and Jackson: Diseases of the Nose, Throat and Ear. W. B. Saunders Co.)

muscles that close the larynx receive innervation from fibers which are in the same nerve as the fibers which innervate the muscles which open the larynx.

The complex character of laryngeal innervation is apparently responsible for misunderstanding in the interpretation of motor paralysis of the larynx. Jackson has simplified this in a sketch (Fig. 118) to illustrate the fundamentals of this innervation.

LARYNGEAL VARIATIONS

The cartilages of the larynx in the newborn are identical in size and shape both for the male and female. These grow at the same rate until the age of five or six when development slows until the onset of puberty. Increased physical activity and a need for increased respiratory exchange stimulate growth again. The larynx begins to grow at a faster rate in the male than in the female. The rate of growth in the male frequently proceeds so rapidly that changes in voice are produced during the period of adjustment as a result of the lengthening of the vocal cords and muscles.

In the infant, the larynx is higher and its angle with the lumen of the trachea is more acute than in the adult. This fact must be considered in the prolonged use of an intubation tube in the infant; the position of the tube may cause pressure necrosis.

CHAPTER XXIII

EXAMINATION OF THE THROAT

An orderly procedure is necessary for a proper study of the patient's throat. This includes the following:

1. A detailed history.

2. A systematic examination of the oral cavity to note the condition of the mucous membrane, orifices of the parotid, submaxillary and sublingual ducts, an inspection of the teeth and gums, observation of the matter of occlusion and the dental "bite," inspection of the hard palate, and finally a study of the tongue.

The tonsils are on the dividing line between the oral cavity and the pharynx and logically are next examined together with the condition of the soft palate.

3. A study of the oropharynx and nasopharynx. As much of the pharyngeal wall as can be visualized with a good light reflected onto this area is next in order. The posterior pillars of the fauces and the soft palate should be gently pushed aside when indicated so as to enlarge the area visualized.

4. Visualization of the nasopharynx noting the condition of the vault of the nasopharynx, the site for Rathke's pouch, Rosenmüller's fossae, the eustachian orifices and the posterior end of the septum, and the choanae.

5. Visualization of the base of the tongue, which includes the lingual tonsils and the site of the foramen cecum, then the valleculae, the tip and laryngeal surface of the epiglottis, the pyriform sinuses, the aryepiglottic folds, the arytenoid prominences, the ventricular bands ("false cords"), the true cords, the anterior commissure, the ventricles of the larynx, as much of the trachea as can be seen, and the esophageal introitus.

6. An inspection of the external neck, front and back, for swelling or other deformity, palpating the laryngeal cartilages and the sites of the cervical lymph glands.

7. X-ray studies when indicated.

HISTORY

The patient with disease in his throat usually complains of one or more of the following symptoms:

1. Sore throat.

2. Discharge in the throat.

3. Sense of lump, or fulness, or swelling.

4. Difficulty in swallowing (dysphagia).

5. Hoarseness.

6. Cough.

When one inquires into the history of the particular symptom or symptoms, there is value in paying attention to specific details. For example, the following detailed inquiry should be made regarding the complaint of sore throat:

Number per month?.... year?.... duration of an attack?.... accompanied by fever?.... discharge?.... expectoration?.... difficulty in swallowing?.... difficult breathing?.... voice change?.... cough?.... location and duration of external swelling?.... Is there any pain reference such as earache?.... which ear?..... Past treatment?....

Discharge in the throat:

Duration?.... Character: mucoid?.... purulent?.... blood stained?..... Amount: profuse?.... scanty?.... Is it coughed or hawked up?.... or does it drop into the postnasal space?.... Is it worse on arising in the morning?.....

Sense of lump, fulness, swelling:

Duration?.... site?..... Is the sensation intermittent or constant?.... painful or painless?..... If painful, is there any reference of pain such as earache?..... Is there any actual difficulty in swallowing?.... breathing?.... Are you nervous?.... worried about cancer?.....

Difficulty in swallowing (dysphagia):

Duration: ....wks. ....mos. ....yrs. Is it increasing?.... Have you any pain?.... How well can you swallow ordinary food?.... Does the obstruction increase when swallowing liquids or solid food?.... Where does the obstruction seem to be (have patient indicate level)?...... Is there any regurgitation?.... odor?.... Have you lost weight?.... amount?.....

Hoarseness:

Duration: ....wks. ....mos. ....yrs. Was the onset sudden or gradual?.... Was your voice completely gone at any time?.... for how long?.... Have you ever been hoarse before?.... when?.... number of attacks?.... Was the attack preceded by a head cold or sore throat?.... Do you experience any discomfort in the region of the larynx?.... do you cough?.... raise much phlegm?.... Is there any pain related to the use of your voice?.... or discomfort in breathing?.....

Cough:

Duration: ....wks. ....mos. ....yrs. In what part of the throat does the cough seem to start?...... What do you cough up?..... What makes the cough worse such as exposure to cold air, smoke, dust, etc.?..... Is it worse at night when lying down?.... or on exercising?.... Have you lost weight?.... how much?.... appetite?.... strength?.....

PHYSICAL EXAMINATION

In describing the examination of the nasal space (page 148), it was stated that it is important to scrutinize the general appearance of the patient's head and neck, noting any abnormalities of color of skin, swelling, and external expression of pain, worry and apprehension, and so on. This also applies to a throat examination. Invariably, the oto-

laryngologist completely examines the nose, throat and ears, whether
or not the patient has a single complaint confined to one of these three
areas. In the description of an examination of the nasal space, the details
of an examination of the oral cavity and of the nasal space were de-

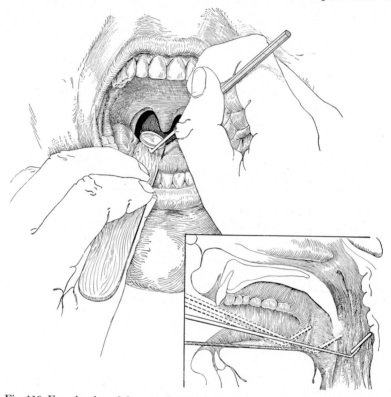

Fig. 119. Examination of the nasopharynx by means of a mirror introduced through
the mouth. The figure shows the various positions in succeeding portions of the
examination. A tongue blade is gently introduced and the tongue pushed downward.
The mirror is slipped along the tongue blade and in many cases does not even touch
the tongue itself. The mirror is held exactly as one holds a pen during writing. The
handle is lowered as the mirror is introduced into the mouth until light is reflected
from the mirror into the nasopharynx. This light returns to the mirror and to the
observer's eye. The mirror is rotated by moving the thumb on the handle so that the
handle turns on its long axis. This permits a panorama view of the nasopharynx.

scribed, since these have important relationships to the areas mentioned.
The same is true in diseases or disorders of the throat and for added
emphasis, these details are repeated here.

Oral Cavity. The condition of the following should be recorded:

Mucosa: .... Duct orifices: (parotid, submaxillary, sub-
lingual)................ Teeth:................ Gums:.................
Hard palate: (describe shape)......................... Occlusion:..........
Soft palate:...................... Tongue:.......................

Tonsils. The most important structures in the posterior part of the oral cavity are the tonsils. The following aspects concerning these should be noted:

Size (grade 1, 2, 3, 4):.... Color.......... Recessed?......... Crypts: (prominent or sealed)................ Expression obtained by pressure or suction: (describe)................ If the patient has had a tonsillectomy and there is some questionable tissue in the fossae: Is the tissue definite faucial tonsil?...... .... lymphoid buds?........... lingual hypertrophy?.......... remains of plica?........... Is there definite evidence of infection?......... Are the pillars intact?........................

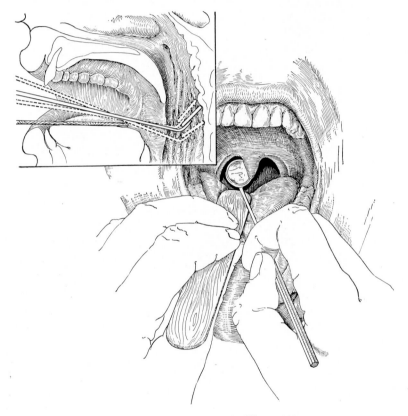

Fig. 120. See caption for Figure 119.

The Posterior Pharyngeal Wall. This is studied next. A considerable portion of it may be seen directly through the oral cavity by gently pushing aside the posterior pillars of the fauces, raising the soft palate and depressing the tongue.

Nasopharynx and Lower Pharynx. Beyond this, mirror inspection of the nasopharynx and the lower pharynx (Figs. 119, 120) is in order. This examination of the nasopharynx is often supplemented by inspection with the nasopharyngoscope (Fig. 121). The lower pharynx is studied with larger mirrors and in certain instances direct inspection with a laryngoscope or an esophageal speculum is indicated. The following details concerning the pharynx should be noted:

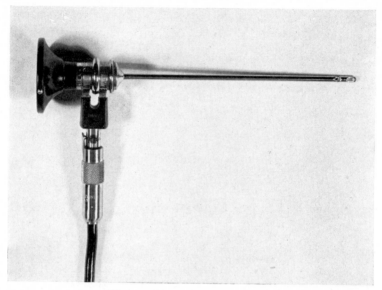

Fig. 121. The nasopharyngoscope.

Appearance: normal, injected, hypertrophic changes, dry. Secretion: mucoid, purulent, adherent, crusts. Are the hypertrophic changes in the nature of granular lymphoid patches?................ lateral pharyngeal bands?................. (grade 1, 2, 3, 4). Is there any other swelling? (describe)................... Mirror view of the nasopharynx: adenoid tissue?...... hypertrophied or atrophied? .... prominent crypts?.......... secretion? (describe)........... Fossae of Rosenmüller:................. Eustachian orifices:..................... adhesions?....................... Is the site of evagination of Rathke's pouch normal?............ Choanae: posterior tips of the turbinates: normal, hypertrophied, injected, pale, "mulberry"; mucosa on the vomer hypertrophied?..... .... secretion? (describe character and location)................... polyps (locate):................................

Lower Pharynx and Larynx. The next examination visualizes the lower pharynx and larynx. An adequate inspection of this area can usually be accomplished with the ordinary laryngeal mirror (Fig. 124), except in small children. The successful use of the mirror requires:

1. A clear reflected light by way of a head mirror.
2. A laryngeal mirror of the proper size. Several sizes should be available. The largest size which can be used is desirable (Fig. 122). It should be heated so that it will not steam, but not so warm as to cause the patient discomfort.

3. The proper position of the patient (Fig. 123).

4. Gentle tension on the patient's tongue, using a strip of gauze to grasp the tongue and gently pull it out. The under surface should be protected against the patient's lower incisor teeth. Carelessness on this point is often a source of considerable discomfort to the patient and makes it difficult for the patient to cooperate successfully.

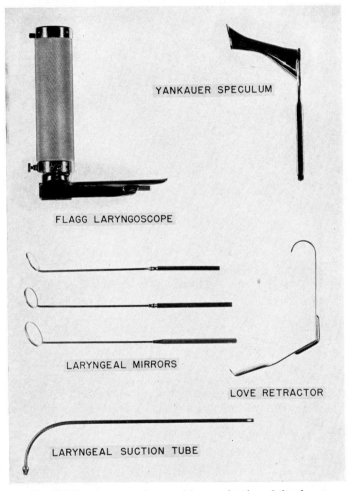

YANKAUER SPECULUM

FLAGG LARYNGOSCOPE

LARYNGEAL MIRRORS

LOVE RETRACTOR

LARYNGEAL SUCTION TUBE

Fig. 122. Instruments often used in examination of the throat.

Many patients start to gag as soon as the mirror is inserted into the oral cavity even though there is no actual contact of the mirror with the palate. It is wise therefore to instruct the patient carefully as to what is expected of him and to have him practice breathing and emitting the sounds Ah-h-h-h and E-E-E-E. When the patient breathes in and out regularly and does not break the rhythm, he will not gag.

There are persons who are amazingly easy to examine and others who present a difficult problem. The muscular person whose neck is short and tongue is big usually offers the most resistance. Occasionally a person is encountered in whom it is necessary to anesthetize the pharyngeal surface.

A small percentage of patients will be encountered in whom the position of the epiglottis obscures a portion of the vocal cords so that the

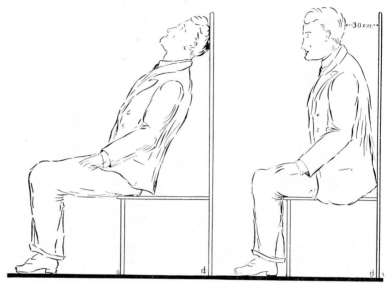

Fig. 123. "Pen sketch showing faulty position in which most patients will place themselves for examination of the larynx. The patient is sitting on the forward edge of the examining chair, the trunk is inclined backward and the head is thrown back as if to have the neck shaved in a barber's chair. It is impossible to get a good mirror view of the larynx with the patient in such a position."

"Pen sketch showing the proper position of the patient in which he should be placed for examination of the larynx with the mirror. *Before* he is asked to open his mouth he should be asked to sit all the way back in the chair. His head and shoulders should then be brought forward so that his vertex is about 30 cm., or more, from the vertical which is shown here as the back of the patient's examination chair." (From Jackson and Jackson: Diseases of Nose, Throat, and Ear. W. B. Saunders Co.)

anterior part of the vocal cords cannot be visualized. In these cases where it is important to visualize the entire glottis, a direct laryngoscopy should be performed.

The technic for examination of the lower pharynx and larynx is illustrated in Fig. 124.

METHOD OF EXAMINATION

Jackson urges a seriatim examination as the best means to insure against overlooking an important abnormality in its early and curable stage. He emphasizes the need of firmly establishing this habit of examination so that it is followed routinely so that there is a mental check-off of each part as it is examined. He suggests the following order of examination:

1. Free edge of epiglottis.
2. Posterior surface of epiglottis.
3. Right glosso-epiglottic fold.
4. Left glosso-epiglottic fold.
5. Right arytenoid eminence.

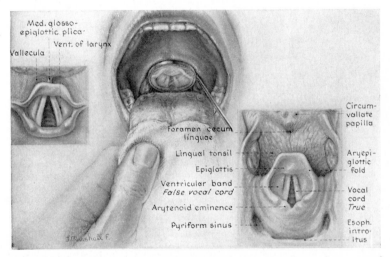

Fig. 124. Indirect laryngoscopy requires a mirror of the proper size, warmed so it will not steam on the patient's exhalation.

Gentle tension should be made on the patient's tongue, using a strip of gauze to grasp the tongue and gently pull it out. The under surface should be protected against the patient's lower incisor teeth. Carelessness on this point is often a source of considerable discomfort to the patient, and makes it difficult for him to cooperate successfully.

6. Left arytenoid eminence.
7. Right ventricular band.
8. Left ventricular band.
9. Glottic silhouette.
10. Right vocal cord.
11. Left vocal cord.
12. Anterior commissure.
13. Posterior commissure.
14. Anterior wall of the trachea.
15. All the foregoing observations are made without asking the patient to do anything, in order to note the condition during quiet

breathing. The patient is now asked to take a deep breath. Glottic silhouette noted.

    16. Movement, right cord.
    17. Movement, right arytenoid.
    18. Movement, left cord.
    19. Movement, left arytenoid.

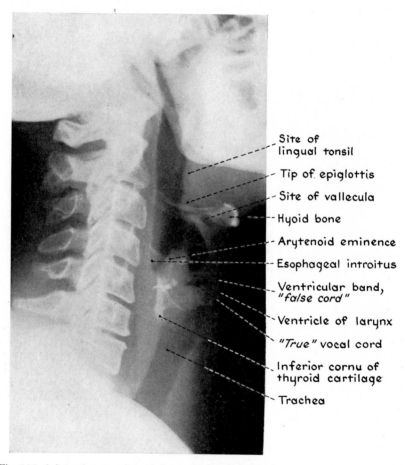

Fig. 125. A lateral x-ray view of the neck showing the airway from the base of the tongue through the larynx.

    20. Patient asked to phonate "E-e-e-e"; preceding four observations repeated.
    21. Repeat during long phonation of "Ah."
    22. Repeat "E-e-e-e", highest pitch.
    23. Repeat "Ah," lowest pitch.
Since a laryngeal mirror of the proper size is needed to study the

lingual tonsils, an examination of the lower pharynx and larynx should begin at this point. The details to be noted are as follows:

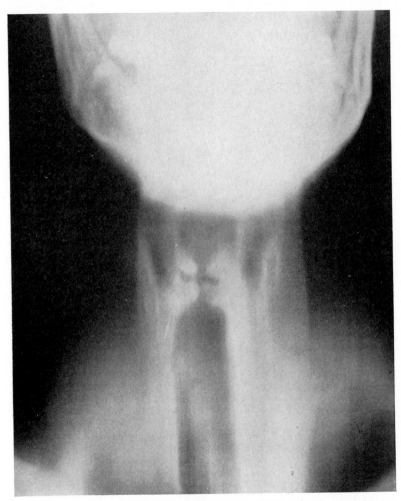

Fig. 126. Planigraph of a normal larynx.

Lingual tonsils: size? (grade 1, 2, 3, 4)........ evidence of acute or chronic infection? (describe).................. Site of foramen cecum: normal?........
.... Valleculae: note any abnormalities such as swelling, secretion, etc
.... Epiglottis: shape?.......... swelling or ulceration?......
.... Pyriform sinuses: retained secretion, swelling or ulceration?......
.... Ventricular bands: (describe any swelling, injection, ulceration or
other surface change)....................... Arytenoid eminences: (describe
any abnormality of movement, edema, or ulceration)......................
Vocal cords: (describe any swelling, injection, ulceration or other surface change)
.... describe any abnormalities of movements..................
Subglottic space:........................

The examination of the throat is completed by careful palpation of the neck noting the character and location of any swellings, palpable glands, tender spots and so on.

Some additional instruments for exposing parts of the throat are shown in Fig. 122. An x-ray study of the lateral pharynx, larynx and upper end

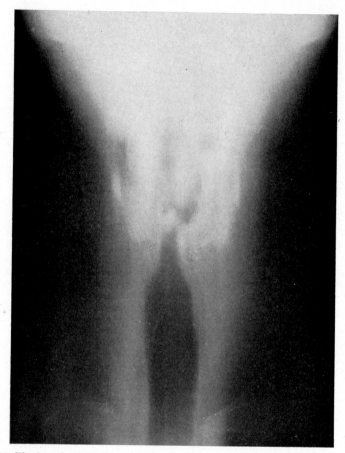

Fig. 127. Planigraph of the larynx shows infiltration of the glottis with malignant disease. The chief value of this is to delineate the subglottic extent of the disease.

of the esophagus (Fig. 125) may outline abnormalities which are revealed chiefly through soft tissue changes. Planigraphs of the larynx (Figs. 126, 127) are occasionally employed.

CHAPTER XXIV

DISEASES OF THE NASOPHARYNX

Robert E. Priest, M.D.

Knowledge of nasopharyngeal anatomy, physiology and pathology is essential to rational treatment of nose, throat and ear disorders. The location of the nasopharynx at the confluence of nasal, aural and pharyngeal air passages, with the base of the skull above and the uppermost cervical vertebrae behind, gives its diseases a special significance. Its tumors and inflammatory processes cause disorders in important neighboring structures. The nasopharynx shares the diseases of the nasal chambers and the oropharynx in addition to having its own maladies.

Nasopharyngeal malignancy often advances unchecked because it produces local symptoms which seem unimportant. When secondary involvement of adjacent structures produces symptoms too grave to be ignored, thorough search brings the primary disease to light. This may occur too late for treatment to be successful. The physician sometimes evaluates the symptoms improperly because he does not think in terms of nasopharyngeal anatomy, physiology and pathology. The nasopharynx is a neglected but important region. To emphasize its importance, an entire chapter of this text is being devoted to it.

APPLIED ANATOMY AND PHYSIOLOGY

The nasopharynx is the funnel-shaped cephalic end of the pharynx. The oropharynx and hypopharynx lie below it. The nasopharynx lies above the soft palate and behind the nasal chambers. The rigid, ovoid choanae open into the nasal chambers through its anterior wall. The posterior end of the nasal septum forms a vertical boundary between the two choanae. The posterior ends of the inferior and middle turbinates and the posterior portion of the nasal lining mucosa are visible through these openings.

The lateral and posterior walls of the nasopharynx are formed by the mucosa-covered upper parts of the superior pharyngeal constrictor muscles. The narrow portions of these fanlike muscles arise laterally from the pterygomandibular ligaments. The broad ends insert into the median raphe behind the cavity of the nasopharynx. The muscles are defective above, and the semilunar gaps are partially filled by the

pharyngeal aponeurosis. The pharyngotympanic tubes leave the pharynx
through such gaps.

Eustachian Tube Orifices. The most prominent features of the
lateral walls of the nasopharynx are the eustachian tube orifices (Fig.
128). They lie behind the posterior ends of the inferior turbinates.
Each is bounded above and posteriorly by a ridge of cartilage known
as the torus tubarius. This cartilage can be seen shining through the
mucosa of the tube openings in ordinary mirror examinations of the
nasopharynx. This cartilaginous ridge is used as a landmark when
placing metal catheters for inflation of the middle ear spaces. The
border of the tube orifices is deficient in front and below. The deep
pharyngeal recesses project laterally beneath the petrous bones above
and behind the tube openings. They are called the fossae of Rosenmüller.
They are clinically important as sites for growth of lymphoid tissue.

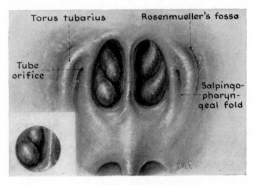

Fig. 128. Nasopharynx as viewed through nasopharyngeal mirror inserted into
the throat through the mouth. Mirror shows amount of nasopharynx indicated
in small insert at each position but by moving mirror entire nasopharynx can be
examined, and information on all parts of nasopharynx shown in larger figure can
be obtained.

This lymphoid tissue interferes with proper ventilation of the middle
ear spaces by narrowing the tube openings.

The position of the eustachian orifices in relation to the nasal chambers
differs in the child and the adult. In newborn infants, the orifices lie
on a level with the nasal floor. As the child grows older, the orifices rise
above the floor to take their adult position behind the inferior turbinates.

The child's tube openings lie directly in the path of purulent nasal
secretion flowing backward from the nasal floor. The straight, short,
almost patulous tubes lead infection to the middle ear. The adult tubes
are longer but not much wider. Their structure makes the adult middle
ear less accessible to infection originating in the nasopharynx.

Muscles. The levator and tensor veli palatini muscles are situated
on the lateral sides of the nasopharynx below the eustachian tube
orifices. These muscles extend downward to their insertion in the soft

palate. Their contraction, in conjunction with that of the superior pharyngeal constrictor, shuts off the nasopharynx from the oropharynx during swallowing. The same contraction opens the eustachian tubes. Normal tubes open with swallowing and yawning, but are closed otherwise. Some people can open their tubes at will by moving their mandibles forward. When normal eustachian tubes are open, there is free passage of air to and from the middle ear cavities. Equal pressure on both sides of each tympanic membrane is maintained. The tympanic membranes are delicately suspended and respond easily to the vibration of air against them.

The muscles forming the anterior and posterior pillars of the faucial tonsils extend downward from the lateral margins of the soft palate. The palatoglossus is in front and the palatopharyngeus behind.

Nerve Supply. The vagus nerves and the medullary portions of the spinal accessory nerves provide motor nerve supply to all of the muscles of the nasopharynx except the tensor veli palatini. The fibers of the spinal accessory nerves and the vagus nerves are distributed by way of the pharyngeal plexus. The tensor veli palatini muscles are supplied by the mandibular divisions of the trigeminal nerves through the otic ganglions. When normal action of the soft palate musculature is interfered with by disease or trauma, speech defects occur and food enters the nasopharynx during swallowing. These conditions are discussed in detail in the portion of this chapter dealing with neuromuscular disorders. The main sensory nerves of the nasopharynx are the glossopharyngeal and the maxillary division of the trigeminal. The great superficial petrosal nerves send sensory fibers via the vidian nerves and the sphenopalatine ganglions. The extensive connections of all these sensory nerves permit pain from nasopharyngeal disease to be referred to a very large portion of the head and neck.

Blood Supply. The blood supply of the nasopharynx is carried by branches of the external carotid arteries. The internal carotid arteries give off no nasopharyngeal branches but pass lateral to the nasopharynx in company with the ascending pharyngeal branches of the external carotid arteries. These arteries are sometimes involved in severe inflammatory processes of the lateral pharyngeal walls. The walls of the affected artery are weakened by the inflammatory process and rupture occurs. The ensuing hemorrhage is very severe and calls for immediate ligation of external, internal, or common carotid arteries.

Hemorrhage may not begin until a large abscess is drained either surgically or spontaneously. The release of pressure on the outside of the vessel by drainage of the abscess leaves the weakened vessel walls unsupported. Motion of the inelastic vessel or pressure of blood within it causes it to burst.

Mucous Membrane. The entire nasopharynx is lined by mucous membrane. This merges anteriorly with the nasal lining and below

11

with that of the oropharynx. This mucosa is stratified squamous epithelium in parts and typical pseudostratified ciliated columnar in other areas. The stratified squamous areas cornify but little. The mucosa is in apposition with lymphoid tissue in many areas. This structural arrangement is important in connection with certain malignant tumors to be considered later.

Roof of Nasopharynx. This begins in front just above the upper choanal margins and rounds over into the posterior wall. The roof is made rigid by portions of the sphenoid, petrous and occipital bones. These bones, together with the bodies of the cervical vertebrae, are points of origin of fibroangiomas of the nasopharynx. These tumors are discussed with other neoplasms later in this chapter.

Adenoid Mass. In the midline just behind the posterior end of the nasal septum is the adenoid mass (Fig. 129). This is sometimes called

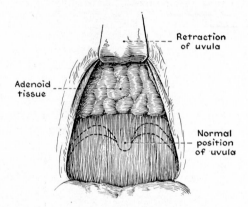

Fig. 129. Adenoid mass as seen at operation and drawn directly from life. A retractor is shown pulling the soft palate and uvula upward to expose the lower portion of the adenoid vegetations. Note the sharp inferior margin of the adenoid mass.

the pharyngeal tonsil. It is connected with the faucial and lingual tonsils by narrow ridges of lymphoid tissue extending down the lateral pharyngeal walls just behind the posterior tonsillar pillars. These ridges are the lateral pharyngeal lymphoid bands.

Tonsils. The pharyngeal tonsil, the lateral pharyngeal lymphoid bands, the faucial tonsils and the lingual tonsil form Waldeyer's ring of lymphoid tissue encircling the body's portal of entry for food and air. From the histologic structure of the lymphoid tissue, it seems probable that it plays a defensive role. The adenoid mass tends to atrophy after puberty. Its disappearance ought to be almost complete by the eighteenth to twentieth year. (For complete description, see Chapter XXVI.)

Pharyngeal Bursa. In the midline of the nasopharynx just behind and below the pharyngeal tonsil, a pit called the pharyngeal bursa is sometimes found (Fig. 130). It results from the ingrowth of epithelium along the course of the degenerating notochord. Clinically it may be important because of cysts which form at its site. Rarely, nasopharyngeal neoplasms arise from remnants of the notochord.

Mucous Blanket. The nasopharynx is the conduit through which inspired air passes from nose to oropharynx. Over its walls flows the mucous blanket carrying particulate matter entrapped as the inspired

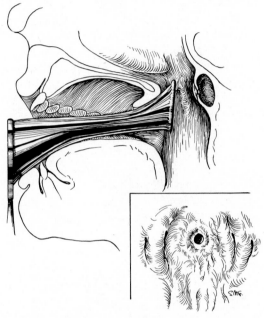

Fig. 130. Sagittal section showing Yankauer speculum in place to give view of nasopharynx illustrated in the small insert of the figure. A nasopharyngeal bursa is seen in both views, with a small round opening near the midline of the pharynx.

air goes through the nasal chambers. This mucous layer, propelled by the cilia, flows as an elastic but continuous sheet carrying particles on its surface like debris floating upon water. Its channels of flow are definite and have been mapped. This mucous layer is believed to be an important factor in protection of the upper respiratory tract against infection. The nasopharynx functions with the nasal spaces and paranasal sinuses as a resonating chamber for the voice.

METHODS OF EXAMINATION

The nasopharynx may be looked at directly by retracting the soft palate, and indirectly with a mirror or an electrically lighted nasopharyngoscope. It may be palpated by the examiner's finger. Radiographic studies are useful, particularly when neoplastic disease is suspected. The commonest method of examination is mirror nasopharyngoscopy. This procedure is successful in a majority of cases when the examiner has developed the proper technic. With practice, the procedure is simple, but to the novice it may seem impossible.

Mirror. A mirror from 1.4 to 1.7 cm. (9/16 to 11/16 of an inch) in diameter mounted at a 75 degree angle on a handle 20 cm. (8 inches) long is used (Figs. 131, 132). Such mirrors are designated as sizes 1 through

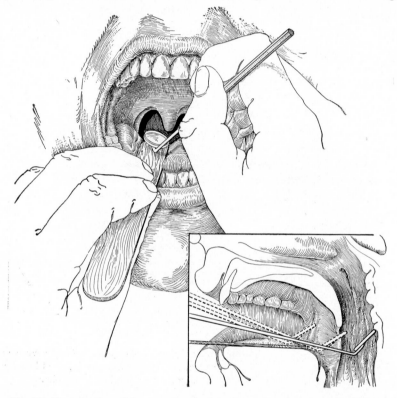

Fig. 131. Examination of the nasopharynx by means of a mirror introduced through the mouth. The figure shows the various positions in succeeding portions of the examination. A tongue blade is gently introduced and the tongue pushed downward. The mirror is slipped along the tongue blade and in many cases does not even touch the tongue itself. The mirror is slightly warmed to prevent fogging during exhalation. The mirror is held exactly as one holds a pen during writing. The handle is lowered as the mirror is introduced into the mouth until light is reflected from the mirror into the nasopharynx. This light returns to the mirror and to the observer's eye. The mirror is rotated by moving the thumb on the handle so that the handle turns on its long axis. This permits a panorama view of the nasopharynx.

3 by medical supply agencies. The mirror is warmed by holding its reflecting side toward the flame of an alcohol lamp or by immersing it in warm water. This warming prevents fogging by condensation of moisture carried in the expired air. The use of water to warm the mirror does not frighten children as does the flame. The warmth of the mirror should be tested against the examiner's hand before it is used.

The tongue is gently depressed with the left hand and light from a head mirror is focused on the pharyngeal wall just below the uvula. The patient is encouraged to go on breathing quietly. The handle of the mirror is held in the examiner's right hand like a pencil. The mirror is gently slipped along the tongue depressor and turned slightly to avoid the uvula. In most patients, the experienced examiner can carry out these maneuvers without discomfort to the patient. Local anesthesia may be necessary in some instances.

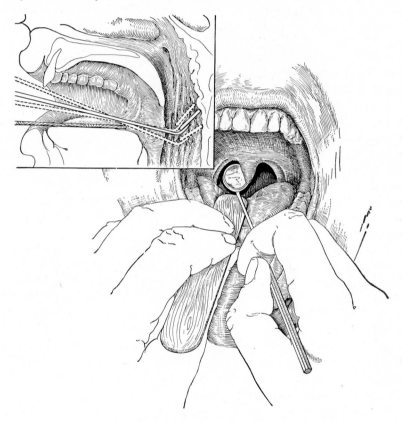

Fig. 132. Same caption as Figure 131.

After the mirror has been insinuated behind the uvula, it is tilted into a more vertical position and moved slowly by twisting the handle. The observer locates the posterior end of the nasal septum, and from this landmark the inspection proceeds. The choanae, the posterior ends of the middle and inferior turbinates, the vault of the nasopharynx with the adenoid mass, and the two eustachian tube orifices are visualized.

Direct inspection is possible only when the soft palate is retracted mechanically or is structurally defective. The tubular Yankauer speculum (Fig. 122) lifts the soft palate out of the way while the examiner makes his inspection through the instrument. An electrically lighted model of this instrument has recently been produced by an American instrument maker. The Love soft palate retractor (Fig. 122) is a properly shaped single blade which accomplishes the same purpose.

The soft palate may be retracted by means of two soft rubber urethral catheters. This method requires anesthesia of the nose, nasopharynx and oropharynx. A catheter is passed through each nostril into the oropharynx where it is grasped by forceps and drawn out the mouth. Each catheter thus forms a loop with one end protruding from the nose and the other from the mouth. Traction on the loops pulls the soft palate out of the way allowing the nasopharynx to be seen. This type of soft palate retraction is employed in operations upon the nasopharynx and is not ordinarily used for routine examination.

Digital Exploration. In children, one may find it necessary to explore the nasopharynx with his finger. This procedure takes only a moment. It is somewhat disagreeable but the child quickly forgets. Sensible parents do not object to this method of examination if they understand the importance of the information to be gained. Care should be taken to prevent injury to the soft palate. A mouth gag or bite block should separate the teeth to protect the examiner. Ordinary tongue depressors turned on edge are adequate. In larger children, several may be piled up and taped together.

Nasopharyngoscope. The nasopharyngoscope is an electrically lighted instrument constructed like a miniature cystoscope (Fig. 121). The instrument is 15 cm. (6 inches) long and 2.5 mm. ($\frac{1}{8}$ inch) in diameter. At one end is a tiny electric incandescent lamp and a lens which is the "eye" of the instrument. The "eye" is on the side of the instrument about 1.2 cm. ($\frac{1}{2}$ inch) from the end. The examiner looks through a lens which caps the opposite end of the instrument. By means of prisms, he inspects a field alongside the "eye" of the nasopharyngoscope. The instrument contains an optical lens system through which one can see structures at right angles to the long axis of the instrument. The nasopharyngoscope is introduced through the nose or mouth and the region above the soft palate is brought into view. This instrument is better suited to the specialist's practice than to that of the general practitioner.

LYMPHOID TISSUE OF THE NASOPHARYNX

The adenoid mass proper and other smaller lymphoid masses of the nasopharynx have long been the object of attack by physicians. At first this attack was not based on clear-cut therapeutic indications. Tonsils and adenoids were removed from a high proportion of American children. Many of the operations were performed without proper surgical indications. As time passed, the universal removal of adenoids ceased and the indications for adenoidectomy became clearer. Even today many children have unnecessary adenoidectomies, but the proportion is diminishing. Hypertrophied lymphoid tissue is usually removed from the nasopharynx because of its harmful influence on contiguous nasal and aural structures.

INDICATIONS FOR ADENOIDECTOMY

The following are indications for adenoidectomy. (For further discussion, see Chapter XXVI.)

Nasal Respiratory Obstruction. The mouth-breathing child usually is cured by removal of adenoids. It should be noted in passing that nocturnal mouth-breathing in adults is a firmly established habit. Ordinarily it is not improved by correcting respiratory obstruction. This does not preclude such correction for its own sake, but one should be cautious about allowing the patient to expect mouth-breathing to stop. Before adenoidectomy is performed in children, other causes for nasal respiratory obstruction must be considered. Nasal allergy, with its intumescent mucosa and polyps, is not cured by adenoidectomy. Nasopharyngeal neoplasms, retropharyngeal abscess and laryngeal obstruction must also be eliminated. A case of adenoidectomy is recorded in which the actual cause for the respiratory obstruction was an open safety pin in the larynx.

Upper Respiratory Tract Infections. Repeated infections in the nasal space or nasopharynx of children usually improve after adenoidectomy. Allergy must be taken into account but does not necessarily contraindicate removal of lymphoid tissue.

Tonsillectomy is generally performed at the same time as adenoidectomy. Some physicians advocate adenoidectomy without tonsillectomy.

Aural Complications of Hypertrophied Nasopharyngeal Lymphoid Tissue. Acute suppurative otitis media in children is nearly always the result of rhinopharyngitis. Enlarged and infected lymphoid masses in the nasopharynx totally or partially block the eustachian tube. Edema of the tube orifice occurs and infection extends through the tubal mucosa to the tympanum. Recurrent purulent otitis media or exudative catarrh of the middle ear constitutes an indication for adenoidectomy.

Acute serous otitis media results from tubal closure. Negative pressure is produced in the middle ear when the air is absorbed by the vessels of the middle ear mucosa. No more air can get in, owing to the failure of the pharyngotympanic tube to open, and fluid transudes from the blood vessels of the tympanic mucosal lining into the tympanic cavity or is secreted by the tympanic mucosa. This fluid is sterile. If pathogenic microorganisms enter, suppuration ensues. Recurrent serous otitis media is an indication for removal or irradiation of nasopharyngeal lymphoid tissue.

Partial tubal obstruction producing hearing defects in children has been studied since 1924 at the otological laboratory at Johns Hopkins

University by Crowe and his co-workers. From their studies, they discovered that many children showed loss of hearing for the higher tones normally audible to the human ear. Some children regained hearing for these tones after adenoidectomy. The observation that hearing did not always return after operation led the investigators to reexamine the upper air passages in search for the cause. Masses of lymphoid tissue were found to have overgrown the eustachian tube orifices in most cases. This lymphoid tissue interfered with proper aeration of the tympanic cavities and the ears gradually ceased to hear the higher tones of the normal auditory range. The tones of human speech are among the lowest heard by the human ear. As the damage progressed from higher to lower portions of the auditory scale, the conversational range was finally invaded. Undetected damage was being done for a long time before the speech range was reached. Such damage was not reversible if it had existed too long.

TREATMENT BY IRRADIATION

The location of the offending lymphoid tissue around and actually within the tube orifices precludes surgical removal without injury to the tubes. The susceptibility of lymphoid tissue to irradiation suggests the use of roentgen rays or radium as a method of treatment. Irradiation in safe doses does not destroy lymphoid tissue but does reduce its size.

Irradiation of the eustachian tubes and the area of the nasopharynx near the eustachian tubes may be accomplished by using a source of irradiation within the nasopharynx or by using a roentgen tube as a source outside the nasopharynx. The irradiation from the tube is applied through the mouth and through the skin.

The offending lymphoid tissue is not scattered along the entire eustachian tube but is situated mainly in the pharyngeal end of the tube. It is easily reached by a nasopharyngeal source of irradiation. When the beam from an outside source passes through the salivary glands, bones and other structures of small children's heads, damage may occur. If small portals are used outside, slight movement of the child gets the beam out of line and prevents accurate cross-firing on the target. If large portals are employed, the proper nasopharyngeal dose is easily reached, but too much treatment is given to other parts of the head. It is an advantage to have nasopharyngeal irradiation applied by the physician studying and treating the ear disorder; but roentgen ray treatments require a trained radiologist for safety. High voltage roentgen therapy is more expensive than the other type.

Applicators. For all these reasons a capsule made of monel metal containing radium salt has been devised for use in the nasopharynx. It depends for its effectiveness on beta rays and must be very accurately placed because these rays travel only a short distance. The beta rays have a power of penetration in tissue of about 8 or 9 mm. ($\frac{3}{8}$ inch). The

50 mg. radium applicator is used for 12 minutes (600 milligram-minutes) in each side of the nasopharynx for three applications given a minimum of two weeks apart (Fig. 42).

The applicator is inserted either without anesthesia or after topical anesthesia of the lower part of the nasal space has been secured. The end of the applicator, containing radium is held next to the lymphoid tissue to be irradiated. Its position is determined by visualization with the nasopharyngoscope inserted through the opposite side of the nose, or by touching the posterior pharyngeal wall with the applicator and withdrawing it to a position opposite to the tube orifice.

Irradiation of nasopharyngeal lymphoid tissue is not a cure-all. Its purpose is to make the local condition of the nasopharynx as favorable as possible for normal functioning of the eustachian tubes. Thus loss of hearing from eustachian tube narrowing or closure may be prevented or minimized. Irradiation of nasopharyngeal lymphoid tissue has been carried out at the University of Minnesota since 1939. The treatment has proved to be a useful adjunct to surgical removal of adenoids, but is not a substitute for surgery.

SURGICAL REMOVAL OF NASOPHARYNGEAL LYMPHOID TISSUE

Proper removal of nasopharyngeal lymphoid tissue is more important than tonsillectomy for many children. The exact surgical technic is taken up elsewhere in this text, but a few comments are appropriate here.

The operation should be conducted with the adenoid mass under the direct vision of the surgeon. The soft palate should be retracted by the Love retractor or by rubber catheters as outlined in the section on methods of examination earlier in this chapter. Anesthesia should be such that the airway is open and free. The surgeon should have enough time to remove the adenoid mass completely.

The practice of discontinuing the anesthesia when the faucial tonsils have been excised, then blindly removing the most prominent part of the adenoid mass by inserting the guillotine type adenotome is poor surgery. The surgeon who assumes that he has performed an adenoidectomy in this manner will be disillusioned if he will visualize the nasopharynx when he has completed his procedure.

The gullotine-type adenotome, the curette, and dissection using scissors and tonsil hemostatic forceps may all be necessary for complete removal of adenoids in many cases. The adenoid tissue can seldom be adequately removed in one piece.

POSTNASAL DRAINAGE

The natural depository for nasal secretions is the nasopharynx. Postnasal drainage, therefore, is normal. The nasal mucosa secretes about a quart of fluid each day, and what is not absorbed by the inspired air as part of the nose's air-conditioning function is propelled by the nasal cilia to the back of the nose and deposited in the nasopharynx with the help of the wiping action of the soft palate. Normally the postnasal drainage is unnoticeable and has no effect on the mucosa of the pharynx. It is nature's intention, apparently, that this secretion should be swallowed.

However, if the nose or the sinuses are infected and the mucous blanket is depositing a continuous load of irritative purulent material in the nasopharynx, the mucous membrane becomes thickened and inflamed as a matter of self protection.

This postnasal drainage and its effect on the pharyngeal mucosa are sometimes the only evidences of the presence of a low grade sinus infection. The lateral lymph structures which course down the side walls of the pharynx on each side of the eustachian orifices can then be seen as red hypertrophic bands behind the posterior tonsillar pillars.

Excessive postnasal drainage may come from causes other than sinusitis. A person who breathes dusty air or irritative vapors into his nose naturally needs more nasal secretion to accomplish his nasal air-conditioning than one not so subjected. So, likewise, should the smoker expect more postnasal secretion than the nonsmoker.

The thick, boggy mucosa of an allergic person also secretes more mucus than is normal because of the irritative nature of the offending allergen. The ability to secrete more mucus to carry away offending materials, whether pollen, smoke, pus, or dirt, is a major weapon of the nose in its attempts to defend itself. Sometimes the offender may be a constant one—a septal spur or marked deviation may be in contact with the turbinate or perhaps be close enough to it that it makes contact when the turbinate becomes larger for some physiological reason. If so, the nose responds in the same manner—it attempts to wash out the offender—and in this case, it becomes a more or less continuous process.

Excessive drainage of this sort may cause chronic cough, hoarseness, or cracking of the voice, especially on tones in the very high and very low registers. Irritation of the larynx and the epiglottis are commonly caused by excessive postnasal discharge. It may cause and keep alive a chronic bronchitis or bronchiectasis.

ETIOLOGY

There are, however, several clinical entities in the nasopharynx which cause postnasal discharge. These are:

Pharyngeal Bursa (Thornwaldt's Disease). Occasionally postnasal discharge is produced by mucoid material draining from a pocket on the uppermost part of the posterior pharyngeal wall. This pocket is called the pharyngeal bursa (Fig. 130). When it is the cause of postnasal drainage, *surgical excision* or destruction by *surgical diathermy* offers an excellent prognosis.

Acute Infectious Nasopharyngitis. Sometimes inflammatory reaction begins in the nasopharynx, causing the patient to feel a hot, burning spot which persists and gradually develops into acute nasopharyngitis. This condition can be treated by local application of 5 to 10 per cent *silver nitrate*. The application should be guided by observation with a nasopharyngeal mirror unless a very weak solution of silver nitrate is used. If the infection extends to the nasal space or downward in the pharynx, and is accompanied by systemic reaction, such as malaise or fever, the use of *penicillin* or a *sulfonamide* is indicated.

Pharyngitis Sicca. Occasionally, extreme dryness of the mucosa of the nasopharynx is found. This condition is analogous to certain chronic dermatoses in some instances and cannot be cured, but can be treated palliatively by *irrigation* with isotonic saline solution (see p. 420) or topical application of such solutions as *Mandl's paint*. The formula for Mandl's paint is:

	Cc.
Iodine	.3
Potassium iodide	.3
Oil of gaultheria	.3
Glycerin	30.0

An applicator with a rather abrupt curve and on which the cotton can be wound securely is used. Two types are illustrated in Fig. 175.

Sometimes pharyngitis sicca results from the drying of secretions produced by infected posterior sinuses or pharyngeal bursae. Pharyngitis sicca is treated by eliminating the cause, if possible, or by palliative treatment if the cause cannot be found. It is a common accompaniment of atrophic rhinitis (see Chapter XX), but may exist alone.

NEUROMUSCULAR DISORDERS OF THE NASOPHARYNX

Lesions of Motor Nerves. The nerves supplying the muscles of the nasopharynx are interfered with in bulbar lesions, peripheral neuritis and tumors encroaching on the nerve trunks. Upper motor neuron lesions occurring in cerebrovascular disease can cause palatal paralysis. However, paralysis may result from hysteria.

Paralysis of the soft palate musculature prevents complete sealing off of the nasopharynx from the oropharynx during swallowing and results in regurgitation of food and fluid into the nasopharynx. This is a most distressing symptom. Speech in patients having soft palate paralysis has a peculiar hollow quality similar to the rhinolalia aperta of cleft palate patients. Enunciation is difficult. The enunciation may be temporarily corrected by closing the nose. The ultimate prognosis of neurologic disorders depends on the cause. Diphtheritic peripheral neuritis may last several months but usually recovers. No general statement of prognosis can be given for paralyses due to tumors or cerebrovascular disease. Hysterical paralysis is usually temporary.

Trauma. Traumatic interference with soft palate musculature by tonsillectomy and adenoidectomy may lead to changes in vocal resonance. When the operation has been properly performed, these changes are unimportant and recovery is prompt. However, the possibilities should be anticipated and understood before operation on singers. Many singers have noted increased vocal resonance after tonsillectomy. The few who believe that their voices are changed for the worse are difficult patients. The surgeon should protect himself by being sure that they understand the situation prior to operation. However, one cannot promise the patient that the voice will not be temporarily altered, but an operation skilfully done in an adult should produce no alteration of the singing or speaking voice.

Permanent or intermittent patency of the eustachian tubes is occasionally encountered. The patient complains that he hears his own breathing and talking. One or both ears may be involved. Changes in position of the head may eliminate the sounds. The patient's breathing is plainly audible to the examiner if he connects his own ear to that of the patient with a rubber tube. The condition usually occurs in persons who have lost weight rapidly. It is seen in young adults as well as debilitated old people. It may be due to interference with the tone of the tubal musculature. As a rule, recovery follows improvement in general health. Palliative treatment consists of insufflating *boric acid*, 3 parts, combined with *salicylic acid powder*, 1 part, into the tube through a eustachian catheter.

Glossopharyngeal Neuralgia. This disease is also called a tic of the glossopharyngeal nerve, and is a true tic douloureux, similar to that occurring in the trigeminal nerve. (See Chapter XVIII.) The very severe pain begins during swallowing, particularly when cold liquids are taken. The pain radiates from throat to ear along the course of the nerve. Sometimes the pain is entirely referred to the ear on the same side. The diagnosis is made by topically anesthetizing the lateral pharyngeal wall and tonsil. This temporarily inactivates the trigger zone. The pain of an attack will then subside and cold liquids may be swallowed without pain. The disorder is incapacitating. The treatment is *intracranial division of the nerve*. If the diagnosis has been correct, the treatment is satisfactory.

TUMORS OF THE NASOPHARYNX

Nasal polyps protruding into the nasopharynx through the choanae are commonly seen. They are more properly considered with nasal conditions. (For additional information, see Chapter XV.) Unusual neoplasms such as chordomas, neuromas, craniopharyngiomas and others do occur. Their diagnosis is made by histologic study. Their general importance is not great because they are so rare.

Two neoplasms do occur in the nasopharynx often enough to justify thorough consideration in this text. These are fibroma and carcinoma.

Nasopharyngeal Fibroma. This tumor, also called vascular fibroma, fibroangioma and juvenile sarcoma, occurs chiefly in males between ten and thirty years of age. It arises from the basi-occipital, body of the sphenoid, medial pterygoid laminae and the anterior surfaces of the first two cervical vertebrae. The tumor does not metastasize or infiltrate. It destroys by pressure necrosis.

Nasal obstruction is the most prominent symptom produced by a nasopharyngeal fibroma. Bleeding as a primary symptom is uncommon. There is little pain. Changes in the voice, and aural symptoms resulting from eustachian tube involvement are frequent. Diagnosis is made by inspection of the nasopharynx. The lesion is not often visible when the oropharynx is inspected through the mouth in the usual throat examination.

Grossly, these tumors are pink or red, resemble nasal polyps in appearance, but bleed freely on slight manipulation. Microscopically, they consist mainly of connective tissue and a large number of blood and lymph vessels. Some areas resemble sarcoma. There usually are areas having the histology of inflammatory tissue or a fibromyxoma or a fibroangioma. The vessels are often cavernous. When this tumor is encountered, care must be taken to prevent excessive bleeding. Radium and electrocoagulation are the agents used to eradicate a tumor of this type. Excision is extremely dangerous because of hemorrhage. However, in competent hands, the mortality from this lesion is very low. When treatment is carried out, the equipment and surroundings must be such that hemorrhage can be dealt with promptly. Only experienced operators should attempt treatment.

Cancer of the Nasopharynx. This disease makes up from 2 to 3 per cent of malignancies of the head and neck. Epidermoid carcinoma is by far the most common type of tumor. A few sarcomas, notochord tumors and adenocarcinomas of salivary gland origin are encountered.

The exact histological classification of carcinomas of the nasopharynx has produced much discussion. These tumors arise from an area covered by stratified squamous epithelium in apposition with lymphoid tissue. The term "lympho-epithelioma" has been advocated. This term has suggested to some observers that the tumors are a form of malignant lymphoma. This view is not widely accepted. The general opinion is that these are highly undifferentiated carcinomas which contain many lymphocytes because of their area of origin. They behave like carcinomas generally.

All malignant neoplasms of the epipharynx must be diagnosed early if treatment is to be of any value. One large series shows that an average of fifteen months elapsed between the first symptoms and beginning of treatment (Furstenburg). Other investigators report that 32 per cent of their patients have had operations such as mastoidectomy and tonsillectomy as a result of erroneous diagnoses (Hauser and Brownell). Thorough inspection of the nasopharynx is the only way in which early diagnosis can be made. Much valuable information can be gained later by roentgen studies of the skull base and of the nasopharynx (Belanger and Dyke).

Carcinomas of the nasopharynx may produce no local symptoms. They metastasize early via the lymphatics. Enlargement of cervical nodes is often the first symptom. Nasal obstruction or epistaxis may lead to diagnosis. Pain in the ear or development of symptoms of eustachian tube closure are common.

The location of the primary tumor adjacent to the base of the skull permits early infiltration of the cranial bones. This produces localized pain and allows the tumor to extend into the foramina of the base of the skull. Symptoms resulting from interference with the structures passing through these foramina are among the most prominent produced by the tumor. Involvement of any or all the cranial nerves occurs. Various combinations of symptoms resulting from paralysis of some cranial nerves with sparing of others are seen.

Treatment. Most authorities agree that the only rational treatment for nasopharyngeal cancer is *irradiation*. A few physicians use electrocoagulation and one large clinic uses actual cautery. Furstenburg believes that treatment by any method is completely futile. New and Stevenson of the Mayo Clinic reported a small proportion of five- and ten-year cures of nasopharyngeal cancer. In their opinion, squamous carcinoma with cervical lymph node metastases offers the worst prognosis, carcinoma without metastasis is next poorest in outlook, and sarcoma has the best prognosis. Their treatment is by irradiation only. They apply radium directly to the tumor as well as using high voltage roentgen therapy from portals on the skin or in the mouth.

It must be emphasized that these highly undifferentiated tumors are very sensitive to irradiation. The initial response is often good. This may give rise to a false sense of security. The recurrences, which almost always occur, are not very radio-sensitive and the prognosis is poor.

The relief of pain in cancer of the nasopharynx is most important. Even though the lesion cannot be cured, the use of neurosurgical measures to make the patient more comfortable is a contribution. That such measures exist must be borne in mind by anyone caring for these patients (Pack and Livingston).

REFERENCES

Belanger, W. G., and Dyke, C. G.: Roentgen Diagnosis of Malignant Nasopharyngeal Tumors. Am. J. Roentgenol., *50:*9, 1943.
Coates, G. M.: The Nasopharynx. Arch. Pediat., *60:*10, 1943.
Crowe, S. J.: The Prevention of Deafness. J.A.M.A., *112:*585, 1939.

Crowe, S. J.: Irradiation of Nasopharynx. Ann. Otol., Rhin. & Laryng., *57*:779, 1946.

Decker, R. M.: Relation of Eustachian Tube to Chronic Progressive Deafness. Arch. Otolaryng., *36*:926, 1942.

Figi, F. A.: Fibromas of the Nasopharynx. J.A.M.A., *115*:665, 1940.

Fisher, G. E.: Use of Radium to Irradiate Lymphoid Tissue Around Eustachian Tube in Conduction Deafness. Ann. Otol., Rhinol. & Laryng., *52*:473, 1943.

Fowler, E. F., Jr.: Nonsurgical Treatment of Deafness. Laryngoscope, *52*:204, 1942.

Furstenburg, A. C.: Malignant Neoplasms of the Nasopharynx. Surg., Gynec. & Obst., *66*:400, 1938.

Godwin, R.: Thornwaldt's Disease. Laryngoscope, *54*:66, 1944.

Hauser, J. J., and Brownell, D. H.: Malignant Neoplasms of the Nasopharynx. J.A.M.A., *111*:2467, 1938.

New, G. B., and Stevenson, W.: End Results of Treatment of Malignant Lesions of the Nasopharynx. Arch. Otolaryng., *38*:205, 1943.

Pack, G. T., and Livingston, E. M.: The Treatment of Cancer and Allied Diseases. New York, Paul B. Hoeber, Inc., 1940, p. 2319.

Proetz, A.: "Postnasal Drip:" The Current American Nightmare. Ann. Otol., Rhin. & Laryng., *54*:739, 1945.

Thompson, C. M., and Grimes, E. L.: Carcinoma of the Nasopharynx. Am. J. M. Sc., *207*:342, 1944.

Wechsler, I. S.: A Textbook of Clinical Neurology. Philadelphia, W. B. Saunders Co., 1947.

CHAPTER XXV

ACUTE AND CHRONIC SORE THROAT

John J. Hochfilzer, M.D.

The throat is considered to be the portal of entry of organisms which cause many diseases, and in some cases the organism enters the body through this portal without causing any noticeable local symptoms. A prompt diagnosis of the cause of a sore throat is important, as it may prevent the outbreak of a serious epidemic for a whole community.

ACUTE SORE THROAT

A list of acute throat infections regarded as clinical entities follows.

Disease	Incidence
Acute tonsillitis	Very common
Peritonsillar abscess	Moderately common
Lingual tonsillitis	Moderately common
Acute pharyngitis without membrane formation	Very common
Acute pharyngitis with membrane or ulceration:	
1. Septic sore throat	Rare
2. Plaut-Vincent angina	Relatively common
3. Diphtheria	Uncommon
Associated with blood disturbances, as in	
4. Infectious mononucleosis	Common
5. Agranulocytic angina	Uncommon
6. Acute leukemia	Uncommon
Retropharyngeal abscess	Uncommon

ACUTE TONSILLITIS

Etiology. A streptococcus, most often the beta hemolytic type, is the causative agent. Occasionally a nonhemolytic streptococcus or *Streptococcus viridans* is cultured, usually from the less severe forms. Nonhemolytic streptococci and *Streptococcus viridans* may be cultured from the throats of healthy persons, and particularly in the winter months and during epidemics of acute respiratory infections, hemolytic streptococci can be found in the throats of apparently healthy persons. It is possible that some of these apparently harmless bacteria may become activated as the result of a new strain of bacteria, a virus infection, or a general lowered resistance of the host.

Pathology. There is a general inflammation and swelling of the

318

tonsil tissue with an accumulation of leukocytes, dead epithelial cells and pathogenic bacteria in the crypts. It is probable that different strains or the virulence of different organisms may account for the variation of such pathologic phases as:

1. A simple inflammation of the tonsil area.
2. Formation of exudate.
3. A phlegmonous cellulitis of the tonsil and its surrounding area.
4. Formation of a peritonsillar abscess.
5. Tissue necrosis.

Symptoms. The patient complains of a sore throat and various degrees of dysphagia. In the severe cases, he is usually disposed to take neither fluid or food by mouth. He may appear to be acutely ill, and certainly he experiences general malaise. The temperature is usually high, sometimes reaching 104° F. The breath is fetid. There may be

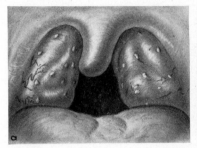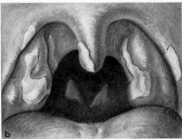

Fig. 133. (a) Acute follicular tonsillitis. (b) Membranous involvement of the tonsils and pharynx.

otalgia in the form of referred pain. Occasionally, otitis media is a complication of the inflammation in the throat. The cervical glands are often tender, but are usually not as enlarged as in the chronic infections.

The appearance of the tonsils is that of edema and injection. They are usually spotted, sometimes covered with an exudate (Fig. 133). This exudate may be grayish or yellow. It may become confluent and form a membrane and in some cases an evident localized tissue necrosis occurs.

In older textbooks, considerable attention was given to the differential diagnosis between acute tonsillitis and a diphtheritic infection. At the present time, diphtheria is a rather well-controlled disease, at least among those who have pediatric care, because of immunization. However, in any municipal or contagious hospital, diphtheria is not uncommon and it occurs frequently enough to make it important for the general practitioner, the pediatrician, or the laryngologist to remember certain differential points. These are:

Acute Tonsillitis	*Diphtheria*
1. Usually an abrupt onset with a sharp rise in temperature accompanied by a chill.	1. Onset and temperature rise more gradual, usually a low temperature.
2. Intermittently, the patient may not seem very sick.	2. Depression marked. Illness is obvious.
3. Lymphadenopathy not marked in the average case.	3. Lymphadenopathy common even in mild cases.
4. Exudate: limited to the tonsils, especially the crypts. It is characterized by not being adherent. It is soft and friable, and ordinarily comes away without bleeding.	4. Exudate: adherent, firm and leathery, can be removed in strips, leaving a bleeding surface.
5. Specific organism (*Corynebacterium diphtheriae*) is absent.	5. *Corynebacterium diphtheriae* is present.

Treatment. In general, the patient with an acute tonsillitis with fever should have bed rest and an adequate fluid intake with a light diet. Local applications, such as throat paints, are considered to have relatively little value. However, the local application of 10 per cent silver nitrate once or twice daily to the surface of the tonsil only, seems helpful in its local effect on the exudate from the crypts and the membrane.

Hot Throat Irrigations. Irrigation of the inflamed area in acute tonsillitis or pharyngitis adds materially to the comfort of the patient and contributes, because of its local effects, to the cleansing and processes of repair.

The equipment required consists of a one-quart container, two or three feet of rubber tubing, a glass or rubber irrigating tip, and a pinchcock to control the flow through the tubing (Fig. 174).

The patient is seated in bed or stands over a washbowl. The container with the irrigating fluid is held at two feet above the patient's head. The irrigating tip (Fig. 173c) is held in the patient's hand so that a stream is directed against the tonsillar area or pharyngeal wall while he breathes quietly through his nose. The flow of the solution is temporarily interrupted in case the patient has to gag, cough or swallow. The temperature of the fluid placed in the irrigating can should be as hot as can be borne on the back of the hand. A total of two quarts of fluid should be used.

The following solutions may be used for irrigation of the pharynx:

		Cc.
1.	Isotonic saline solution	
2.	Sodium bicarbonate, sodium chloride, āā..........	4.0
	Water (1 pint)...............................	500.0
2.	Liquor antisepticus N.F......................	120.0
	Water (1 pint)...............................	500.0

Formula for liquor antisepticus: Cc.

Boric acid	25.0
Thymol	1.0
Chlorthymol	1.0
Menthol	1.0
Eucalyptal	2.0
Methyl salicylate	1.2
Oil of thyme	0.3
Alcohol, distilled water, āā	q.s. ad 1000.0

An ice collar adds to the patient's comfort.

Gargles. The effectiveness of gargles has been questioned. It is true that the act of gargling does not bring much of the fluid used in contact with the pharyngeal wall. In most instances it does not go beyond the fauces. However, clinical experience would indicate that gargling performed with a certain routine is useful to add to the patient's comfort and probably influences to some extent the course of the disease.

Unless a patient is specifically instructed, he will probably feel that the treatment is finished when he has used up a glassful of lukewarm gargling solution. This is inadequate. The patient should be instructed to use three glassfuls of the gargling solution at one time. The first glassful should be as warm as he can comfortably stand it. The second and the third glassfuls can be hotter. It is well to give the patient specific instructions to use the gargling solution every two hours. It is practical to write on a prescription pad the hours on which he is expected to gargle and to ask him to cross off the time as he finishes each treatment. This will insure to a great extent his carrying out of the instructions given him.

It is probable that the heat of the gargling solution is more effective than its medical content.

The following solutions are useful:

1. Isotonic saline solution ($\frac{1}{2}$ teaspoonful of table salt to 1 full glass of hot water).

2. Sodium perborate powder (1 teaspoonful to the glass of hot water). This is useful in "Vincent's infections" or "trench mouth."

3. Dobell's solution.

The formula: Cc.

Sodium borate	15.0
Sodium bicarbonate	15.0
Liquefied phenol	3.0
Glycerin	35.0
Distilled water	q.s. ad 1000.0

(1 part of this solution to 1 or 2 parts of hot water.)

4. Alkaline aromatic solution (liquor aromaticus alkalinus, Seiler's formula).

The formula:

	Gm. or cc.
Potassium bicarbonate	20.0
Sodium borate	20.0
Thymol	0.5
Eucalyptol	1.0
Methyl salicylate	0.5
Tincture cudbear	20.0
Alcohol	50.0
Glycerin	100.0
Distilled water	q.s. ad 1000.0

(1 part of this solution to 1 or 2 parts of hot water.)

This medication may be conveniently purchased in tablet form as Seiler's Tablets. Dissolve three or four tablets in a glass of hot water for gargling.

5. Troches and powders. Medicated troches have long been used to treat throat infections. Their exact value is questionable except in the more recent use of penicillin medications, which apparently are effective in some instances. These are prescribed as follows:

Penicillin troches, 1000 to 2500 units. Dissolve one between cheek and teeth every two to three hours.

Sulfathiazole gum (each piece contains $3\frac{3}{4}$ grains or 0.25 gm. of sulfathiazole). It seems doubtful that the small amount of sulfonamide in the gum could really be very effective. The patient is given directions to chew two tablets for ten to twenty minutes every three hours.

Powders for analgesic effect are ethyl amino benzoate (benzocaine) and orthoform. One of these powders may be applied lightly to the throat with a powder blower or inhaled through a glass tube from a small saucer.

Today, penicillin is the most effective drug to use in checking an attack of acute tonsillitis. It is most effective when given parenterally in adequate doses.

PERITONSILLAR ABSCESS

Etiology. Occasionally, the infection of the tonsil extends through the capsule to form an abscess in the surrounding tissue. It may occur early or late in the course of an acute tonsillitis. It is usually unilateral and is rare in children.

Pathology. A suppurative infiltration of the peritonsillar tissue occurs most often in the supratonsillar fossa. It causes edema of the palate on the involved side and displacement of the uvula. The swelling often extends to adjacent tissues causing painful swallowing, trismus, and so on.

Symptoms. In a moderately severe case, there is usually a marked dysphagia, pain referred to the ear of the involved side, increased salivation and trismus. The swelling interferes with articulation and, if marked, the patient speaks with difficulty. The fever usually is around 100° F., although it occasionally goes considerably higher. A thorough inspection of the swollen area may be difficult because of the patient's inability to open his mouth. The examination causes the patient considerable discomfort. There can be little doubt about the diagnosis in a typical case when the examiner views the reddened peritonsillar swelling of the soft palate, the edema of the uvula and the bulging of the swollen tissues toward the midline. Peritonsillitis may, of course, occur without abscess formation. Complications caused by a spread of the infection have occurred, such as edema of the glottis, or a thrombophlebitis of the veins in the neck.

Treatment. The modern treatment of acute tonsillitis with the *sulfonamides* or *penicillin*, or their combination, has apparently reduced the incidence of peritonsillar abscess. When an abscess forms, it should be drained surgically (Fig. 134). An incision made with a thin, sharp

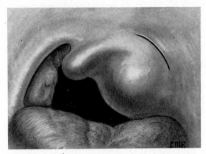

Fig. 134. Peritonsillar abscess (Quinsy). Site for incision for drainage.

blade at the point of greatest bulging will usually provide dramatic relief as soon as the pus escapes. A small, blunt hemostat gently inserted into the incision should be spread to aid evacuation of the abscess. Surgical drainage of a peritonsillar abscess is performed in large children and adults without any anesthesia except a local application of 10 per cent cocaine to the site of the incision and a similar application to the area of the sphenopalatine ganglion which will allow greater freedom in opening the mouth. Small children need a general anesthetic. After induction, a mouth gag is inserted and the head lowered. The contents of the abscess should then be promptly aspirated by suction as soon as it is opened.

LINGUAL TONSILLITIS

The lingual tonsils do not have the complex crypt arrangement, nor are they as large as the faucial tonsils. This accounts for acute infections of the faucial tonsils being more common. Rarely are the lingual tonsils acutely inflamed along with the faucial tonsil. As a clinical entity, lingual tonsillitis is more common in tonsillectomized patients and in adults.

The etiology and pathology are much the same as those of an acute inflammation of the faucial tonsils. The symptoms usually are soreness on swallowing, a sense of lump in the throat, malaise, a slight amount of fever and, in some cases, cervical adenopathy with tenderness. Inspection of the lingual tonsils with the aid of a laryngeal mirror and reflected light reveals a reddened, swollen lingual mass with whitish spots dotting the surface of the tonsil, similar to those in an acute tonsillitis involving the faucial tonsils.

The use of *penicillin* or *sulfonamides* is effective, and 10 per cent *silver nitrate* applied directly to the lingual tonsils once daily for two or three applications also seems to have a beneficial effect.

ACUTE PHARYNGITIS

Some form of acute pharyngitis is a common disorder. Numerous attempts have been made at classifications of an acute inflammation involving the pharyngeal wall. It probably is most logical to group a

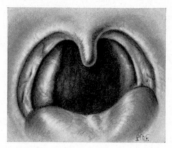

Fig. 135. Chronic pharyngitis characterized by marked hypertrophy of lateral pharyngeal bands. This is also referred to as a "lateral pharyngitis."

number of these affections under the relatively simple title of "acute pharyngitis." This would include acute pharyngitis occurring in the ordinary head cold, as a result of acute infectious disorders such as the exanthemas, influenza, and so on, and from the uncommon miscellaneous causes, such as is seen in herpetic manifestations, thrush, etc.

Etiology and Pathology. The cause of acute pharyngitis may vary from an organism producing a simple exudative or catarrhal change to one which produces edema and even ulceration. The organisms found include various streptococci, pneumococci, the influenza bacillus, and so on. In the early stages, there is hyperemia, then edema and increased secretion. The exudate is at first serous but becomes thicker or mucoid, then tends to become dry and may adhere to the pharyngeal wall. With the hyperemia, the blood vessels of the pharyngeal wall become dilated. Small plugs, white, yellow, or gray in color, form in the follicles of lymphoid tissue. In the absence of tonsils, attention is usually focused on the pharynx and it is observed that lymphoid follicles or plaques on the posterior pharyngeal wall or localized more laterally, are inflamed and swollen. This lateral wall involvement, when isolated, has been referred to as "lateral pharyngitis" (Fig. 135). It is possible, of course, even in the presence of tonsils, to have the pharynx involved alone.

Symptoms and Signs. At the onset, the patient often complains of a dryness or scratchiness of the throat. Malaise and headache are common. There is usually some elevation of temperature, although it is not marked. The exudate in the pharynx invariably thickens. It may be dislodged with some difficulty, causing a rasping, hawking effort and cough. A certain amount of hoarseness is present if the inflammatory process involves the larynx. In severe cases, there may be dysphagia chiefly as the result of pain, referred pain to the ear, cervical adenopathy and tenderness and so on. The pharyngeal wall is reddened. It may appear dry, with a glazed appearance and a coating of mucoid secretion. The lymphoid tissue usually appears red and swollen.

Diagnosis. The diagnosis is usually made without difficulty, particularly in the presence of the symptoms and signs just described. However, it is well to consider an acute pharyngitis as a symptom rather than a disease entity because it may represent the onset of a disease.

Treatment. The use of antibiotics and chemotherapy has changed the routine of treatment of an acute pharyngitis in recent years. This has resulted in a shortening of the disease and a lessening of the incidence of complications. *Penicillin* should be given parenterally in therapeutic doses.

The use of *hot throat irrigations* (see p. 420), a local application of 10 per cent *silver nitrate*, and *supportive care* in the matter of an adequate fluid intake, a light diet and elimination when indicated, is still important to hasten the recovery, in spite of the fact that a sudden dramatic improvement in the course of the disease often occurs with the administration of penicillin or sulfadiazine.

MEMBRANOUS PHARYNGITIS

Membranous pharyngitis has been described as a clinical entity, but a membrane formation occurs as part of several forms of acute pharyngitis which are distinct entities but which more or less resemble one another clinically. These are septic sore throat, Vincent's infection, diphtheria, the throat involvement accompanying certain blood disturbances, and the pseudomembranous character of a variety of throat disorders, such as is seen in the exanthemas and pneumococcus infections.

Septic Sore Throat

The laity and some physicians often refer to a "strep sore throat" as a particular form of throat malady which is identified with considerable morbidity either in the course of the disease or as an aftermath. This is obviously a misnomer, since streptococci usually can be cultured from most cases of an acute infection involving the structures in the throat. There is, however, a form of an acute primary infection of the tonsils and pharynx appearing in epidemic form and traceable to milk, which at one time was and still is in certain instances, designated as "streptococcus sore throat." The agent, a hemolytic streptococcus, is destroyed by pasteurization, so the epidemics of disease caused by this organism can only result from the use of raw milk in which the organism is present.

The symptoms are relatively sudden in onset. Fever, chills, pain on swallowing, malaise, headache and prostration are the usual manifestations. The throat is red and edematous. Spots or grayish surface patches may be seen. Complications were likely before the advent of penicillin or sulfonamides.

The treatment consists of *isolation* of the patient, *general supportive care, hot saline throat irrigations* (see p. 420) and therapeutic doses of *penicillin* parenterally.

Plaut-Vincent's Angina

This infection of the pharynx with fusiform bacilli and spirochetes characteristic of the disease is often referred to as "Vincent's infection" or "trench mouth." It is more often encountered in a limited form without systemic reaction than in the more severe form and it may be associated with other throat inflammations. The disorder usually originates as a focus in a tonsil or a carious tooth.

Symptoms. These depend on the severity of the disease. When localized, a dirty, sloughing, almost "punched out" ulceration is seen. Soreness, salivation, headache and low grade fever are the usual manifestations. When extensive, the febrile reaction and other constitutional symptoms are more marked. Adenopathy, particularly of the submaxillary glands, is common. The breath is foul. A grayish pseudomembrane rather dirty in appearance coats the involved surface. When it is removed, the under surface bleeds easily.

Diagnosis. Certain diagnosis is made by finding a practically exclusive amount of the characteristic organism in a smear made directly from the pseudomembrane. These organisms can normally be found in small amounts in the mouth and throat in ordinary gingivitis, and in the crypts of tonsils. In differential diagnosis, the possibility of the pseudomembrane found in cases of agranulocytic angina, leukemia and acute phases of pernicious anemia, must be considered. Diphtheria, syphilis, tuberculosis and malignant disease should also be ruled out.

Treatment. Topical applications of 10 per cent *salvarsan* in glycerin are beneficial. *Gargles* and *mouth washes* with either hydrogen peroxide (half strength) or sodium perborate (1 teaspoonful to the glass of hot water) are effective. *Penicillin* given parenterally is specific. It should be supplemented by the use of penicillin troches.

Diphtheria

The pharynx is the most common site for this infection. The diagnosis should be considered in all cases of sore throat with membrane. This is the most characteristic feature of the disease. When tonsils are present, the membrane usually starts on the tonsils and spreads to adjacent structures. At the onset, the membrane is white but usually becomes gray in color. It is adherent to the surface, which bleeds when the membrane is stripped off.

Symptoms. This disease may occur in a mild form in which there is relatively little toxicity from the disease except for that manifested in some malaise, headache, backache and sore throat accompanied by a slight fever. In the severe forms, chills and vomiting may occur suddenly with high fever and prostration. The membrane tends to spread rapidly in the severe cases. There is a peculiar fetid odor to the breath. Physicians accustomed to handling these cases often suspect the disease on the basis of this respiratory fetor.

Diagnosis. Smears made from nasal and pharyngeal secretions, and particularly the membrane, should be stained and studied at once while a culture is incubated. If the smears show *Corynebacterium diphtheriae*, the antitoxin should be given at once.

Treatment. The dosage for an average patient is from 20,000 to 30,000 units of *antitoxin*. The more severe cases require 50,000 units. *Isolation* is important. When there are laryngeal symptoms, it is important that the physician be alert to the possibility of serious respiratory obstruction. *Removal* of a laryngeal and tracheal membrane may be all that is indicated. *Intubation* or *tracheotomy* (see Chapter XXVIII) may, however, be necessary for safety and drainage if the obstruction becomes marked.

Penicillin or the sulfonamides are not in themselves particularly effective in the treatment of this disorder. As a supplement to antitoxin therapy, it would seem logical, however, to use penicillin for its effect upon possible complications in which secondary bacterial disorders play a role, such as otitis media and pneumonia.

Aside from the complications requiring intubation or tracheotomy, cardiac failure and muscular paralysis (involving the palate and larynx), are the most feared. An extension of the inflammation to the ears, causing an otitis media, or to the lungs, causing a pneumonia, is not uncommon.

Blood Disorders

Several diseases, which are essentially blood disturbances, produce a sore throat, at least in their acute stages, and an exudate which represents more or less of a membrane formation. These are acute leukemia, agranulocytic angina, and infectious mononucleosis.

Acute Leukemia. The onset is abrupt and the picture consists of angina, anemia, bleeding from mucous membrane surfaces, stomatitis and cervical adenitis. There is a tendency toward a gangrenous change in the involved mucous membrane surfaces. Fetor is prominent. Fever is present and prostration develops. A positive diagnosis is made by examining the blood, and the bone marrow. The treatment is palliative, supporting the patient by fluids, food and blood transfusions.

Agranulocytic Angina. There are two characteristic changes of this disorder: ulceration of mucous membranes of the body, most often in the mouth or throat, and an alteration of the bone marrow. The cause is unknown. The striking change in the blood and marrow is granulocytopenia. The ulcerations are characterized by an absence of the usual inflammatory reaction of the border of the lesion which is in keeping with the fact that the ulceration is not produced by inflammation but rather that it is a trophic change due to a lack of tissue resistance.

The disorder is more common in females. In an acute phase, the onset is abrupt and is characterized by high fever, chills, toxicity and prostration. A definite diagnosis is made by examination of the blood and the bone marrow.

Treatment. In the acute form, the disease has a high mortality. *Supportive care, blood transfusions* and injections of *pentose nucleotide* to stimulate the formation of leukocytes is considered to be the most effective treatment. Liver extract and the extract of yellow bone marrow have been recommended recently.

Infectious Mononucleosis. This is an acute infectious disease of unknown origin characterized by fever, lymph node enlargement and a blood picture in which there is a lymphocytosis ranging from 10,000 to 40,000 total leukocytes with 10 to 90 per cent monocytes.

Symptoms. These are similar to acute pharyngitis or tonsillitis. Fever, chills and malaise accompany an acute sore throat. The lymphoid tissue of the pharynx becomes enlarged and often ulcerates. Often this tissue in the nasopharynx becomes so enlarged that it blocks the postnasal space, obstructing the nose and the eustachian tubes.

The cause of the disease is unknown; it is thought to be due to a filtrable virus.

The course of the disease is usually protracted but ends in recovery. Relapses of fever are characteristic, in which this symptom seemed to be passed but recurs without demonstrable reason.

Treatment. There is no effective treatment which aborts or seems to hasten the recovery. The symptoms should be treated to give comfort to the patient. *Mouth and throat irrigations,* and *ice collar* to the neck and *rest* in bed while febrile are in order. The use of *penicillin* or a *sulfonamide* seems to have little effect upon the course of the disease, but may prevent complications.

RETROPHARYNGEAL ABSCESS

Etiology. This is essentially a disease of infants or small children. There is an accumulation of pus between the posterior pharyngeal wall and the bodies of the vertebrae. It results from a suppuration and breaking down of lymph glands in the retropharyngeal tissue. In older children and adults, these glands have practically disappeared. For that reason, a retropharyngeal abscess caused by ordinary pyogenic organisms is practically seen only in infants and small children.

The disease is secondary to an acute pharyngitis but is less common than it was a decade or two ago, probably due to a better control of infection with penicillin and the sulfonamides.

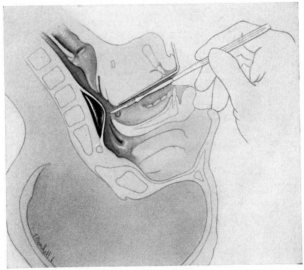

Fig. 136. Position of patient for incision of a retropharyngeal abscess. A mouth gag is usually employed to maintain an open mouth so that aspiration can be readily performed. (Redrawn from Hirsch.)

Symptoms. The disease should be suspected in an infant or young child when an unexplained fever follows an upper respiratory infection and there is loss of appetite and difficulty in swallowing. Stridor occurs when the abscess is large, or edema extends downward to involve the larynx.

Diagnosis. In the small infant, the swelling of the pharyngeal wall may not be readily detected by inspection or palpation. In these cases, a lateral x-ray of the neck may reveal a marked increase in the soft tissue shadow between the pharyngeal airway and the bodies of the vertebrae.

Treatment. As soon as a diagnosis is made, the abscess should be drained. This can usually be accomplished and with greater safety without anesthesia. A mouth gag should be inserted and gently opened, the head lowered so that escaping pus will not be aspirated, and a small pointed scalpel blade used to make a short vertical incision at the point of greatest swelling (Fig. 136). As a factor of safety, the knife may be passed along an index finger placed on the abscess as a guide. If pus does not escape, a small closed hemostat may be inserted into the wound and gently pushed to a deeper level and spread. As soon as pus escapes, the infant should be turned over with face down and lowered so as to prevent aspiration.

Continued postoperative use of *penicillin* or a *sulfonamide* hastens convalescence and usually avoids the necessity of repeated drainage.

Complications. Asphyxia and hemorrhage are the two feared complications of a retropharyngeal abscess. The former has occurred when a mouth gag has been inserted for examination and drainage, or from sudden rupture of a large abscess flooding the larynx with pus. When hemorrhage occurs, the bleeding is usually profuse and involves a pharyngeal branch of the internal carotid artery. Though a clot may form and the hemorrhage seem temporarily controlled, there is usually a second or third episode of bleeding which is fatal. The internal carotid artery on the involved side needs ligation.

CHRONIC SORE THROAT

The complaint of sore throat of a chronic nature is occasionally encountered when no evidence of local disease can be found to account for it. In some cases, some constitutional factor may be uncovered which may seem to be important in the occurrence of this symptom. Such factors as a secondary anemia or a hypothyroidism seem to explain the symptom in some instances. A proportion of patients with chronic arthritis complain of sore throat without evidence of an infection in the pharynx, or involvement the tonsils if present.

The following chronic throat disorders are clinical entities:

Disease	Incidence
Chronic tonsillitis	Common
Granular or hypertrophic pharyngitis	Common
Carcinoma	Moderately common
Syphilis	Uncommon
Tuberculosis	Uncommon
Fungous infections	Uncommon

CHRONIC TONSILLITIS

Diagnosis. This is undoubtedly the most common of all throat diseases. The picture varies. The diagnosis is made largely upon inspection. In general, there are two rather widely differing pictures which seem to fit into the category of chronic tonsillitis. One is the enlarged tonsil, with evident hypertrophy and scarring in which the crypts seem partially stenosed but from which an exudate, often purulent, can be expressed; or in which from one or two crypts, which are usually enlarged, a considerable amount of "cheesy" material or "putty-like" material can be expressed. A chronic infection, usually of a low grade, is obvious in this type of tonsil. The other is the small tonsil, usually recessed and often referred to as "buried," in which the margins are hyperemic and in which a small amount of thin, purulent secretion can often be expressed from the crypts. Cervical glands less often are associated with the large tonsil than with these smaller ones except in children. The small, fibrous tonsil which is recessed is thought to be the most potent in the matter of focal infection relationships. Both types of chronic tonsil infection may exist without soreness but at times may flare up in an acute attack of tonsillitis. Cultures from tonsils with chronic disease usually show several organisms of relatively low virulence. At times, pathogenic streptococci may be cultured, particularly during the winter months, even though the patient is apparently well.

Treatment. Medical treatment of chronic tonsillar infection consists in *aspiration of the crypts* and the application of weak solutions of *silver nitrate*. Aspiration is performed with spot suction or with a tonsil suction tube, the enlarged end of which covers the tonsil to produce negative pressure (Fig. 181). The immediate effect of this treatment is usually an improvement. Rarely are permanent results obtained. The one certain cure for chronic tonsillitis is a *surgical removal* of the tonsil.

HYPERTROPHIC PHARYNGITIS

Patients are frequently encountered who complain of a chronic sore throat and who exhibit, on examination, prominent lymphoid granules studding the pharyngeal wall or bands or plaques of tissue laterally, sometimes partially hidden by the posterior pillars of the fauces. Many writers have expressed the belief that an important causative factor in the production of these lymphoid structures is a nasal condition in which the secretion drains postnasally and irritates the pharyngeal wall. Mouth breathing is also held responsible to some extent for stimulation of this tissue to grow.

When the patient complains of frequent sore throats in the presence of prominent lymphoid tissue on the pharyngeal wall, the removal of this tissue by cautery or by excision is indicated. Small granules or follicles may be destroyed by applying a cautery point directly to the follicles. A prominent lateral pharyngeal band should be removed with biting forceps, excising it level with the surface of the pharyngeal mucosa. For palliative treatment, from 5 to 10 per cent *silver nitrate* applied topically, produces a temporary improvement. *X-ray therapy* may also produce symptomatic relief.

ATROPHIC PHARYNGITIS

A condition which is just the opposite of hypertrophic pharyngitis is not uncommon. Varying degrees of atrophy of the mucosal elements of the pharynx are frequently encountered. In the mild cases, the mucosa appears thin and glistening or glazed, with an absence or but few of the lymphoid collections which are seen in an average pharynx. On careful inspection, one can usually see that the blanket of mucus, which is normally transparent, seems thicker and semitransparent. It may be raised off the surface in spots.

In the advanced form of atrophic pharyngitis, the dryness is striking, the mucous coating is glue-like in its consistency and at times an actual crust is seen. When this secretion is removed, the underlying mucous membrane has a dry, furrowed appearance. This advanced stage of atrophic pharyngitis has been termed "pharyngitis sicca" and is usually associated with an atrophic rhinitis or "rhinitis sicca." (See Chapter XX.)

Etiology. The cause of atrophic pharyngitis is not definitely known. It has been claimed that it is due to the fact that the air is not sufficiently warmed and humidified by the nasal mucosa, as would occur in chronic mouth breathing and in the instances of atrophic rhinitis in which the air-conditioning role of the nose is not functioning. There are apparently, however, trophic changes in the mucosa which result in a hyposecretion of mucus which are influenced by some factor which is not understood.

Symptoms. The symptoms of atrophic pharyngitis are a sense of dryness and thickness in the upper pharynx. The patient's attempt to dislodge the adherent secretion consists of frequent attempts to clear the throat, usually by "hawking." Varying degrees of soreness are not uncommon. Hoarseness of a mild degree may accompany this disorder, owing to an extension of the process to the larynx and the irritation of frequent attempts to clear or cough out the sticky secretion. In some instances, there is fetor.

Treatment. When an atrophic rhinitis is present, this should receive the first attention (see Chapter XX). Local application of *Mandl's paint* is beneficial:

	Cc.
Iodine	0.3
Oil of gaultheria	0.3
Potassium iodide	0.3
Glycerin	30.0

The effect of this medication is to simulate secretion. *Potassium iodide* may be given internally too for the same effect. An average dose is 10 drops of a saturated solution three times daily with meals. A combination of the local application of a throat paint and the internal administration of the iodide is desirable. The breathing of warm moist air, such as can be accomplished by placing a hot moist turkish towel across the nose and mouth helps to moisten the inspissated secretion. Twenty or thirty minutes of this once or twice a day is desirable. Attention to matters of general health should, of course, receive consideration.

CARCINOMA

When a chronic soreness persists in the throat, it is important to scrutinize the pharyngeal wall in all its aspects thoroughly and repeatedly if an early diagnosis of cancer is to be made. The subject of tumors of the throat is covered in Chapter XXXI. Malignant lesions causing a complaint of sore throat are usually squamous cell carcinomas. These begin as a small ulceration which persists and increases in size. The lateral pharyngeal wall, the margin of the epiglottis, the aryepiglottic fold and pyriform sinus and the base of the tongue are the common sites in the early stages. The soreness is usually localized and is more of an irritation than a really painful discomfort. The patient usually complains of a feeling as if something was scratching or "feels raw," as might be experienced from a toothbrush bristle or a fine fish bone sticking into some wall of the pharynx. Accompanying this, there is usually an increased secretion of mucus in the pharynx. The patient clears his throat frequently in an attempt to get rid of this mucus. There are cases, however, in which the early local symptoms are slight and in which attention is not centered on the throat until a gland is found in the neck. This is more common with lympho-epithelioma or lympho-sarcoma, the surface of which does not tend to ulcerate while the tumor is small.

The diagnosis is not difficult to make *if the possibility of a malignant disease is suspected,* and looked for. Any chronic ulceration of the pharynx should be suspected of malignancy. Biopsy and microscopic study made the diagnosis certain.

SYPHILIS

In private practice, a syphilitic lesion of the throat is relatively rare. In free clinics or dispensaries in larger cities, all stages of syphilis involving the throat are occasionally encountered, though not as often as once was the case. The primary stage, a chancre, may be seen on the tonsil and adjacent pharyngeal wall, or the soft palate. In secondary syphilis, mucous patches and erythematous areas are more or less generalized in the throat and may cause hoarseness and cough in addition to the sore throat. The gumma of the tertiary form shows a predilection for the tonsil and soft palate and less often involves the pharyngeal wall. Healing is often associated with scar formation. On a routine examination of the pharynx, when scarring is observed, the experienced observer raises the question of a previous syphilitic infection or a tubercular process. The routine check on the changes in the blood by blood studies (Wassermann and Kline) should always be made in cases of chronic soreness with membrane formation and ulceration. Combinations of disease, ordinary infection and specific lesions often obscure the picture. In an acute process, the dark field examination offers a more rapid diagnosis.

TUBERCULOSIS

As with syphilis, tuberculosis of the throat is uncommon in private practice. The tubercular lesions which occur in the throat are seen not infrequently in large public clinics and among those hospitalized in sanatoria.

In the oropharynx, a tuberculous lesion is more likely to be found involving the tonsils, the adenoids, the pillars of the tonsils and the palate. Primary tuberculosis of the tonsils is believed to be due to a bovine type of infection. Other tubercular throat infections are usually associated with a positive pulmonary picture. Ulceration is usually present in pharyngeal involvement.

The epiglottis is commonly involved in affections of the lower pharynx. A chronic laryngitis in which the picture of injection and slight swelling of the vocal cords exists should always be suspected of tubercular origin whenever it persists. It has been estimated that as high as 30 per cent of tubercular patients in sanatoria have acute, subacute, or chronic laryngeal injection from the underlying pulmonary tuberculosis below.

Tuberculosis of the throat is a relatively painful disease, as compared with syphilis and carcinoma. In an advanced stage, otalgia via the glossopharyngeal nerve or the vagus nerve is common. Dysphagia, increased salivation, loss of appetite, fever and cachexia are common, as they also are in malignant disease.

Lupus as a chronic tuberculosis of the pharynx is rare. The most common site is on the soft palate, particularly on the anterior pillar of the fauces. When a diagnosis is made, general treatment is of first importance. Modern therapy of tuberculous lesions involving the throat points to *streptomycin* as the drug of choice in chronic lesions.

FUNGOUS INFECTIONS

A fungous infection as a cause of sore throat is rare. In the form of a hyperkeratosis, which is believed to be associated with a mycotic infection, this disorder is not uncommon, but in most instances does not cause an actual sore throat.

Hyperkeratosis of the pharynx is characterized by little white or yellow cone-shaped elevations, sometimes as large as a grain of rice, studding the lymphoid tissue of the faucial and lingual tonsils and the lateral pharyngeal wall. It is a disorder of the entire lymphoid ring of the pharynx. The small raised conical projections on microscopic examination show fungi of the mycosis type, usually *Leptothrix buccalis*, with a mixture of dead epithelial cells, nonpathogenic microorganisms and an absence of pus cells.

This disorder often exists without symptoms. In some patients, however, a scratchiness is experienced accompanied by a spasmodic cough. The diagnosis is rather easily made when one sees these whitish cone-shaped projections resembling on casual inspection an acute follicular tonsillitis except that other signs of inflammation are absent. These areas of keratosis are tenaciously adherent in spite of the fact that they are superficial. There is no bleeding on removal.

The best treatment is to grasp each projection with a fine forceps and pull it off the surface to which it is attached. There is no medical therapy which is effective. Spontaneous disappearance of these growths has occurred.

Actinomycosis and blastomycosis have been described, involving the tonsils and pharynx.

REFERENCES

Bloomfield, A. L.: Differentiation of the Common Varieties of Sore Throat. Stanford M. Bull., *1*:199, 1943.

Clodfelter, H. M.: Treatment of Severe Acute Tonsillitis with and without Sulfonamides. Ohio State M. J., *41*:819, 1945.

Figi, F. A.: Dermatologic Conditions of the Ear, Nose and Throat. Ann. Otol. Rhin. & Laryng., *48*:81, 1939.

Freedman, L. M., and Hirsch: Complications of a Peritonsillar Abscess. *Ibid.*, *51*:133, 1942.

Hochfilzer, J. J.: Phlegmon of the Neck and Osteomyelitis of the Mandible following Tonsillectomy. Arch. Otolaryng., *17*:697, 1933.

Hochfilzer, J. J.: Retropharyngeal Abscess and Massive Hemorrhage. Minnesota Med., *28*:644, 1945.

Hopp, E. S.: Penicillin in the Oral Therapy of Vincent's Angina and Acute Follicular Tonsillitis. Arch. Otolaryng., *44*:409, 1946.

Kuttner, A., and Krumwiede, E.: Observations on Epidemiology of Streptococcic Pharyngitis and Relation of Streptococcic Carriers to Occurrence of Outbreaks. J. Clin. Investigation, *23*:139, 1944.

Lillie, H. L.: The Clinical Significance of Compensatory Granular Pharyngitis. Arch. Otolaryng., *24*:319, 1936.

Marcotte, R. H.: Chronic Granular Pharyngitis. Ann. Otol., Rhin. & Laryng., *51*:400, 1942.

Pewters, J. T.: Epidemic of Acute Pharyngitis Due to Hemolytic Streptococci. Bull. U. S. Army M. Dept., *4*:579, 1945.

Rantz, L. A. : Natural History of Hemolytic Streptococcus Sore Throat. California Med., *65*:265, 1946.

Rosenberg, A.: Penicillin in Peritonsillar Abscess and Peritonsillar Phlegmon: Report of Penicillin Therapy in 25 Cases. Arch. Otolaryng., *44*:662, 1946.

Salinger, S., and Pearlman, S. T.: Hemorrhage from Pharyngeal and Peritonsillar Abscesses. *Ibid.*, *18*:464, 1933.

Schenck, H. P.: Chronic Infections in the Pharynx: A Pathological Study. *Ibid.*, *24*:299, Sept. 1936.

Schenck, H. P.: Histopathological Changes Occurring in Chronic Infections of the Pharynx. Ann. Otol., Rhin. & Laryng., *50*:817, 1941.

Shea, J. J.: Mycotic Infections of the Throat. Arch. Otolaryng., *34*:1171, 1941.
Endemic Exudative Pharyngitis and Tonsillitis: Etiology and Clinical Characteristics. J.A.M.A., *125*:1163, 1944.

CHAPTER XXVI

TONSILS AND ADENOIDS

Inflammation, acute or chronic, involving the lymphoid tissue of the throat is the most common disease in this area and probably of all diseases. The surgical treatment of tonsils and adenoids represents, in its incidence, about one-third of the number of surgical operations performed in the United States in any year. These facts indicate the great importance of the tonsils and adenoids, both from the standpoint of morbidity and also from the economic aspect.

The question, what are tonsils and adenoids? cannot be fully answered. In older writings, a number of theories have been advanced, none of which is entirely satisfactory. The most accepted theory of tonsil physiology is the one which contends that the tonsil plays an important role in immunizing the body against the invasion and multiplication of virulent microorganisms. Early in life, the first invasion of pathogenic organisms reaches the tonsils. From the resulting localized infection, the body is vaccinated against further invasion. The position of the Waldeyer ring at the entrance to the lower respiratory tract and the alimentary tract might lend support to the idea of this protective function. The fact that this function, if a function it actually is, should be so frequently lost in childhood through inflammatory change or excessive hypertrophy need not be an argument against this theory. The purpose could still have been fulfilled in the age period (infancy and early childhood) when the need may be greatest.

ANATOMY OF THE WALDEYER RING

The component parts of this ring of lymphoid tissue are the palatine or faucial tonsils, the linguals, the adenoids and the lymphoid tissue of Rosenmüller's fossa. These all have the same basic structure, a lymphoid mass supported by a framework of connective tissue reticulum. The adenoid (pharyngeal tonsil) has its lymphoid structures arranged in folds; the palatine tonsil has its lymphoid arrangement around crypt-like formations. The complex system of crypts in the palatine tonsil probably accounts for the fact that it becomes diseased more frequently than any of the other components of the ring. These crypts are more tortuous in the upper pole of the tonsil, become plugged with food particles, mucus, desquamated epithelial cells, leukocytes and bacteria, and are an excellent place for the growth of pathogenic bacteria. During an acute inflammation, the crypts may fill with a coagulum which produces a characteristic follicular appearance on the surface of the tonsil.

The lingual tonsils have small crypts which are not particularly tortuous or branched as compared to the palatine tonsil. The same is true of the adenoids and there is less marked crypt or crevice formation in other lymphoid collections in Rosenmüller's fossa and on the pharyngeal wall.

The most important of the structures in Waldeyer's ring is, of course, the palatine tonsil. The anatomical details of its relationships are very

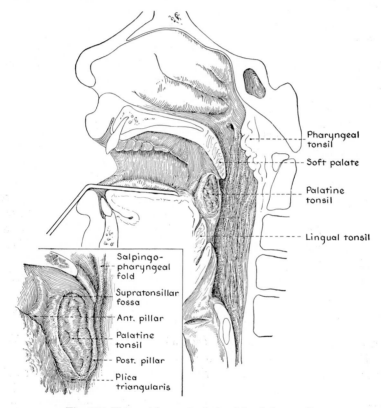

Fig. 137. The position and relationship of the tonsil.

important in its surgical treatment (Fig. 137). The tonsil surgeon must have a clear knowledge of the following:

1. The structure of the two pillars; the palatoglossus muscle (anterior pillar), and the palatopharyngeus muscle (posterior pillar).

2. The lateral boundary of the tonsillar fossa, the superior constrictor muscle.

3. The relationships of the plicae, particularly the plica triangularis.

4. The blood supply, which is derived from five arteries: dorsalis linguae from the lingual artery; the ascending palatine and the tonsillar,

both from the external maxillary; ascending pharyngeal from the external carotid; descending palatine from the internal maxillary.

Anomalous blood vessels in this area may offer certain difficulties in tonsillar surgery.

The main lymphatic drainage from the palatine tonsils leaves the fibrous trabeculae of the tonsil to pass through the capsule to the superior constrictor muscle of the pharynx. Several trunks form at this site, pierce the buccopharyngeal fascia and enter glands of the deep cervical chain from which drainage reaches the thoracic duct and then enters the general circulation. There has been no proof that there are effective afferent lymphatic vessels to the tonsils.

BACTERIOLOGY OF THE TONSILS

An extensive literature has developed on the bacteriology of tonsils. Cultures made within twelve hours after birth are almost always sterile; organisms begin to appear soon after nursing commences. Some of the micrococcus (staphylococcus) group are found first. These correspond to the organisms recovered from the skin of the nursing mother. Nonhemolytic streptococci begin to appear within twenty-four hours. It is assumed that these are derived from the throats of attendants. Other organisms recovered are gram-negative cocci and a few diphtheroids. Hemolytic streptococci are not found in the throats of well infants, but are frequently found in healthy adults from whose throats nonhemolytic streptococci, gram-negative cocci and diphtheroids are constantly recovered. Influenza bacilli and pneumococci are also found in relative frequency.

Nakamura reported a bacteriologic study of 2048 tonsils removed at the Mayo Clinic. These were removed because of recurring attacks of tonsillitis, but more often because they were believed to be foci of infection in a variety of conditions. Of a group of 1250 tonsils, 52 per cent revealed hemolytic streptococci, 58 per cent *Streptococcus viridans* and 18 per cent indifferent streptococci alone or with other types. Other organisms were also found. The virulence of these streptococci was of a relatively low order. A relative increase in the number of hemolytic streptococci occurred in December and persisted throughout the winter months.

VALUE OF SURGERY

The literature on tonsils and adenoids is tremendous and an expression of viewpoints and experiences still goes on. In the five years from 1942 to 1946 inclusive, there has been an average of over 100 papers per year concerning tonsils listed in the Quarterly Cumulative Index, and this in spite of war years, when medical literature was less voluminous than in ordinary times.

The most comprehensive survey in recent years is presented in a book by Kaiser, a pediatrician, who recorded a clinical evaluation of the problem under the title "Children's Tonsils, In or Out." Observations were made on 2200 tonsillectomized children, checked three years after operation and again ten years after the operation. The health of this group was compared with a control group in whom tonsillectomy had been recommended but not performed. The conclusions were as follows:*

1. The real value of removal of the tonsils and adenoids cannot be definitely established in a few years. Apparent benefits during the first few postoperative years are not so evident over a ten year period.

2. Outstanding benefits are apparent in influencing the incidence of sore throats over a ten year period.

3. Substantial benefits are apparent in rendering individuals less susceptible to scarlet fever and diphtheria.

4. Acute head colds and otitis media, though definitely lessened over a three year period, are not essentially influenced over a ten year follow-up.

5. Cervical adenitis is decidedly reduced in tonsillectomized children over a ten year period.

6. The respiratory infections such as laryngitis, bronchitis, pneumonia, not only are not benefited, but actually occur more frequently in tonsillectomized children.

7. First attacks of rheumatic manifestations occur about 30 per cent less often in tonsillectomized children. The greatest reduction occurs in children tonsillectomized early. Recurrent attacks are not benefited at all.

8. Incomplete tonsillectomies do not offer the same protection against the usual throat complaints and infections as complete removal of tonsils.

9. The hazards of tonsillectomy must be considered in evaluating the end results. Considering this hazard, the late results seen in 2200 children ten years after operation are evident only in the reduction of sore throats, cervical adenitis, otitis media, scarlet fever, diphtheria, rheumatic fever and heart disease.

With the advent of the sulfonamides and the antibiotics, these agents might have influenced a reduction in the indications for tonsil and adenoid surgery. It is my observation that this has not occurred to any noticeable extent. These drugs are effective in controlling acute infections involving the lymphoid structures of the pharynx and certainly have reduced the incidence of complications from these infections. However, the sulfonamides and penicillin are not effective in curing chronic infections of the lymphoid structures or reducing the physical factor of obstruction from hypertrophy whether the latter is the result of infection or some other factor.

Indications for Surgical Intervention. Today, the thoughtful pediatrician, internist, laryngologist and general practitioner who examines critically the tonsil and adenoid situation in his patients will find the indications for tonsillectomy included in three categories as follows:

1. Repeated attacks of tonsillitis.
2. Hypertrophy to the extent of obstruction.
3. Evidence of persistent chronic infection.

* Kaiser, A. D.: Children's Tonsils, In or Out. Philadelphia, J. B. Lippincott Co.

There should be little argument concerning the first and second indications. Simple tonsillar hypertrophy is common in early childhood and in itself is not a need for tonsillectomy. When the hypertrophy is excessive, the child is invariably a mouth breather, even though the adenoid may not be obstructive. Also, he eats poorly. In a majority of these instances, a considerable weight gain is experienced after the tonsils and adenoids have been removed.

The third category is one in which there is often the element of chance that tonsillectomy will not relieve a condition in which a focus of infection is thought to be a factor in the morbidity. However, the chance seems worth taking.

There are many aspects of this third category concerning which the pros and cons could be discussed. Not infrequently patients are encountered in whom the family or the doctor are interested in tonsillectomy to prevent head colds. When the tonsils and adenoids are obstructive or obviously diseased, the benefits from tonsillectomy and adenoidectomy in the prevention of colds not of virus origin are in most cases very obvious. When the tonsils and adenoids are within normal limits and removal is advised as a prophylactic measure, the end results are often disappointing. Some physicians have expressed a belief that removal of tonsils and adenoids has rendered a child more susceptible to head colds. It is possible that a protective function of the tonsils and adenoids does play a role in this respect. However, the fact is often overlooked that the early school age is usually the child's most susceptible period in the matter of respiratory infections, a period in which he may be developing some immunity, and that the removal of his tonsils and adenoids in a preschool period may have little to do with the relatively increased frequency of upper respiratory tract infections after he is exposed to the infections so prevalent in the early years of school life. (For additional information, see Chapter XXV.)

Adenoids. In most discussions on tonsils and adenoids, the attention is usually focused on the tonsils, and the adenoids receive secondary consideration. In the removal of tonsils in children, it is the common practice to remove the adenoids routinely. If the rest of Waldeyer's ring could be easily removed, it is probable that that would be done, even though the lingual tonsils or lymphoid tissue of Rosenmüller's fossa did not apparently share in the morbidity caused by the tonsils and adenoids. In recent years, increased attention has been given to the role of lymphoid hypertrophy in the pharynx as a cause of morbidity in the upper respiratory tract, including the eustachian tubes and middle ear. It is recognized that lymphoid tissue is an integral part of the mucosa of the pharynx in all persons, but in some persons the location of certain accumulations of this tissue, especially when infected, may result in morbidity related to hearing loss, attacks of bronchitis and asthma, and so on. The amount of morbidity caused by these accumulations is not in direct proportion to the amount of tissue present but rather to its location and to the apparent susceptibility of the patient to the infection. However, adenoid tissue when large in amount tends to block the eustachian orifices and the choanae so that nasal obstruction

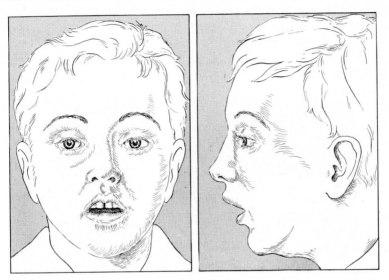

Fig. 138. The "adenoid facies" characterized by the open mouth, dull expression, and apparently short upper lip.

is experienced. An obstructive adenoid mass, in addition to being a prominent cause of mouth-breathing and the so-called "adenoid facies" (Fig. 138), may affect the appetite of children, since it is uncomfortable to swallow when the nasopharynx is blocked.

OPERATION OF TONSILLECTOMY AND ADENOIDECTOMY

General Considerations. The technics for tonsillectomy and adenoidectomy vary with the operator. Obviously, the aim is to remove the tonsils and adenoids cleanly with the minimum of trauma and bleeding.

In children, the use of a guillotine type of instrument, as initiated by Sluder and those who have modified his instrument, is popular. Others prefer the routine dissection and snare. Regardless of the method used, the skill and experience of the operator plays an important part.

Adenoidectomy is usually done with the LaForce type of basket adenotome or with the sharp curet. The latter is considered more traumatizing, but in experienced hands is a satisfactory method. Incomplete or traumatizing adenoidectomy is often the result of a hasty operation without proper inspection of the nasopharynx.

Careful attention to hemostasis (and the requirements vary with each patient) will, in almost all cases, prevent hemorrhage within the immediate postoperative period. However, regardless of the skill and care with which tonsils and adenoids are removed, troublesome hemorrhage may occur. This calls for prompt and adequate control of the bleeding point by local hemostasis.

At the end of the first postoperative week, the membrane lining the tonsillar fossae and adenoid space separates, and there is a slight tendency toward bleeding.

The tonsil and adenoid operations are classified in most hospitals as minor operations. In some instances, these may be relatively simple procedures. In others, the morbidity approaches or is greater than that of

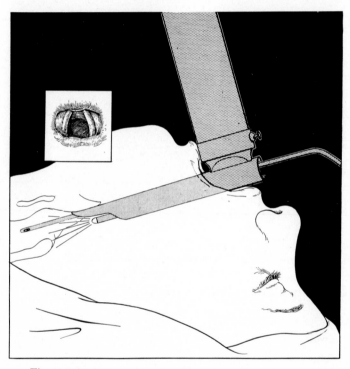

Fig. 139. Aspiration of trachea through the direct laryngoscope.

the average major operation. It has occasionally happened that this operation has ended fatally. I was once consulted on five cases within a year's time to express an opinion as to the fault in deaths associated with tonsillectomy. Three of these seemed to be anesthetic deaths and two could be blamed on hemorrhage.

Modern anesthesiologists remark that statistics indicate that the tonsil anesthetic as usually administered with ether is the most hazardous of general anesthetics.

Requirements. Skilful tonsil and adenoid surgery requires:

1. Complete visualization of the operative field by reflected light or illumination from a bright head light.

2. Exposure of the site with mouth gag and tongue depressor.

3. Placid anesthesia with free airway in those patients receiving a general anesthetic. Complete freedom from pain during dissection of a tonsil in those operated under a local anesthetic.

4. Systematic control of hemorrhage as the tonsil is dissected free. Prompt hemostasis by sponge and hemostat in the cases in which the tonsil is enucleated in one maneuver with a guillotine.

5. Thorough completion of hemostasis using a tie or suture when indicated.

6. Inspection of the adenoid space by retracting the soft palate after the adenoidectomy is completed. It is common to find chunks of remaining adenoid tissue and it is wise to clamp any free bleeding points with a hemostat.

7. Finally, it is desirable to have the tonsil fossae and the adenoid space very dry and free of clots when the operation is completed. Also, it is well to aspirate the pharynx and trachea with a laryngeal suction tube applied through a direct laryngoscope (Fig. 139).

INSTRUMENTS AND TECHNICS

The instruments commonly used for tonsil and adenoid surgery are shown in Fig. 140. There are two basic technics for tonsil surgery; one is a dissection method, usually completed with a snare; and the other is with a form of guillotine.

Dissection and Snare Technic. Figure 141 illustrates the principal maneuvers in this technic. The sites for injection of a local anesthetic, the usual method with adults, are illustrated. Otherwise, the steps are the same whether the patient receives local or general anesthesia. These are as follows:

1. The tonsil is grasped and pulled slightly out of its bed.

2. Incision is made at the junction of the anterior pillar and the tonsil near the upper pole.

3. I prefer scissors for dissection and use a Lillie model. The upper pole is loosened and then the pillars are freed.

4. Dissection is then continued to free the attachments of the tonsil to the bed of the fossa.

5. Hemostasis is secured as bleeding is encountered.

The base of the tonsil is dissected free and its attachment with the plica triangularis may be cut across with scissors or a snare applied to this base to complete the separation.

Guillotine Technic. The enucleation of the tonsil with a guillotine is performed by engaging the posterior margin of the tonsil at its junction with the pillar against the distal rim of the fenestra of the guillotine. The guillotine is then pressed outward against the ramus of the mandible and the tonsil is everted through the fenestra of the guillotine (Fig. 142). The blade of the guillotine is then closed. This action practically splits the tonsil free from its bed in the fossa. If correctly done, the tonsillar fossa is left smooth and the margins of the

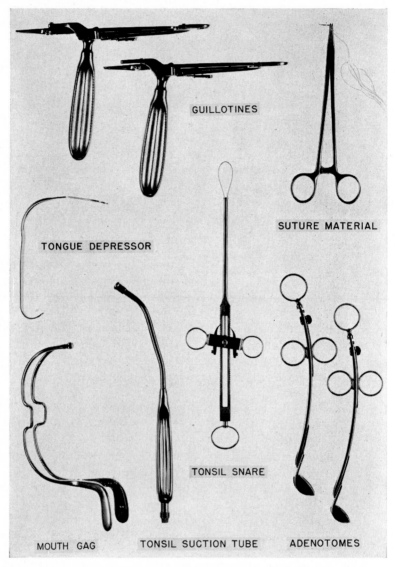

GUILLOTINES

SUTURE MATERIAL

TONGUE DEPRESSOR

TONSIL SNARE

MOUTH GAG   TONSIL SUCTION TUBE   ADENOTOMES

Fig. 140. Instruments commonly used for tonsillectomy and adenoidectomy under general anesthesia.

pillars intact. Moderately brisk bleeding from the vessels which have been cut across often occurs. This can usually be controlled without difficulty by filling the fossa with a soft sponge clamped in a sponge holder. If it does not completely cease, the bleeding points should be clamped with a hemostat. If this is not sufficient, ties and even sutures should be used.

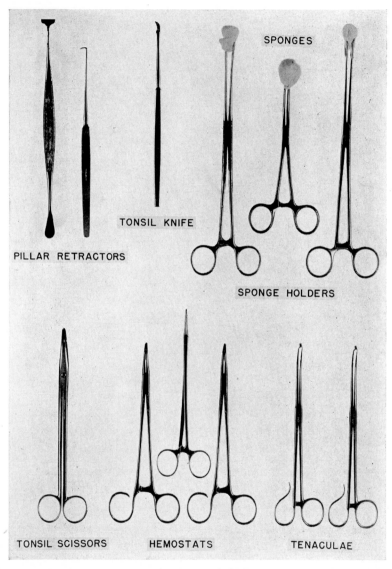

Fig. 140 (*Continued*). Instruments commonly used for tonsillectomy and adenoidectomy under general anesthesia.

I prefer a guillotine with an oval or round fenestra utilizing a single blade of medium sharpness. There are guillotines with square fenestra and double blades, one blade being used to crush a thin layer of tissue and the second one to cut loose the tonsil.

If the plica triangularis is well developed, a considerable piece will often escape the guillotine. It should be grasped with a tenaculum,

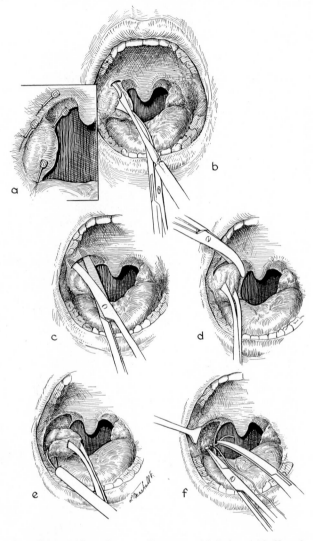

Fig. 141. A method of dissection tonsillectomy: (a) Points of infiltration for local anesthesia. (b) Start of incision with tonsil knife at attachment of anterior pillar to the tonsil superiorly. (c) Separation by scissor dissection of the superior pole of the tonsil. (d) Continuation of dissection of tonsil from its attachment to pillars and bed of tonsillar fossa. (e) Separation of the tonsil by snare at the lower pole, including the plica triangularis. (f) Hemostasis.

loosened by incision at its junction with the pillars and removed with a snare.

Removal of a completely enucleated tonsil by guillotine technic is illustrated in Fig. 143. When the tonsil is not cleanly and completely removed, the usual sites for a piece of the tonsil that is left are shown in Fig. 144. When the fossa has healed, these remnants or "tags" appear as illustrated in Fig. 145.

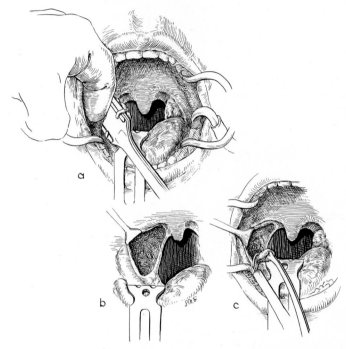

Fig. 142. Tonsillectomy by guillotine. Several types of instruments employing the guillotine principle are in use for enucleation of the tonsil. This instrument employing this principle was first introduced into this country by Sluder. Most of the instruments in use today employing this principle are modifications of Sluder's original instrument. The open fenestra of the gulliotine is pressed against the tonsil which everts through the fenestra as the tonsil is pressed laterally against the ramus of the mandible. (a) Pressure by the index finger of the free hand against the anterior pillar aids this eversion. As the blade of the instrument is closed, the tonsil is split loose. Skillful use of this instrument allows a clean enucleation of the tonsil. (b) With the original technic this was rapidly done and dependence for hemostasis was placed on the natural contraction of bleeding vessels. Many operators who use this technic today take time to secure hemostasis by hemostat and tie or ligature if prompt cessation of bleeding does not occur. Also many operators prefer to remove an additional amount of the plica triangularis by snare (c).

Suction Treatment for Cleaning Tonsils. Occasionally there is a need for ridding a tonsil of debris which clogs the tonsil crypts. A tonsil suction tube (Fig. 181) fits over the tonsil and negative pressure exerted on the surface of the tonsil will withdraw debris from the crypts and may even demonstrate considerable liquid pus. Following several trials of the suction tube, a fine cotton-tipped applicator is used to apply

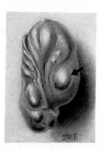

Fig. 143. A large, soft tonsil cleanly enucleated with the guillotine. The enlargement (indicated by the arrow) which bulges the capsule may be cut across by the guillotine. (Boies, L. R.: Tonsillectomy in the United States. Ann. Otol., Rhin. & Laryng., 57:352.)

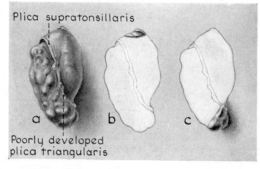

Fig. 144. A large, soft tonsil cleanly and completely enucleated. The supratonsillaris is intact. In this type of tonsil development, the plica triangularis is usually poorly developed. Occasionally guillotine enucleation misses a piece of tonsil at the upper pole (b) or cuts across a portion of the lower pole (c). The tonsil should be carefully inspected for a defect of this type as soon as it has been enucleated. (Boies, L. R.: Tonsillectomy in the United States. Ann. Otol., Rhin. & Laryng., 57:352.)

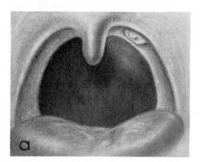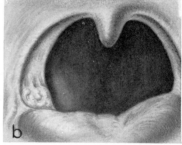

Fig. 145. Completely healed fossas with hypertrophy of the remnants in instances of tonsil pieces left in guillotine tonsillectomy (a) at the left upper pole and (b) at the base. (Boies, L. R.: Tonsillectomy in the United States. Ann. Otol., Rhin. & Laryng., 57:352.)

5 per cent silver nitrate to the crypts. The benefits of this treatment are often prompt but may be only temporary.

Adenoidectomy. Adenoidectomy is performed with the basket type of adenotome or a curet. I prefer the former because it is less traumatic. It is inserted open and in some cases the complete central mass is

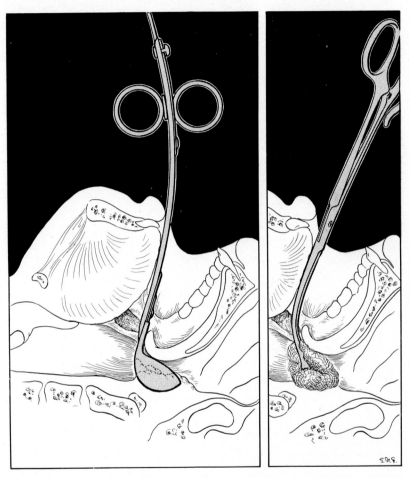

Fig. 146. The principle of adenoidectomy with the LaForce adenotome requires insertion of the opened adenotome in the midline followed by additional insertion of the adenotome in lateral positions on either side of the midline. The advantage of this instrument is that it is less traumatic than the curette, the depth of incision is better controlled and the adenoid removed is safely caught in the basket of the adenotome. After the adenoid is removed or during phases of its removal, there is value in holding a sponge in the nasopharynx to control the bleeding so that the site of removal can be repeatedly inspected to insure thorough removal of the adenoid mass and to visualize bleeding points on which to apply a hemostat.

enucleated intact in one maneuver. In other cases, the whole mass cannot be engaged intact and two or three maneuvers are necessary. I prefer to take the central mass first, then the lateral areas, and finally to make another search rather high in the midline (Fig. 146). Afterward, or interspersed between these steps, a sponge on a curved forceps is inserted into the nasopharynx to exert pressure as the bleeding points retract and the pharynx becomes dry. Final inspection with the soft palate retracted is advisable.

A special mouth gag (Fig. 147) is used on large children and adults under general anesthesia. It has the advantage of easily keeping the airway free by lifting the tongue and lower jaw as ether is insufflated

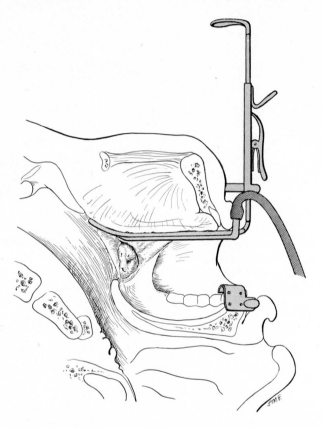

Fig. 147. The Davis mouth gag is an efficient instrument for holding up the lower jaw and tongue in large children or adults under general anesthesia. It allows easy maintenance of airway. Many operators prefer the Rose position with head extended when operating with this gag.

through a tube attached to the tongue blade and directed posteriorly beyond the base of the tongue. Some surgeons prefer the Rose position when using this mouth gag or whenever general anesthesia is used. In this position, the head is extended as far as possible and the operator sits at the head of the table and sees the tonsil in an upside down position. The purpose of this position is to avoid aspiration of blood into the trachea.

With the newer developments in anesthesia, an intratracheal tube is becoming popular. It prevents obstructed breathing, avoids troublesome gagging and swallowing without deep anesthesia, and lessens the chance of aspiration of blood into the trachea.

REFERENCES

Anderson, J. J.: Poliomyelitis and Recent Tonsillectomy. J. Pediat., 27:68, 1945.

Boies, L. R.: Tonsillectomy in the United States. Ann. Otol., Rhin. & Laryng., 57:352, 1948.

Campbell, E. H.: Local Results of Tonsillectomy. Arch. Otolaryng., 30:863, 1939.

Collins, S. G.: An Epidemiological and Statistical Study of Tonsillitis. Pub. Health Bull. No. 175, 1927.

Diamant, M.: Problem of Focal Infection. Acta oto-laryng., 5:109, 1944.

Editorial: Tonsil Stumps. J.A.M.A., 134:698, 1947.

Editorial: Tonsillectomy in the United States. Ibid., 91:1195, 1928.

Ehrich, W. E., and Harris, T. N.: The Site of Antibody Formation. Science, 101:28, 1945.

Howard, R.: Relationship of Poliomyelitis and Tonsillectomy. Ann. Otol., Rhin. & Laryng., 53:15, 1944.

Kaiser, A. D.: Children's Tonsils, In or Out. Philadelphia, J. B. Lippincott Co., 1932.

Kelly, J. D.: Choice of Operations in Tonsillectomy. Laryngoscope, 47:7, 1937.

Leshin, N., and Pearlman, S. J.: Are Tonsil Recurrences Due to Faulty Operative Technic? Arch. Otolaryng., 13:37, 1931.

Meyer, O.: The Mechanism of Oral Focal Infection in Arthritis. M. Rec., 158:604, 1945.

Rhoads, P. S., and Dick, G. F.: Efficacy of Tonsillectomy for the Removal of Focal Infection. J.A.M.A., 91:1149, 1928.

Roberts, E. R.: Tonsillectomy and Poliomyelitis. Ann. Otol., Rhin. & Laryng., 55:592, 1946.

Sputh, C. B., Jr., and Sputh, C. B.: The Tonsil Stump and Its Removal. J. Indiana M. A., 30:401, 1946.

CHAPTER XXVII

HOARSENESS

Hoarseness is a symptom and not a disease. It is one of the most important symptoms in throat diseases, because, in its chronic form, it may be an early warning of serious disease in the larynx and elsewhere.

Hoarseness may be defined as a rough, harsh quality of voice which is lower in pitch than is normal for a person (Jackson).

Etiology. The physiologic action of the vocal cords has been described in Chapter XXII. Any disease or disorder which will interfere with the *approximation, tension,* or *vibration* of the cord or cords will cause a hoarseness. This interference may result from any of the following:

1. Tumor, inflammatory swelling and secretion interfering with approximation of the cords, as well as of the tension alone in some instances.

2. Paralysis of the muscles which adduct the cords or produce tension. These paralyses are often associated with paralysis of the abductor function.

3. Cicatricial concavity of the margin of a cord, as may result from disease, surgical procedures on the vocal cords and so on.

4. Fixation of the range of movement of the crico-arytenoid joint.

5. Usurpative function of the ventricular bands ("false cords").

TUMORS, INFLAMMATORY SWELLINGS, SECRETIONS

Pathology. The common benign tumors which cause hoarseness are papillomas, polyps, hematomas and vocal nodules. Less common to rare are fibromas, angiomas, neurofibromas, myxomas and chondromas. Jackson has pointed out that the majority of benign tumors of the larynx are not true neoplasms but that the term has been applied quite generally to lesions which are tumor-like in appearance and symptoms but which are really of inflammatory origin and do not show histologically the characteristics of a neoplastic process. He points out, too, that several of our common diagnoses are incorrectly applied. For instance, the most common tumefaction causing hoarseness is a hematoma resulting from voice strain. It appears as a roundish, reddish mass of tissue on the margin of the vocal cord and causes hoarseness because it interferes with the normal approximation of the cord. In time, this small reddish mass undergoes organization; in the early stages, it simulates an angioma and later a fibroangioma or fibroma. Because of the presence of blood cells and blood vessels in the structure, this tumor is often designated in the pathologist's report as an angioma or fibroangioma. These terms, if they are to be used correctly, should be reserved for true neoplasms which arise from blood vessels.

The common malignant tumor to cause hoarseness is the squamous cell carcinoma. When it begins on the margin of the cord, the warning in hoarseness is an early one, allowing a cure at this stage by relatively simple means. When a carcinoma begins on a ventricular band, the epiglottis, or any other part of the rim of the glottis (extrinsic location), hoarseness is one of the late symptoms (see Chapter XXXI). Other types of malignant disease are relatively much less common. Sarcomas are rarely encountered.

Swelling of the vocal cords as a cause of hoarseness is commonly encountered in acute infectious laryngitis, such as occurs as a part of the common cold, in laryngitis accompanying specific diseases such as the exanthemata, pertussis, influenza, and in stages of chronic laryngitis. The swelling need not be marked to interfere with the physiologic actions which determine the pitch of the voice. The mucosa and submucosa are involved in the tissue changes common to acute or chronic inflammations. There is increased activity of the glands of the mucosa in the acute phases and lessened activity in the chronic phases. This accounts for interfering secretions playing a role in the symptom of hoarseness. Thick, stringy secretions in chronic laryngitis and the gluelike secretions in laryngitis sicca (which is part of an atrophic picture) offer obvious mechanical obstruction to the normal action of the cords in voice production.

Chronic laryngitis may result from repeated attacks of acute laryngitis or severe damage in a first attack. In all chronic states, infections above in the nasal space or pharynx, as well as irritation coming from below, such as may occur with pulmonary disease, should be considered.

Treatment. Removal of the common benign tumors of the larynx is accomplished through the direct laryngoscope or suspension laryngoscopy with reflected light. The aim is to remove the tumor with as little of the vocal cord margin or structure as possible. A simple scalping off of the tumor mass followed by diathermy cauterization of the site of attachment provides a cure in most cases. In certain instances, such as in the removal of vocal nodules, cauterization is unnecessary and should be avoided, since a removal of the swelling which is the result of irritation will, under vocal rest and avoidance of irritation, be cured with the maximum preservation of function.

Multiple Papillomas. Occasionally, multiple papillomas of the larynx are seen in children. There is some basis for the belief that these are caused by a virus infection. Implantation may result from expression of tissue juices during the act of removal. There is some basis for a belief that the maturity of the epithelium of the vocal cord may have something to do with the tendency of papillomas in children to recur. Observations have been reported that maturation of this epithelium by local application of an estrogenic substance prevents this recurrence.

Large Benign Tumors. Large benign tumors might require operative removal by an external route, a splitting of the thyroid cartilage, through which opening the new growth could be completely and safely removed.

Malignant Lesions. Malignant lesions causing hoarseness must be treated radically. A small percentage which are diagnosed early and are confined to the margin of a cord, can be safely treated through a suspension laryngoscope. Another small group can be treated by a relatively simple operation—thyrotomy, or laryngofissure. (See Chapter XXXI, Fig. 169.) A third group requires total laryngectomy (Fig. 170). When the lesion is on the rim of the larynx (extrinsic) or invades the pharynx, surgery has little to offer and irradiation is palliative in a majority of cases.

Swelling and Secretions. Inflammatory swelling and secretions, acute or chronic, as a cause of hoarseness, are very common. The treatment is based on certain very definite principles. Of primary importance is rest of the voice. Many of the cases will be cured on this basis. The addition of warm, moist air ranks second in importance. Local medications have a limited value, especially in acute phases. In chronic cases, a stimulating effect apparently has some value. Jackson has favored a formula containing mono-*p*-chlorophenol, camphor and liquid petrolatum (Pilling). A few drops are instilled with a laryngeal syringe or spray at two or three day intervals.

In considering causative factors, it is important to detect and control any irritative factors from below such, as tracheitis, bronchitis and tuberculosis, and such conditions as chronic pharyngitis, tonsillitis and sinusitis from above. The irritation to the pharynx and larynx caused by smoking and by the ingestion of alcohol must also be considered.

VOCAL CORD PARALYSIS

Some form of motor vocal cord paralysis as a cause of hoarseness is relatively common. There are various pictures in this paralysis according to the muscles affected. The paralysis may be unilateral or bilateral, spastic or flaccid. There are three main classes according to the muscle groups affected. These are adductor, abductor, or tensor. The actions of the muscles concerned with these functions has been described in Chapter XXII.

Unilateral Midline Paralysis. The most common type of motor paralysis of the larynx is one in which the paralyzed cord is in the midline and does not abduct on inspiration. This constitutes a unilateral midline paralysis. It occurs more commonly on the left side than on the right because of the longer course of the left recurrent laryngeal nerve, making it more vulnerable to injury. On inspiration, the paralyzed cord remains in the midline and the healthy one moves out normally (Fig. 148). On phonation, the two cords approximate in midline and it may

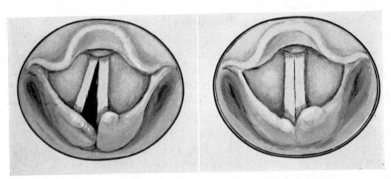

Fig. 148. "Reflected image seen in unilateral midline laryngeal paralysis. On inspiration, the right cord moves outward normally, while the left cord remains in the midline. The arytenoid eminence on the paralyzed side is tumbled over forward, giving a tumor-like appearance on inspiration but it is jostled back into place on phonation by the impact of the active arytenoid. Phonation is good in such cases." (Jackson.)

be difficult to detect any abnormality in their appearance during the act of phonation. An experienced observer will, however, note a tendency of the active cord to push against the paralyzed cord, and to "jostle" the arytenoid on the sound side (Jackson). He will also notice that the

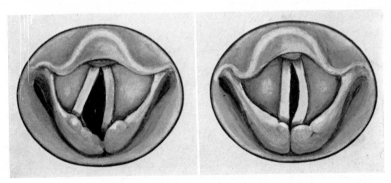

Fig. 149. The reflected appearance of left incomplete unilateral paralysis. The right cord (left) moves outward on inspiration, leaving the paraboloid left cord motionless. Voice is poor with air waste because of paralytic defective approximation (right). (Jackson.)

slit of the glottis is slightly askew from the sagittal line, and that the mound of the arytenoid is more prominent, tends to seem limp and may droop slightly forward. The inexperienced observer may mistake this appearance for a swelling or tumor.

In this type of paralysis, there is usually a mild degree of hoarseness at the onset of the paralysis, but there is usually a compensatory adjustment in the actions of the normal portions of the larynx to provide apparently normal phonation. The treatment is that of the causative lesion, if indicated.

Unilateral Incomplete Paralysis. This occurs when all of the laryngeal muscles of one side except the arytenoideus are paralyzed. This muscle is incapable of unilateral paralysis because it has bilateral innervation.

The characteristic appearance is shown in Fig. 149. The edge of the affected cord is concave, and it is in a position midway between phonation and approximation, thus producing a paraboloid silhouette of the glottis on inspiration. On phonation, the sound cord crosses the midline to meet the disabled cord and jostles the sound arytenoid. An expiratory blast of air will displace the edge of the flaccid paralyzed cord slightly upward. A husky voice results from this type of paralysis but improves with the adjustments which are made in time. Treatment is directed toward finding the cause and instituting appropriate therapy for it. Recovery of the paralysis is doubtful, although adjustment to a degree of satisfactory function is not uncommon.

Bilateral Midline Paralysis. The most frequent cause is said to be goiter surgery. Jackson remarks that in his experience, an overlooked preoperative unilateral paralysis has been present in most cases deemed postoperative.

The injury from thyroid surgery may be due to postoperative swelling or later cicatrization as well as actual cutting of the nerves.

Other causes along the circuitous course of the inferior laryngeal nerves are a compression or involvement of these nerves by adenopathy, tumors, aneurysms and any disease that may cause enlargement of structures in the neck and upper mediastinum. Central causes of paralysis are found in such disorders as disseminated sclerosis and tabes.

The characteristic of midline bilateral abductor paralysis is that the larynx is paralyzed shut (Jackson). When this occurs, the outstanding manifestation is the obstruction to inspiration. When the glottis is visualized, it is seen that on phonation it is closed with the cords practically in contact. On inspiration, the cords remain in the midline position and the patient experiences difficulty in drawing in air unless the cords are at a different level and a considerable chink which is invisible exists between the two levels (Fig. 150).

The voice in bilateral midline paralysis is usually good because of approximation of the cords on phonation. An inexperienced observer might doubt the presence of paralysis because of a relatively good voice.

The only condition which may simulate midline paralysis is a fixation of the crico-arytenoid joints in a midline position. This can be determined by the experienced laryngologist who performs a passive

mobility test through the direct laryngoscope and ascertains whether
or not the joints are fixed by pushing on the arytenoids with a blunt
probe such as a closed laryngeal forceps.

The most serious complication of a bilateral midline paralysis is
asphyxia. When this is imminent, tracheotomy is necessary. After
tracheotomy is performed, the patient's chief concern is when can he

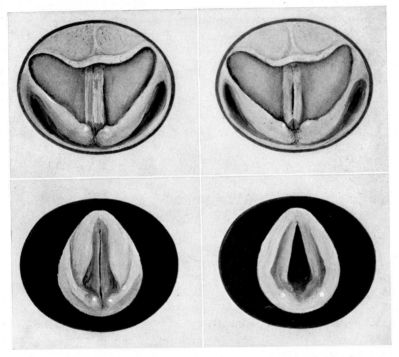

Fig. 150. At the left, above, is the reflected appearance on inspiration in a case of
midline paralysis, the cannula being corked. The cords are forced tightly together,
instead of being widely separated as they would be normally. At the right, above,
is the position on expiration; the cords are slightly blown apart by the expiratory
current. The voice was good; but both postici were paralyzed, so the patient could
not open his glottis for breathing. At the left, below, is the appearance on direct
laryngoscopy. At the right, below, is shown the position to which each arytenoid, in
turn, could be displaced in the passive mobility test. The closed forceps with which
the passive mobility was demonstrated are omitted so as to give an unobstructed
view of the range of passive mobility. (Jackson.)

get rid of his tube. Nerve anastomosis was used in the past, but was
rarely successful. Submucous resection of the cords which were then
sutured outward provided an adequate airway but left the patient
aphonic or with a poor voice. More recently, an external operation which
transfixes an arytenoid laterally or removes it, has developed. This
provides a glottic chink posteriorly which is adequate for respiratory
exchange and preserves the anterior half of the larynx for phonation.

A number of modifications of the original King operation have been suggested. Success in the matter of providing an adequate airway and preserving a useful voice has been attained. It represents one of the most useful advances of recent years.

Bilateral Incomplete Paralysis. Next in frequency of paralysis to the unilateral midline paralysis, unilateral incomplete paralysis, and bilateral midline paralysis, is bilateral incomplete paralysis. In this condition, all of the laryngeal muscles except the arytenoideus are paralyzed. It may follow goiter surgery and may be transitory or permanent. It also has been described (Jackson) following surgery in other parts of the body, apparently the result of circulatory disturbances.

The picture is shown in Fig. 151. The vocal cords appear to be motionless midway between the position of deep respiration and that of phona-

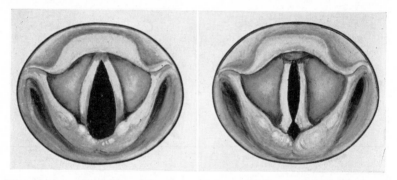

Fig. 151. At the left, is shown the reflected appearance of a bilateral incomplete paralysis. The cords have concave edges and are motionless in a position midway between the midline and that of extreme abduction. This position is often wrongly called "cadaveric," and "complete." The proper name for it is "incomplete," because, obviously, there remains some power of movement in the arytenoideus. This form of paralysis may disappear, but usually it becomes a midline paralysis. The right hand drawing shows complete paralysis. This appearance always means that the abductors, adductors, tensors and tonus are all gone. (Jackson.)

tion. The edges are symmetrically concave, and the glottic chink tends to be ellipsoidal and remains practically unchanged when the patient inspires, expires and attempts to phonate.

Air waste, a husky voice, wheezing on attempts to cough and difficulty in raising secretion are characteristics of this picture.

There is no local treatment for this condition. The cause should be found when possible and treatment instituted. Syphilis is said to be one of the most frequent causes in cases not related to goiter surgery. Spontaneous cure occurs in some cases. In others, the cords may assume the midline position. If this occurs, relief by tracheotomy is usually required.

Complete Paralysis. This bilateral condition is pictured in Fig. 151. The immobility of the cords and arytenoids has given rise to a description of the image as "wooden." The voice is husky, there is considerable air waste and it is difficult to raise secretions. The prognosis for recovery is poor. The causative lesion and the complications from pulmonary infection are serious.

There are three additional types of laryngeal paralysis which are rarely seen as distinct clinical entities but often occur as part of some of the other types just described. These are adductor paralysis, thyro-arytenoid paralysis and cricothyroid paralysis.

Adductor Paralysis. A sole condition, this is a supranuclear lesion involving the fibers of both sides. The larynx is paralyzed open and there is an aphonic voice with air waste. Two forms of adductor paralysis may be seen; one, in which the arytenoideus is functioning and the glottis closes posteriorly, and the other, in which only arytenoideus ceases to function. In the latter, there is a triangular glottic chink posteriorly and the voice is good.

The treatment is usually general and directed at the causative lesion.

Thyro-arytenoid Paralysis. This disorder has been described both as a unilateral and bilateral condition. It is uncommon except as part of a complete paralysis. The picture in bilateral paralysis shows a glottic chink on phonation between the two cords with the arytenoids in approximation. There is, of course, a hoarseness and a low-pitched voice. If the lesion is unilateral, the involved cord bows slightly on phonation. The hoarseness and low pitch of the voice is not as marked as in the bilateral condition.

Cricothyroid Paralysis. An isolated lesion of the superior laryngeal nerve, this type of paralysis is rare. It may be unilateral or bilateral. The laryngeal picture shows normal abduction and adduction, but the margins of the involved cord are wavy. This is more marked when the paralysis is flaccid. The wrinkling or waviness is due to the action of the thyro-arytenoid muscle, which is innervated by the inferior laryngeal nerve.

Anesthesia of the larynx accompanies the motor paralysis in bilateral involvement. The voice is weak and rough. Fluids, oral secretions and food may drop into the anesthetic larynx and cause cough.

CICATRICIAL CONCAVITY OF THE MARGIN OF A CORD

This condition is relatively rare. In destructive lesions involving the cord or cords, healing or cure by surgery will, of course, produce scarring. Tuberculosis or syphilitic lesions are not as common as they once were, and scarring from these causes will probably not be encountered often in the future. The removal of tumors as in laryngofissure (see Chapter XXXI) invariably leaves a defect in a cord. Fulguration or other forms of cautery destruction, as used in the treatment of certain benign tumors, will in some instances produce cicatricial changes causing hoarseness. The condition is not amenable to treatment.

FIXATION OF RANGE OF MOVEMENT OF THE CRICO-ARYTENOID JOINT

The crico-arytenoid joint may become partially or wholly fixed in its normal range of movement by inflammatory processes involving it from adjacent infection, trauma, or in an arthritic process such as may occur in any other joint. If the involvement is unilateral, there may be relatively little interference with phonation and thus only a slight, if any, hoarseness.

The diagnosis of fixation is determined by testing the passive mobility of the arytenoid. This is done by palpating it with a blunt instrument through the direct laryngoscope. In cases of an obstructive bilateral fixation, the joints may be mobilized through surgery.

USURPATIVE FUNCTION OF THE VENTRICULAR BANDS

Phonation with the ventricular bands (false cords) instead of the vocal cords is known as dysphonia plicae ventricularis and was first desecribd by the Jacksons in 1935. This usurpative function of the ventricular bands may start when the voice is forced during temporary impairment of the vocal cords in an acute laryngitis. A small tumor mechanically propping the cords apart may cause the ventricular bands to take on this vicarious function.

In surgical defects involving the vocal cords, this function of the ventricular bands is the result to be desired.

This disorder can also be congenital. Hoarseness is present, even in the mild cases and is the only symptom. Treatment consists of removing the cause and avoiding forcible or strained use of the voice.

REFERENCES

Auerbach, O.: Laryngeal Tuberculosis. Arch. Otolaryng., *44*:191, 1946.

Boies, L. R.: Papilloma of the Larynx. Laryngoscope, *53*:601, 1943.

Broyles, E. N.: Treatment of Laryngeal Papilloma in Children. South. M. J., *34*:239, 1941.

Cody, C. C.: Associated Paralysis of the Larynx. Ann. Otol., Rhin. & Laryng., *55*:549, 1946.

Jackson, C., and Jackson, C. L.: The Larynx and Its Diseases. Philadelphia, W. B. Saunders Co., 1937.

Jackson, C., and Jackson, C. L.: Dysphonia Plicae Ventricularis. Chapter IV in The Larynx and Its Diseases. Philadelphia, W. B. Saunders Co., 1937.

Negus, V. E.: Significance of Hoarseness, New York State J. Med., *39*:9, 1939.

Riseman, B., and Aagesen, W.: Laryngeal Neurosis Incident to Military Service. Arch. Otolaryng., *43*:22, 1946.

Ullmann, E. V.: On the Etiology of the Laryngeal Papilloma. Acta-otolaryng., *5*:317, 1923.

CHAPTER XXVIII

LARYNGEAL OBSTRUCTION

Definition. Laryngeal obstruction is an obstruction to the normal free passage of air through the glottis.

ETIOLOGY

Laryngeal obstruction may be caused by the following:
1. Inflammations
   Acute laryngitis either in the form of laryngotracheobronchitis or epiglottitis.
   Diphtheria.
   Tuberculosis.
   Syphilis.
2. Tumors—malignant and benign.
3. Abductor paralyses.
4. Foreign bodies.
5. Edema due to allergic reactions or instrumentation.
6. Congenital weakness of laryngeal structures, malformations (web), etc.
7. Spasm of laryngeal muscles.

Acute inflammation is the most common cause of a serious, rapidly, developing laryngeal obstruction. The pediatrician sees this not uncommonly. It is a fairly frequent condition in the large municipal hospital with a busy contagion service (Fig. 152).

PATHOLOGY

The narrowest portion in the lumen of the respiratory tract between the pharynx and bifurcation of the trachea is at the valve-like glottis. Just above and below the edge of the glottis, the mucosa is vascular and loose, especially in the subglottic area. Especially is this true in the infant. Inflammations involving the larynx may produce serious edema in this area. In the infant, the width of the larynx at the subglottic level narrows down to about one-fifth of its superior diameter.

Obstruction by tumor forms slowly. The most frequent tumor to cause a definite respiratory obstruction is carcinoma. Occasionally, multiple papillomas and other benign growths are encountered.

Paralysis of one side of the larynx may cause only a very mild obstruction or none at all. Bilateral abductor paralysis produces a serious obstruction to respiration.

361

Foreign bodies causing laryngeal obstruction must be large enough to lodge in the larynx. Occasionally a tracheotomy is necessary to remove a foreign body from the trachea.

Edema of a serious degree owing to instrumentation occasionally occurs after bronchoscopy.

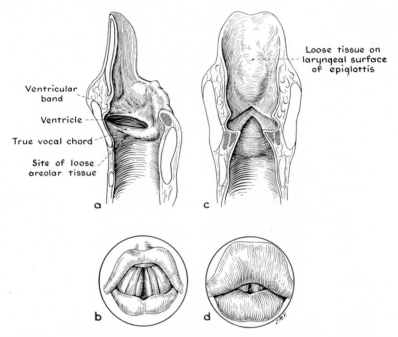

Fig. 152. There are two sites in the mucosa of the larynx at which there is loose areolar tissue that is prone to swell easily when inflamed. One is subglottic just below the vocal cords (a). The swelling is characteristic at this site in acute laryngotracheobronchitis (b) or after prolonged instrumentration as in bronchoscopy with a relatively tight fitting bronchoscope. The other site is on the laryngeal surface of the epiglottis (c), which swells rapidly when acutely inflamed as part of the picture of supraglottic inflammation (d).

Allergic reactions of a serious degree are not common.

Laryngeal obstruction in the newborn, young infant, or child, may be caused by weakness of the structure of the larynx, neuroses, or anomalies.

SYMPTOMS AND SIGNS

The earliest symptom of a gradually developing laryngeal obstruction of inflammatory cause is an inspiratory dyspnea. This may be both seen and heard. It is a stridor that is heard. Often, attention has been focused on the larynx previous to the onset of the dyspnea because of hoarseness and cough. As the dyspnea increases, retraction of the supraclavicular and epigastric soft parts on inspiration is noted. Cough is usually present and of a brassy character. The victim, usually a small child, exhibits anxiety. In the gradually developing obstruction, cyanosis is not a prominent sign, and when the obstruction becomes marked it is usually a "pale cyanosis," indicating exhaustion.

The picture just described characterizes the development of croup in the child. When laryngeal obstruction develops from chronic inflammatory processes, such as tuberculosis and syphilis and from tumors, a stridor is usually the first sign of obstruction, associated with dyspnea on exertion. Evidence of laryngitis is invariably present in the symptom of hoarseness. Cyanosis which is not marked, and the use of accessory muscles of respiration are only evident when the obstruction reaches a serious degree. This picture may also be characteristic of an interference with normal respiratory movement of the cords, such as may develop when an edema from inflammation on the external surface of the larynx interferes with normal arytenoid action.

Paralysis of Vocal Cords. Paralysis must be bilateral to cause a serious obstruction. It may come on suddenly, as after bilateral injury in neck surgery, or the onset may be gradual. Foreign bodies, trauma and allergic reactions cause a relatively sudden onset of obstruction.

Congenital Causes. These are occasionally seen. A weakness of laryngeal cartilages allows the aryepiglottic folds and arytenoids to be pulled into the laryngeal cavity and the epiglottis to fold on itself during inspiration. This causes an obstruction manifested by a high-pitched, crowing inspiratory stridor, particularly on exertion. Cyanosis and actual dyspnea may occur during crying. A rare congenital malformation in the form of a web between the anterior part of the vocal cords may be a cause of laryngeal obstruction. The extent of this diaphragm determines the symptoms, which may include hoarseness, aphonia, dyspnea on exertion and, in infants, asphyxial attacks.

Muscle Spasm. Spasm of the laryngeal muscles which close the glottis occurs in infants and young children, with sudden onset, abrupt termination and without fever. It is usually considered to be a manifestation of tetany. The onset of the obstruction may suddenly follow a fit of crying, anger, or emotional excitement. There is a crowing inspiration, the child stops breathing, and becomes cyanotic for a number of seconds, and a whistling inspiration follows with resumption of normal breathing within a few moments.

TREATMENT

Medication. There is no medication which is reliably effective in lessening obstructive edema of an inflammatory process. Certain drugs are definitely contraindicated, such as atropine and morphine. The former has a drying effect on the secretions and this is undesirable. Morphine lessens the cough reflex, which should be preserved to rid the respiratory tract of obstructing secretions.

In simple croup in a small child, a teaspoonful of *syrup of ipecac* may be given in a little water every fifteen minutes until vomiting occurs. This medication has an expectorant as well as an emetic action.

Control of Oxygen, Temperature and Humidity. An obstructive laryngitis caused by bacterial infection should receive penicillin or a sulfonamide, or their combination. This therapy is supplemented with oxygen and controlled humidity. The old-fashioned croup tent provided increased humidity, but also increased the temperature of the patient's environment to an uncomfortable point. Consider the lack of comfort one experiences on a warm day in the presence of a high humidity and an inkling may be had of what one would experience in the 90° F. temperature of a croup tent, with the relative humidity markedly increased over normal surroundings.

The modern therapy tent (Fig. 184), in which a humidity of 90 degrees in a temperature of approximately 22° C. (72° F.) is maintained and in which oxygen in varying amount can be introduced, has proven to be one of the most effective measures in the treatment of obstructive laryngitis, particularly laryngotracheobronchitis. Combined with the sulfonamides, antibiotics, and relief of the obstruction by intubation or tracheotomy, the once high mortality of acute obstructive laryngitis has been markedly reduced when the condition is recognized early and is promptly treated.

Often in a case of obstructive laryngitis, there is prompt relief after the administration of the antibiotics or chemotherapy combined with oxygenation and increased humidity. When this relief does not occur, surgical procedures should be considered.

Two methods for relief from the laryngeal obstruction are available: intubation and tracheotomy.

CHOICE OF METHOD OF SURGERY

When the cause of serious obstruction is a tumor, paralysis, a congenital anomaly, or a chronic infection producing stenosis, tracheotomy is the unquestioned procedure in view of the prolonged treatment necessary. To relieve an obstruction due to an acute inflammation, the edema which occasionally results after instrumentation, an allergic reaction, and so on, intubation may be adequate, but there are definite situations in which tracheotomy is the procedure indicated.

The following considerations are important:

1. Intubation is a relatively simple procedure quickly accomplished in the hands of an experienced operator. However, it demands that an experienced intubator be quickly available to put the tube back once it is coughed out.

2. Repeated intubations or prolonged use of an intubation tube produce an irritation in the subglottic area which may cause stenosis.

Tucker believes that tracheotomy conserves the laryngeal structure better than intubation in infants.

3. A small infant may not take food or fluid by mouth satisfactorily with an intubation tube in place.

4. In the presence of an infection producing a membrane below the glottis, as in acute laryngotracheobronchitis, an intubation tube is inadequate. Tracheotomy, in addition to providing an adequate airway, facilitates removal of the inspissated secretions and offers drainage. The factor of drainage provided by tracheotomy in the acute fulminating infections has probably been overlooked.

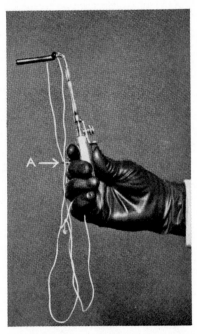

Fig. 153. An instrument for indirect intubation assembled and ready for insertion. The very important traction hook, A, is back of the index finger with which traction anteriorward is to be made at the proper moment. (Jackson and Jackson: The Larynx and Its Diseases, W. B. Saunders Co.)

5. The fact that a tracheotomy opening does not admit air warmed and moistened in the upper respiratory tract has been shown from clinical experience to be an unimportant consideration. The use of a warm humidified air in the acute stage is a satisfactory substitute.

Technic of Intubation of the Larynx. This procedure has usually been done in the past by the indirect method. A tube is chosen of the proper size for the age of the child (Fig. 153). The patient is placed in supine position. A side mouth gag is inserted and the forefinger of the free hand is passed over the tongue to feel the tip of the epiglottis (Fig. 154). This is pushed forward. The prominences of the arytenoids are felt. The intubation tube, fitted to the introduction forceps and with a loop of silk thread anchored in the flange of the tube, is then inserted into the larynx. The tip of the tube points posteriorly, resting on the

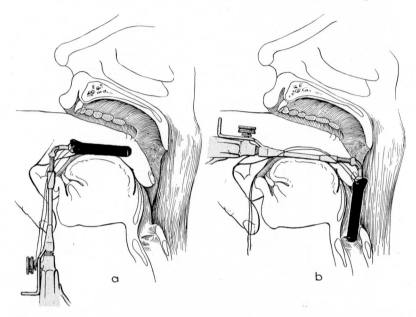

Fig. 154. The principal maneuvers in the act of intubation consist of palpating the tip of the epiglottis with the index finger of the free hand (a) and then introducing the intubating instrument along side the tip of this finger to place the tube in the glottis (b). It finally rests between the vocal cords with its superior lip resting on the arytenoid eminence.

arytenoids. The palpating finger holds the tube in place while the introduction forceps is withdrawn. As soon as it has been determined that the tube will remain in place, the silk thread may be cut and removed.

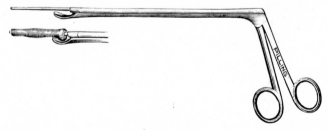

Fig. 155. Mosher's forceps for introducing an intubation tube under direct vision through a laryngoscope.

Direct intubation with a special forceps used through a direct laryngoscope is often preferred by laryngologists, since it can be done under direct vision with a minimum of trauma (Fig. 155).

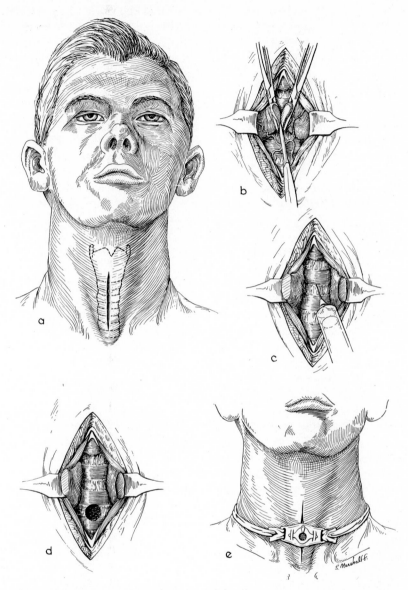

Fig. 156. Important in the technic for orderly tracheotomy are (a) an adequate incision; (b) careful hemostasis when the isthmus of the thyroid has to be divided, (c) injection of a few drops of 5 per cent cocaine into the trachea a few minutes before the trachea is opened, (d) removal of a disk of tissue below the second tracheal ring in an average case. This disk should be just slightly larger than the diameter of the lumen of the tube to be used so that it will slip in and out easily, and (e) avoidance of sutures in the tracheotomy wound except possibly at the ends. Air is invariably coughed out around the tube within the few hours after tracheotomy and if the wound is closed snugly, emphysema of the soft tissues invariably develops and more or less reaction in the wound.

13

Technic of Tracheotomy. The position of the patient is important. A sandbag should be placed beneath the shoulders so that the head and neck are fully extended. Local anesthesia is secured by injection of the skin and soft tissues from the lower border of the thyroid cartilage to the jugulum and on either side of the trachea. The cricoid cartilage is then palpated and the skin incision is made precisely in the midline from the lower border of the cricoid cartilage down almost to the jugulum (Fig. 156). It is then deepened until the white line of the fascia between the muscle groups is exposed. This is also cut precisely in the midline. As the front of the trachea is exposed from the cricoid cartilage downward, the isthmus of the thyroid gland as it lies across the trachea is identified and pushed downward or is clamped and divided as is required for proper exposure of the first three or four rings of the trachea. Careful hemostasis is secured. If tracheotomy is orderly, time is taken to inject a few drops of cocaine (5 per cent) by hypodermic syringe into the trachea through the first interspace. This prevents undue irritation on insertion of the tracheal cannula.

The trachea is then opened in the midline by incising the second and third, and, if needed, the fourth tracheal rings.

Type of Incision. We prefer the removal of a disk of cartilage slightly larger than the tube to be inserted. The incision, unless unusually long, is not sutured. Drainage around the tube is important and suturing causes more reactions and a tendency to emphysema. Experimental work (Richards and Glenn) has shown that this type of opening does not interfere with the patency of the tracheal lumen after the tube is removed and healing has taken place. It seems illogical to insert a tube through a narrow longitudinal slit with the resultant tension on the margins of this slit. An adequate opening facilitates exchange of tubes with the least amount of irritation. It also facilitates the matter of drainage from the trachea.

There seems to be a tendency to use too small a tube. Clinical observation indicates that the size of the lumen is not a factor in producing irritation in the trachea. In this respect, only the length of the tube is important. The larger the lumen of the tube, the less the tendency for it to clog with mucus to an extent to interfere with an adequate airway. A larger lumen is also easier to keep clean.

Classification of Tracheotomy. The old descriptive terms of "high," "median," or "low" tracheotomy have been discarded. All tracheotomies should be low except those preliminary to laryngectomy when conservation of as much of the trachea as is possible is important.

Tracheotomies may be conveniently classified as "emergency" or "orderly"; some writers prefer the terms "necessary" and "elective." Emergency tracheotomies may still be orderly in cases of extreme dyspnea. The use of a bronchoscope or Mosher life-saving tube (Fig. 157) inserted through the glottis changes the procedure from an acute emergency to an orderly one and produces a more satisfactory and a safer technical effort.

Nursing care of tracheotomized patients by those experienced in the management of this type of care is extremely important.

Tracheotomy wounds tend to heal promptly without surgical interference even though tubes have been worn for months.

Patients are surprisingly comfortable in permanent tracheotomy. Tracheitis and bronchitis are uncommon after the variable amount of this reaction present in the first few days after the operation has subsided. There seems to be no increased susceptibility to pneumonia. Thomson and Wood have each reported a case of tracheotomy tube worn over 70 years. Wood remarked that his patient claimed that she had never had bronchitis.

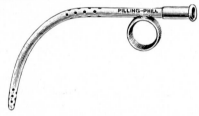

Fig. 157. Mosher's tube for temporary intubation (commonly known as a "life-saving tube").

Emergency Tracheotomy. Fortunately, it is an uncommon occasion when a physician is faced with an emergency tracheotomy which must be accomplished in a matter of minutes. Jackson states that "the best procedure, in dealing with an asphyxiating patient, is to insert a bronchoscope, establish regular respiration through it, and then perform a low tracheotomy in an orderly manner." However, if an emergency tracheotomy has to be performed without establishing an airway, and usually without the desired equipment, a knife and a pair of trained hands may have to be enough. No local anesthesia is used. General anesthesia would be fatal with an obstructed airway.

The two-incision Jackson technic should be followed. The proper position of the patient is to have the neck thrown into prominence by pushing a roll of blanket or a pillow under the shoulders. If these are not available, the neck may be brought above the left knee of the operator, who is in a sitting position.

Technic. If the physician is right-handed, the thumb and the index finger of the operator's left hand are utilized to press the large vessels back under the respective sternomastoid muscles. This also throws the trachea into prominence. The notch of the thyroid cartilage ("Adam's apple") then becomes the important landmark. An incision is then made from this notch almost to the suprasternal notch. It is carried completely through the skin and subcutaneous tissues.

In the next step, the left index finger of the same hand which is repressing the danger lines in the neck burrows by sense of touch down along Adam's apple over the cricothyroid membrane and two rings of the trachea, easily felt as corrugations. The knife slides along the palmar surface of the left index finger to make the tracheal incision.

The lips of the incision need to be spread apart. Then a cannula is inserted. If none is available, the tracheal incision needs to be held apart until one is obtained. If respiration has ceased, artificial respiration must be performed and an oxygen and carbon dioxide mixture should be administered. During these procedures, bleeding may be troublesome and alarming. Temporary control may be effected by packing gauze firmly into the wound and around the cannula. As soon as it can be accomplished, ties or sutures should be employed to secure good hemostasis. Afterwards the usual dressing technic is followed.

ACUTE LARYNGOTRACHEOBRONCHITIS

This condition is now regarded more or less as a clinical entity.

Age is a predisposing factor. The small child three years of age or under has a relative abundance of loose areolar tissue in the larynx, particularly in the subglottic area. A virulent organism which is not specific for this disease supplies an important second factor. Hemolytic streptococci often predominate, yet other bacteria such as *Streptococcus viridans*, pneumococci, *Staphylococcus haemolyticus* and *Hemophilus influenzae* have been reported in pure culture.

The initial symptoms begin as a cold in the head, followed by hoarseness and a croupy cough. Fever is usually slight at the beginning and moderate until advanced stages.

As the disease progresses, stridor develops, then restlessness, air hunger and signs of obstructive laryngeal dyspnea. Cyanosis as ordinarily observed is not a prominent feature. The experienced observer, however, recognizes the pale cyanosis as the gray pallor of exhaustion.

Direct examination of the larynx with the laryngoscope reveals a deep red injection of the laryngeal mucosa which is not quite as marked on the cords, with evident subglottic swelling (Fig. 152b). This subglottic swelling appears as a semi-elliptic fold below each cord. These swellings are peculiar to children and are the result of the swelling of the loose connective tissue in the conus elasticus. As the disease progresses, a membrane forms which is first serous, then mucoid, and finally thick and tenacious and almost like partially dried glue. This tenacious exudate extends down the trachea and into the bronchi producing obstruction, atelectasis, pneumonia and death if unchecked.

Treatment. Treatment consists of early relief of the laryngeal obstruction by tracheotomy, providing an atmosphere of high humidity with comfortable temperature (above 90 degrees humidity in 70° F.) (see p. 430), the use of penicillin or a sulfonamide in therapeutic dosage, and adequate fluid intake. Reference has previously been made regarding the avoidance of opiates which lessen the cough reflex and atropine which dries the secretions (see p. 363).

The mortality used to be extremely high but has been markedly reduced with the treatment just outlined. In addition, care by nurses experienced in the management of tracheotomized patients and the laryngologist's ready presence is important. A short bronchoscope may be needed to remove the tenacious secretions in the trachea and bronchi if signs of obstruction develop. The bronchoscope is inserted through the tracheotomic orifice and suction or forceps employed to free the airways.

With modern advances, the course of this disease has been shortened to a week or slightly longer.

ACUTE EPIGLOTTITIS

There seems to be a clinical entity in the development of symptoms of obstructive laryngitis coming on in three or four hours or less and in which the laryngoscopic view reveals a markedly swollen, deeply injected epiglottis (Fig. 152d). Usually, *Hemophilus influenzae* is found on the culture. There may be complicating influenzal pneumonitis. The picture is more common in older children. Tracheotomy is needed to relieve a serious obstruction. When a diagnosis of infection with *Hemophilus influenzae* is made, streptomycin in therapeutic dosage is indicated, combined with penicillin. The other supportive measures such as oxygenation, humidity, and fluid intake, are important.

LARYNGEAL DIPHTHERIA

Since immunization has lessened the general incidence of diphtheria, and antitoxin has made laryngeal involvement as an extension from the pharynx, less common, laryngeal diphtheria is a rare condition. For that reason, it sometimes goes unsuspected. Every case of laryngitis with obstructive dyspnea should have the benefit of laryngoscopy, indirect or direct, so that the glottis can actually be visualized. Diphtheritic laryngeal involvement can exist without evidence of an involvement of the pharynx or the nasal space. Smears and cultures should always be made when there is any possibility of the inflammation being diphtheritic, and antitoxin should be administered early.

OTHER CAUSES OF LARYNGEAL OBSTRUCTION

Laryngeal obstruction due to tumors, tuberculosis, and syphilis have been described in the chapter dealing with new growths and also in the one concerned with hoarseness.

Laryngeal obstruction due to paralysis of the vocal cords means a bilateral involvement with loss of abductor function. This usually is the result of injury to both recurrent nerves as in such procedures as thyroid surgery although it may result from the effects of trauma, new growths, toxic neuritis, or involvement of the centers controlling the action of the recurrent nerves (see Chapter XXVII). The voice in bilateral abductor midline paralysis is good, but the airway is inadequate for normal respiration, with dangers of asphyxia. If one cord happens to be a little higher than the other, however, there is enough of a glottic chink to allow the victim a sufficient respiratory exchange to get along on limited activity. The paralysis may not be permanent, but if it clears, it usually does so in a few months. After nine months, the paralysis is usually considered permanent.

Treatment. The modern treatment for bilateral abductor midline paralysis is to remove one arytenoid and attach the posterior end of the cord from which the arytenoid is removed outward so as to produce a posterior glottic chink adequate for easy respiration in which the function of the anterior one-half of the vocal cords in phonation is preserved. Thus, the patient retains a useful voice. Since King first described an operation for bilateral abductor midline paralysis, there have been several modifications of the idea which have simplified the procedure. One of the most useful is that of De Graff Woodman.

Laryngeal obstruction due to edema from allergic reaction may be relieved by a dose of epinephrine. Edema due to instrumentation sometimes follows bronchoscopy. A severe case may need relief by intubation or even tracheotomy.

LARYNGISMUS STRIDULUS

This condition, also known as spasmodic croup, is a clinical entity which is usually associated with abnormal calcium metabolism. It is most common between the ages of two and six. Characteristically, a child may awaken from a peaceful sleep, exhibit a croupy cough then a crowing inspiration and, following that, a typical inspiratory obstructive dyspnea. Usually this frightens the child, which increases the symptoms. Cyanosis follows and then the attack gradually subsides. Tracheotomy has been performed on these patients, but probably unnecessarily. Insufflation of oxygen, if available, may shorten or stop the attack. Reassurance and quieting of the child's fear go far toward the relief of the symptoms.

CONGENITAL LARYNGEAL STRIDOR (LARYNGOMALACIA)

This is not an uncommon disease of the newborn. A flabbiness of the epiglottis and aryepiglottic folds allows an indrawing or infolding of these parts during inspiration, producing stridor and dyspnea. A characteristic picture is seen on direct laryngoscopy, which is often indicated to rule out some congenital defect such as a web, or cyst. Usually no treatment is indicated. As the infant grows, the flabby structures at fault strengthen and mature and the infant has outgrown the condition by two years of age.

REFERENCES

Brewer, D. W. and Rambo, J. H. T.: Influenzal Laryngitis. Ann. Otol., Rhin. & Laryng. 57:96, 1948.

Davis, H. V.: Obstructive Laryngitis in Children Caused by Hemophilus Influenzae Bacillus, Type B. J. Kansas M. Soc., 48:105, 1947.

Davison, F. W.: Acute Laryngotracheobronchitis: Further Studies on Treatment. Arch. Otolaryng., 47:455, 1948.

Galloway, T. C.: Danger of Unrecognized Anoxia in Laryngology. Ann. Otol., Rhin. & Laryng., 55:508, 1946.

Jeffrey, F.: Epidemic of Acute Laryngotracheobronchitis. Canad. M.A.J., 53:562, 1945.

Kelly, J. D.: A Supplementary Report on Extralaryngeal Arytenoidectomy as a Relief for Bilateral Abductor Paralysis of the Larynx. Ann. Otol., Rhin. & Laryng., 56:628, 1943.

King, B. T.: A New and Function-Restoring Operation for Bilateral Abductor Cord Paralysis. Tr. Am. Laryng. Assn., 61:264, 1939.

Miller, A. H.: Hemophilus Influenzae Type B. Epiglottitis or Acute Supraglottic Laryngitis in Children: Laryngoscope, 58:514, 1948.

McLorinan, H.: Sixteen Cases of Supraglottic Edema. M. J. Australia, 2:220, 1946.

Morgan, E. A., and Wishart, D. E. S.: Laryngotracheobronchitis: Statistical Review of 549 Cases. Canad. M.A.J., 56:8, 1947.

Schwartz, L.: Congenital Laryngeal Stridor (Inspiratory Laryngeal Collapse). Arch. Otolaryng., 39:403, 1944.

Woodman, De G.: The Open Approach to Arytenoidectomy for Bilateral Paralysis. Ann. Otol., Rhin. & Laryng., 57:695, 1948.

CHAPTER XXIX

DYSPHAGIA DUE TO DISORDERS
OF THE ESOPHAGUS

KENNETH A. PHELPS, M.D.

Dysphagia means difficulty in swallowing. The degree of dysphagia may vary from obscure, indefinite sensations to a total inability to swallow anything, even saliva.

The cause of difficulty in swallowing may be located in the oral cavity, the pharynx, the esophagus, the mediastinum, or the nervous system. This chapter will deal only with dysphagia due to disorders of the esophagus.

APPLIED ANATOMY AND PHYSIOLOGY OF THE ESOPHAGUS

The esophagus has an anatomic sphincter at its upper end, the cricopharyngeus muscle, which is at the level of the cricoid cartilage or the 6th cervical vertebra. It has a physiologic sphincter at its lower end where it joins the stomach—40 to 45 cm. (15.7 to 17 inches) from the incisor teeth. There are two other narrow areas, one at the level of the arch of the aorta and the other at the crossing of the left bronchus (Fig. 158).

The function of the esophagus is to convey food, fluids and secretions from the pharynx to the stomach. This is the involuntary phase of deglutition. It begins after food is masticated and moistened in the mouth and passed back into the pharynx, where the normal swallowing reflex must be set up in order to relax the cricopharyngeal sphincter and open the esophagus.

The squeezing action of the pharyngeal constrictor shoots the bolus extremely rapidly through the pyriform sinuses and over the dorsum of the epiglottis into the esophagus.

Solid food is carried through the esophagus by peristalsis, and liquids more or less by gravity. The action of the longitudinal fibers shortens the esophagus and pulls it over the bolus, and also strengthens the inner circular layer. This circular layer really is elliptical in the upper two-thirds and corkscrew-like in the lower one-third.

The lower end of the esophagus is opened to let food through to the stomach. It is not thoroughly understood exactly how this takes place. It is thought that stimulation of the vagus opens the cardia while stimulation of the sympathetics closes it. Other factors are the muscles of the diaphragm, the liver and the twist in the esophageal muscle fibers which is like the twist of a tobacco pouch.

The mucosa of the esophagus is not insensitive, but it is not always possible for a patient to localize his symptoms exactly. Lesions in the lower one-half are apt to be localized at the epigastric region; lesions in the upper one-half are localized at the level of the larynx.

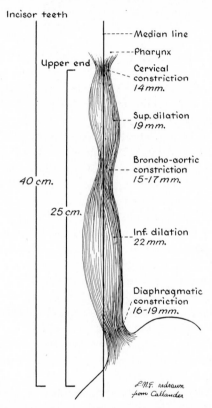

Fig. 158. The sites of narrowing in the esophagus.

The esophagus reacts very poorly to trauma or infection. This fact, together with its location, has led surgeons in the past to hesitate operating upon the esophagus. However, it will stand considerable abuse in cases of cardiac, aortic, or mediastinal lesions which may push it in any direction and to nearly any degree without interfering seriously with its function.

EXAMINATION FOR THE CAUSES OF DYSPHAGIA

Symptoms. The symptoms associated with dysphagia have significance as follows:

Regurgitation: This occurs in esophageal obstruction with retention.

Differentiation from vomiting is made by finding no gastric contents in the material regurgitated.

Respiratory symptoms: Choking and coughing, especially when eating, are due to overflow from the esophagus into the air passages directly, or through an esophagotracheal fistula.

Pain: Seen in ulceration, inflammation, distention, penetrating foreign body. It is rare in early cancer.

Pain on swallowing (odonophagia): Suggests a peri-esophageal extension of inflammation or infiltration, hiatal hernia, or penetrating foreign body.

Weight loss, hemorrhage and anemia are late manifestations.

Diagnosis. Reference has been made to the details of the history and the examination in Chapter XXIII, for one complaining of dysphagia. For emphasis, however, certain details will be repeated here.

A careful history alone will make a diagnosis in about 90 per cent of the cases. The most important points in this history are as follows: age, sex, onset and duration of dysphagia, type of food causing the greatest difficulty, localization of lesion by the patient, regurgitation, respiratory symptoms, loss of weight and pain. These points will become more obvious as the characteristics of each esophageal disorder causing dysphagia are discussed in detail.

In the matter of physical examination, direct inspection of the oral cavity and fauces with reflected light should, of course, reveal a cause for dysphagia in these areas. Inflammatory lesions and the ulceration of neoplasms, are, as a rule, very obvious. Paralyses involving the tongue, soft palate and constrictor muscles of the pharynx, singly or combined, will cause a degree of difficulty in the swallowing. These can usually be detected on direct examination supplemented by indirect examination of the lower pharynx by means of the laryngeal mirror. Examination of the esophagus is limited to x-ray study and direct inspection through the esophagoscope.

The x-ray study usually makes the diagnosis and locates the lesion. The roentgenologist should be requested to use as little barium as possible, particularly if an esophagoscopy is to follow, as is invariably performed in the case of a foreign body.

Esophagoscopy is rarely required for diagnosis. It is usually a confirmation of the diagnosis made by other means.

FOREIGN BODIES

This cause of dysphagia is discussed in the next chapter in a consideration of foreign bodies in the air and food passages.

CARCINOMA

Carcinoma of the esophagus in the past was 100 per cent fatal. It was a hopeless and helpless disease. Now, however, the thoracic surgeon is able to cure some of these patients. With the improvement in surgical technic and the aid of chemotherapy and the antibiotics, the prognosis is changing. Early diagnosis is of great importance, because the earlier it is found, the greater chance the patient has of

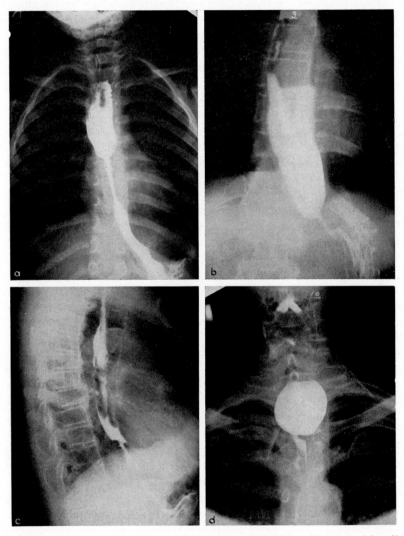

Fig. 159. Strictures in the esophagus from (a) corrosives, (b) cardiospasm, (c) malignant disease, (d) the filling of a diverticulum.

recovery. The patient should be encouraged and educated to seek medical advice upon the first appearance of dysphagia. His physician should insist on a complete examination, including esophagoscopy, in the earliest stages of the disease.

Symptoms. Difficulty in swallowing solid food is the first and only early symptom of carcinoma of the esophagus. This difficulty is often first noted when the patient eats solid food in a hurry. After experiencing such difficulty, the patient is apt to chew his food better and swallow more slowly so this symptom may not recur for some time.

"Queer sensations" in the throat or a feeling of a lump in the throat are not early symptoms of cancer. On the other hand, difficulty in swallowing solid food is rarely complained of by neurotic patients.

Carcinoma is the most frequent disease causing dysphagia. It is a disease occurring in men five times more frequently than in women. It is very rare before forty years of age. It occurs in hard-working men with poor teeth who eat rapidly and irregularly and who may use alcohol to excess.

The lesion is usually located at the level of the cricopharyngeus muscle in females, while in males it is more often near the lower end of the esophagus. Esophageal cancer is pathologically a highly malignant tumor.

Late symptoms are weight loss, pain, vomiting, cough, hoarseness, hiccough and bleeding.

Diagnosis. History and x-ray will usually make the diagnosis (Fig. 159), but the patient should have an esophagoscopic examination for biopsy, particularly when the symptoms and findings are not definite.

Treatment. The advanced case can be palliatively treated by dilating the obstruction by passing a metal dilator along a previously swallowed thread. High-voltage x-ray therapy and radium are not satisfactory. Our only hope of a cure lies in the early diagnosis and the radical surgical treatment.

CICATRICIAL STENOSIS

Cicatricial stenosis is caused by the formation and contraction of scar tissue developed to heal a burn or infection of the esophagus which has invaded the muscle layer.

The most common cause is the accidental swallowing of lye or other caustics by a child. Such an accident occurs much less frequently today, since the label "poison" is legally required on all containers of lye and other caustics.

The strictures are often multiple and may involve the stomach. They are located most frequently at the narrow areas of the esophagus. They are eccentric rather than concentric, with some normal esophageal wall remaining intact. Other causes are: complications of surgery on the esophagus, healed peptic ulcer, tuberculosis and syphilis.

Symptoms. Immediately following the ingestion of a caustic, there is distress from burns of the lips, mouth, tongue, palate and pharynx. Later, dysphagia due to burns and secondary infection, develops.

These symptoms may improve in about ten days. One should not be misled into believing this to be recovery. Unless preventative treatment is started at this stage, stenosis will occur in about six weeks and the patient may not be able to swallow even water. Sudden complete obstruction usually means a foreign body is in the stricture, usually in the form of some food.

Treatment. The immediate treatment should consist of *fluids, sedatives,* and *olive oil* in large amounts.

The preventive treatments should begin as soon as the acute symptoms subside. This consists of passing a nasal feeding tube through the esophagus and leaving it in place several hours every day for six weeks. Inspection of the lesion with the esophagoscope should then be made, and many patients will have no stenoses.

Patients in whom the preventive treatment is neglected will nearly all develop a stenosis which requires dilatation.

A variety of instruments for dilatation have been developed. These include bougies made of rubber or silk, a rubber bougie filled with mercury which gives it weight and plasticity, olive-tipped bougie points of silk (Jackson) on a metal handle for direct vision passage through an esophagoscope, metal olive tips attached to a handle (Plummer) and passed over a previously swallowed thread, and retrograde bougies to be passed through a gastrostomy opening from below upward by pulling on a previously swallowed thread.

Prognosis. Cicatricial stenosis of the esophagus may require dilatations at intervals for the rest of the patient's life. In severe cases, dilatation may be relatively unsuccessful and the patient's food may be restricted to liquids. Eventually, a proportion of cases perforate. However. if treated promptly, many patients develop satisfactory cures.

CARDIOSPASM

Cardiospasm (achalasia) is the name of an esophageal condition characterized by failure of the cardiac end of the esophagus to open and a dilatation of the esophagus proximal to this obstruction. It may be present at birth.

The exact cause is unknown. Some investigators have reported the finding of periesophageal fibrosis. Others have found no fibrosis. Neurogenic changes in the vagus and overaction of the sympathetic nerves as a cause of closure has been claimed. The recent operation of vagotomy (cutting both vagi) may give us more knowledge regarding this function of this nerve.

Since there is not a spasm or other organic stenosis at the cardia, it seems most logical that this condition is due to faulty nervous control of the cardia. It does not open normally—rather than that, it is abnormally closed. The dilatation results from retention of foods. Infection of the mucosa and even muscular structure may occur in the late stages.

The disorder is not on a neurotic basis. It occurs more commonly in the male sex in the proportion of three to two, and usually without any associated diseases.

Symptoms. Dysphagia, epigastric pain and regurgitation are the characteristic symptoms.

The dysphagia is often sudden in onset and worse with cold foods. There may be a total inability to swallow. Usually a patient can tell when the food goes through and can locate the level of obstruction. Some patients take a deep breath, thus increasing the intrathoracic pressure and can force food down.

The pain may simulate coronary disease, radiating to the jaw, neck, ears, or back and arms. It frequently awakes the patient at night and rarely bothers at mealtime. It is worse in early stages of the disease.

Before dilatation develops, the regurgitation occurs soon after eating, but later the patient can hold his esophagus full for hours. It may occur at night when the patient lies down and may be associated with choking and aspiration into the trachea.

Diagnosis. The x-ray picture of a smooth obstruction with marked dilatation is an almost certain diagnosis of cardiospasm (Fig. 159). However, esophagoscopy may be necessary to rule out cancer.

Treatment. There is no medical treatment which seems to be effective. Antispasmodics apparently help some mild cases. Mechanical dilatation with an olive-tipped bougie, guided over a silk or linen thread which has been previously swallowed, is effective, particularly so if the No. 60 French size can be passed. As high as 70 per cent good results have been reported with the use of a bougie of this size. If this is not effective, dilatation with a bag which can be inflated with air or water so as to produce a measured pressure will produce successful results in an additional percentage of the victims of this disorder.

Spasm. Spasm is a closure of the cardia by real spasm and may occur as reflex secondary to abdominal disease, as an ulcer, cancer, cholecystitis and so on. These patients have intermittent pain and dysphagia, but no regurgitation. Usually they are relieved when a primary condition is found or when a dilator is passed. Rarely, the spasm is diffuse and involves a larger area of the esophagus.

DIVERTICULA

Diverticula are sacculations projecting from the wall of the esophagus. They are said to be congenital. However, no case is on record as having been diagnosed in infancy. There are two types: (1) the pulsion type, which is located just above the cricopharyngeus muscle at a congenitally weak point and is really pharyngeal rather than esophageal in origin, and (2) the traction type, which is smaller and lower down and usually requires no treatment.

As a rule, diverticula occur in people over fifty years of age. Mastication is less thorough, as the teeth are apt to be poor. Hurried eating with the gulping of larger boluses of food, is an additional factor which increases the likelihood of a diverticulum developing.

Symptoms. The diagnosis of diverticulum may often be made by history alone. Choking and coughing attacks coming on after eating and associated with difficulty in swallowing, are the most frequent symptoms.

After the sac has appeared, it is filled with food during each swallowing act. The food must get out again in order to enter the esophagus. This slows down the movement of the bolus, so a portion of it very frequently remains in the sac. When the glottis reopens and the cricopharyngeus muscle contracts, some of the retained food may enter the larynx, causing choking and coughing. Now the patient observes that food seems to stick in his throat. He frequently recovers fragments of food several hours after eating. The sac may fill with air and gurgling noises occur during the swallowing act. These sounds may be quite embarrassing to the patient, as others can hear them too.

Diagnosis. An x-ray study will demonstrate the sac and makes the diagnosis (Fig. 159).

When the esophagoscope is passed, it usually enters the sac very easily and the blind end is quickly encountered. However, the sub-diverticular orifice of the esophagus may be very difficult to find.

The treatment is surgical. One or two stage operations are very effective.

HYSTERICAL DYSPHAGIA

(Plummer-Vinson Syndrome)

This is a peculiar disorder characterized by an inability to swallow solid food although there is no obstructive lesion in the esophagus. In the course of the dysphagia, there usually develops an anemia, glossitis, a palpable spleen and, in some cases, a hypothyroidism. Vinson has found that it occurs most frequently in Scandinavian women about forty years of age.

Other investigators object to the use of the term "hysterical" and consider the dysphagia as due to an atrophic change in the pharynx, or some find webs and true spasm at the orifice of the esophagus. Vinson believes that the anemia is secondary to the dysphagia, while others discredit that idea.

All agree, however, that passing a dilator regardless of size through the esophagus cures most of the patients, whether it dilates a stricture or spasm, or relieves the hysteria by suggestion.

There is a mild form of functional dysphagia known as "globus hystericus." It is very common, particularly in women who complain of a sense of a lump in the throat and an indefinite dysphagia. The diagnosis is made by the history, an apparently emotional instability on the part of the patient, and the absence of any disease in the pharynx and upper esophagus.

HIATAL HERNIA

A hiatal hernia may cause dysphagia. This is a disorder in which a portion of the stomach slides through the diaphragmatic hiatus and lies along side the lower end of the esophagus. It is sometimes called a peri-esophageal hernia. The herniated portion of the stomach may be movable or incarcerated. The symptoms are mostly a fulness after eating and a chest pain somewhat like an attack of angina. X-ray studies usually make the diagnosis. The treatment is surgical if the hernia is large enough and the symptoms are troublesome.

CONGENITAL ANOMALIES

The esophagus develops in early fetal life as a groove in the foregut from which originates the pharynx, larynx, trachea and lungs. An abnormal development may result in one or more of the following defects:

Esophagotracheal Fistula. In this, the upper segment of the esophagus is a blind pouch ending usually at the level of the larynx. The lower segment leads from the stomach to the trachea. This is the most frequent of all congenital defects. If the swallowing difficulty seems limited to the nursing act, it is important to rule out choanal occlusion.

The diagnosis is usually made by x-ray, which demonstrates the blind end of the upper segment. Bronchoscopy will demonstrate the fistula in the trachea.

The prognosis is improving, as the thoracic surgeons now report many babies who have successfully survived a surgical correction.

Web or Stricture. This produces partial or complete obstruction at the upper or lower end of the esophagus. It may not be noticed, however, until the child takes more solid food. It is treated by dilatation and often with satisfactory results.

Other Developmental Defects. These are:

Upper and lower cul-de-sacs with solid cord connecting.

Double esophagus.

Simple esophagotracheal fistula.

Congenital shortening of the esophagus with thoracic stomach—the esophagus opens into the apex of the stomach. At one stage of embryological development, the stomach is above the diaphragm. The right half closed before the left and explains why more hiatal hernias are on the left side.

There may be a partial thoracic stomach. Frequently there is a constriction at the cardia, and the most common symptom is obstruction to swallowing.

Cardiovascular anomalies may compress the esophagus and cause dysphagia.

REFERENCES

Clerf, L. H., and Putney, F. J.: Cricopharyngeal Spasm. Laryngoscope, *52*:944, 1942.

Gelis, S., and Holt, L. E., Jr.: Treatment of Lye Ingestion by the Salzer Method. Ann. Otol., Rhin. & Laryng., *51*:1086, 1942.

Harrington, S.: Pulsion Diverticulum of Hypopharynx at Pharyngo-Esophageal Junction. Surgery, *18*:66, 1945.

Holinger, P., and Hara, H.: Cancer of the Esophagus. Laryngoscope, *52*:968, 1942.

Hurst, A.: Nervous Disorders of Swallowing. J. Laryng. & Otol., *58*:60, 1943.

Leegaard, T.: Corrosive Injuries of the Esophagus with Particular Reference to Treatment of Acute Corrosive Esophagitis. *Ibid.*, *60*:389, 1945.

Leven, N. L., and Lannin, B.: Congenital Atresia and Congenital Tracheo-Esophageal Fistula. Journal Lancet, *65*:179, 1945.

Mosher, H. P.: Infection as a Cause of Fibrosis of the Esophagus. Ann. Otol., Rhin. & Laryng., *50*:633, 1941.

Phelps, K. A.: Congenital Anomalies of the Esophagus. *Ibid.*, *39*:364, 1932.

Phelps, K. A.: Early Treatment of Chemical Burns of the Esophagus. Journal Lancet, *58*:237, 1938.

Richardson, J.: New Treatment of Esophageal Obstruction due to Meat Impaction. Ann. Otol., Rhin. & Laryng., *54*:328, 1945.

Sweet, R.: Surgical Management of Carcinoma of Mid-Thoracic Esophagus. New England J. Med., *233*:1, 1945.

Templeton, F. E., and Kredel, R. A.: Cricopharyngeal Sphincter. Laryngoscope, *53*:1, 1943.

Uhde, G.: Chemical Burns of the Esophagus. Ann. Otol., Rhin. & Laryng., *55*:795, 1946.

Viets, H. R.: Diagnosis of Myasthenia Gravis in Patients with Dysphagia. J.A.M.A., *134*:987, 1947.

Wangensteen, O., Merendino, K., and Varco, R.: Displacement of Esophagus into a New Diaphragmatic Orifice in the Repair of Para Esophageal and Esophageal Hiatus Hernia. Ann. Surg., *129*:186, 1949.

14

CHAPTER XXX

FOREIGN BODIES IN THE AIR AND FOOD PASSAGES

Kenneth A. Phelps, M.D.

Foreign bodies are accidentally swallowed or inhaled very frequently. Many of them are coughed out at once or pass on through the intestinal tract and do not become lodged. The newspapers almost daily refer to some such accident and occasionally report the death of the victim before medical aid could be obtained. This publicity undoubtedly increases the fear and anxiety of patients and their relatives when a foreign body is aspirated. As a matter of fact, once the foreign body has become lodged, the patient is rarely in an emergency condition. Ill advised attempts to remove the foreign body are more likely to cause disaster than the presence of the foreign body itself. Before the days of the x-ray and bronchoscope, statistics seemed to prove that a foreign body in the bronchus or esophagus had best be left alone, because more patients recovered when no attempt at removal was made.

Today we expect foreign bodies to be safely and promptly removed. Because this is being done so successfully, we are losing our fear of manipulations carried on within the trachea and bronchi. Obstetricians catheterize the newborn baby's trachea to aspirate secretion; the anesthesiologist inserts tubes to deliver his anesthetic intratracheally and he aspirates the bronchi quite routinely after prolonged anesthesia; the roentgenologist drops iodized oil (lipiodol) into the bronchi; the chest physician and the chest surgeon are using the bronchoscope more and more frequently and possibly the intern or nurse may soon be doing routine bronchial aspirations. The presence of a foreign body, however, provides mechanical problems which demand special technic if the procedure is to be safely performed. It is a performance not without a hazard, particularly in the case of a foreign body in the esophagus.

The study of foreign bodies has contributed a great deal to our knowledge of anatomy and pathology of the bronchi and lungs. It has been pointed out that each branch of the bronchus supplies ventilation and drainage to a definite segment of the lung. A generally accepted terminology is being worked out at present which will correlate the site of a bronchial lesion with the peripheral distribution of its effect.

We now recognize that lung disease produced by a foreign body is due to bronchial obstruction. The knowledge of the definite effects on the lung, produced by bronchial obstruction, has considerably influenced the diagnosis and treatment of pulmonary disease.

The following table summarizes my experience.

ANALYSIS OF 698 FOREIGN BODIES

NUMBER OF CASES	FOOD					METALLIC			
	Mealtime			Not Mealtime		Safety pins	Coin	Dental	Others
	Bones	Meat	Other	Peanuts	Others				
Children									
245 Air Way	2	0	2	109	74	13	2	1	42
165 Esophagus	6	6	1	0	3	40	59	0	50
Adults									
27 Air Way	4	0	0	1	10	1	0	6	5
261 Esophagus	181	51	7	0	2	4	2	4	10

From this table, certain facts may be established. More foreign bodies occur in children than in adults. Foreign bodies are found in the air passages of children nearly ten times as frequently as in adults, while foreign bodies become lodged in the esophagus of adults more often than in children—about two to one.

Food eaten at mealtime may contain a foreign body, such as a bone. This type of foreign body is found almost exclusively in adults. They often masticate poorly, usually because of poor dentistry, and swallow hastily. Children's food is carefully prepared and they are watched while eating.

Nuts, seeds, or other vegetable objects, not swallowed at mealtime, occur almost entirely in children under two years of age. Of 199 such objects, 186 were in children and only 3 were in the esophagus. Peanuts were 109 of these objects. There is no specific reaction produced by peanuts. Any foreign body in this group may set up as violent a reaction.

Metallic objects, as coins or pins, are swallowed about ten times more frequently by children than by adults. They become lodged in the esophagus about twice as often as in the bronchi (Fig. 160). Youngsters pick up these objects and put them in their mouths; adults do not.

FOREIGN BODIES IN THE ESOPHAGUS

A foreign body becomes lodged in the esophagus because it is large; has sharp points or serrated edges which catch in the folds of the esophagus; or because the esophagus is narrowed as a result of pre-existing disease, such as spasm, stricture, or tumor. The symptoms are substernal discomfort, difficulty in swallowing, or pain on attempting to do so. A scratch caused by a foreign body in passing, frequently results in pronounced dysphagia, but rarely persistent pain. This is of considerable

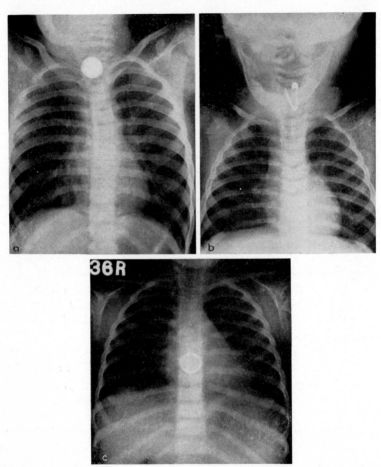

Fig. 160. Common types of esophageal foreign bodies in children. (a) Coin at the cervical narrowing ("upper pinchcock"). (b) Safety pin arrested at the same site as in (a). (c) Campaign button arrested temporarily in the lower one third of the esophagus.

diagnostic importance. It is rare for a foreign body to remain in the esophagus for years, as may occur in the bronchi.

Perforation of the esophagus may result from a foreign body. The symptoms vary according to the level at which the perforation occurs. If in the neck, subcutaneous emphysema may be the only symptom or mediastinitis may develop. If lower down, the pleural cavity may be directly involved, resulting in a pneumothorax or pyothorax. A tracheo-esophageal fistula may occur.

Subcutaneous emphysema in the neck or mediastinitis demands prompt surgical treatment. The use of sulfonamides or the antibiotics

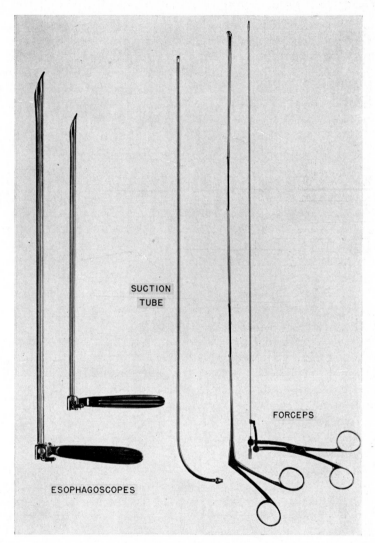

SUCTION
TUBE

FORCEPS

ESOPHAGOSCOPES

Fig. 161. Adult and infant esophagoscope (Jesberg Model), grasping and biopsy forceps, suction tube.

makes this complication less hazardous than it once was, but it is still considered desirable to perform mediastinotomy and pack the wound open for drainage.

Diagnosis. The diagnosis of a foreign body in the esophagus and its location is a simple matter with x-ray in the cases of an opaque substance. When the foreign body is nonopaque, a barium capsule when swallowed may give the clue. Occasionally, inspection through the esophagoscope provides the diagnosis.

The technic of handling a foreign body through the aid of esophagoscopic visualization varies with the particular problem. Local anesthesia is commonly used in adults and, if the esophagoscope (Fig. 161) is skilfully inserted, the amount of trauma is negligible. Some foreign bodies can be grasped and drawn into the lumen of the esophagoscope; others require manipulations to dislodge the foreign body and sometimes even to rotate it as may be the case with a safety pin. These procedures demand the utmost in skill and judgment.

FOREIGN BODIES IN THE AIR PASSAGES

One group of foreign bodies originates from within the chest itself. Mucous plugs occur in postoperative atelectasis, acute laryngotracheobronchitis or other infections, and after the removal of foreign bodies. Diphtheritic membrane, blood from a pulmonary hemorrhage, and ruptured peribronchial lymph nodes containing broncholiths or granulation tissue act as foreign bodies. Also, a tumor may slough and act in a similar role.

Foreign bodies originating from outside the lung and aspirated include stomach contents, particularly during anesthesia or intoxication, and dental objects such as plates and dentures.

Small metallic objects, such as straight pins, do not cause obstruction of the bronchus. Quite often no symptoms are noticed and the object may remain many years without the patient realizing it. Eventually these objects may cause some local reaction which will obstruct the bronchus and produce symptoms such as hemoptysis and cough. A lung containing an unknown foreign body may not recover from an infection in the usual manner. Usually the foreign body is discovered as a result of an x-ray examination.

Large foreign bodies will cause obstruction of varying degree. Sudden complete obstruction results in atelectasis. Complete occlusion of the trachea with bilateral atelectasis is fatal. If the main bronchus is obstructed, unilateral atelectasis results. The most common object causing this is a navy bean which swells rapidly and is perhaps the most dangerous of all foreign bodies. If the foreign body totally obstructs a secondary bronchus, one lobe of the lung may become atelectatic.

Partial obstruction is much more common than complete obstruction. It results in the well-known obstructive emphysema. Air can get into but not out of the lobe or lung and becomes trapped, owing to the valve-like action of the foreign body. X-ray films taken at the end of expiration show that the obstructed part of the lung contains more air than the unobstructed portion because the air cannot get out (Fig. 162). This finding is positive proof of obstruction in the bronchus.

If bronchial obstruction persists, drowned lung, abscess, bronchiectasis, or gangrene develop. True pneumonia is rare.

Symptoms. By far the most constant symptoms are cough, wheeze and dyspnea. The cough is often intermittent and noisy, and shifting of the foreign body may increase it. The wheeze can be heard at the mouth and is both inspiratory and expiratory. Jackson refers to this symptom as an "asthmatoid wheeze."

Any patient who chokes on a foreign body and then develops a cough and a wheeze, is almost certain to have the foreign body lodged in his air passages.

Dyspnea is an increase in the breathing effort. It may result in the ventilation of the lung being normal, increased, or decreased. The clinical

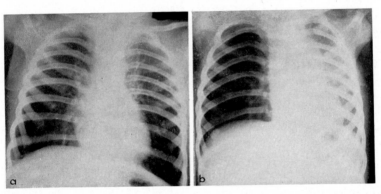

Fig. 162. Obstructive emphysema in a three-and-one-half-year-old child with a foreign body (peanut) in the right main bronchus. On inspiration (a), the bronchus enlarges and air passes around the foreign body to "pump up" the right lung. On expiration, the air escapes normally from the left lung but the right bronchus closes tightly around the foreign body, keeping the air trapped on the right side. There is a mediastinal shift to the left (b).

recognition of early anoxia is not possible, but when shallow and rapid breathing occurs, together with evidence of fatigue and exhaustion, it is time to do something in a hurry. Cyanosis, pain, hemoptysis and other symptoms are less frequent.

Physical Signs. The most constant sign is limited expansion of the affected lung. This is present even in the nonobstructing, symptomless, small foreign body deep in the lung.

Impaired breathing sounds over the obstructed area is a most reliable sign and quite frequently present. The temperature, pulse and respiration are not diagnostic.

Diagnosis. The history is invaluable and can be obtained in almost every case. The x-ray is also invaluable and often makes the diagnosis. When the history and symptoms are suggestive and the physical signs are confirmed by x-ray, bronchoscopy is always indicated. When the history is suggestive and no symptoms, signs, nor x-ray findings are present, bronchoscopy may be performed, but it will usually be negative. Even bronchoscopy may not demonstrate a foreign body which is present. Foreign bodies of long standing may produce symptoms suggestive of almost every chest disease and should always be ruled out as a possibility.

Foreign bodies that have become lodged do not require emergency treatment, unless asphyxia is threatened. This may occur at once with immediate death. Usually the foreign body is aspirated into one bronchus and a period of relative comfort follows. Should it be dislodged and coughed into the trachea or glottis or fall back into the previously unobstructed bronchus, both bronchi may be closed off. The foreign body itself may swell to such a size as to close off the trachea. A general rule is to remove all large foreign bodies and all organic ones immediately. Small metallic objects do not require emergency treatment. It is not advisable to wait for the foreign body to be coughed out, as this occurs in only about 2 per cent of cases. Neither is it recommended that the patient be inverted, as the foreign body may become impacted in the glottis.

Complications due to perforation of the air passages by foreign bodies may result in subcutaneous emphysema, pneumothorax, hydrothorax, or pyothorax. Traumatic laryngitis in young children may occur, for which a tracheotomy may be required. A drowned lung or bronchiectasis is a most frequent sequella of a foreign body remaining in a bronchus.

Technic of Treatment. In children, a general anesthetic is usually used. Complications practically never develop as a result of ether. In some cases, the lack of anesthesia causes the operator to traumatize his patient, resulting in exhaustion and greater shock.

The occasional bronchoscopist is entitled to every advantage he can obtain. With his patient relaxed and under perfect control, he can work much easier and more gently. It is bound to be more comfortable for a child to be asleep while bronchoscopy is being performed. Contraindications to general anesthesia are cyanosis of marked degree and lung abscess or stricture of the esophagus when repeated treatments are necessary.

Local anesthesia in adults is quite satisfactory. The procedure is usually surprisingly comfortable for the patient. Plenty of preliminary sedation is helpful and in certain cases intravenous morphine is very satisfactory. Local applications of a 10 per cent cocaine solution to the gums, pharynx and larynx, as well as instillation into the trachea is routine. This is best done with the patient in the upright position. General anesthesia may be necessary, pentothal sodium with curare being satisfactory.

Frequently the bronchoscope (Fig. 163) can be passed directly into the trachea without using the laryngoscope to expose the glottis. A laryngoscope and a short forceps should always be handy to remove a foreign body if it should be stripped off at the glottis, as it is being extracted.

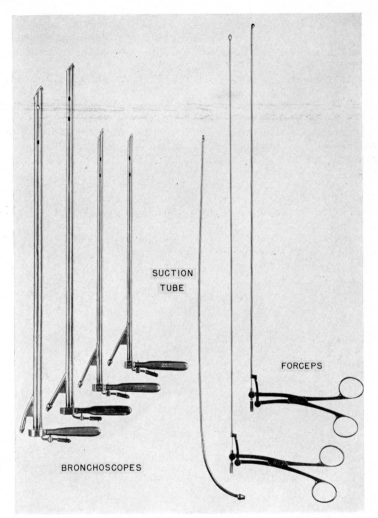

Fig. 163. Bronchoscopes of several sizes. The two larger are the Jackson models, the two smaller the Jesberg models. Forceps and suction tubes.

After the foreign body is removed, a second examination should always be made to be sure that no fragment remains. A thorough aspiration of all pus and other secretions should be performed at this time.

Good equipment is necessary, such as suction, batteries and lights.

Elaborate technic is not needed nor are numerous instruments required. A biplane fluoroscope is rarely essential, but when it is needed, nothing can take its place.

The diagnosis is made earlier nowadays, so neglected cases of long standing are seldom seen. This means complications and fatalities are becoming quite rare.

REFERENCES

Hagens, E.: Anatomy of the Tracheobronchial Tree from the Bronchoscopic Standpoint. Arch. Otolaryng., *38*:469, 1943.

Holinger, P., Andrews, A., and Rigby, R.: Foreign Bodies in Air and Food Passages. Eye, Ear, Nose & Throat Monthly, *22*:415, 1943.

Jackson, C., and Jackson, C. L.: Foreign Bodies in the Air and Food Passages Roentgenologically Considered. New York, Paul B. Hoeber, Inc., 1934.

Jackson, C., and Jackson, C. L.: Bronchoscopy, Esophagoscopy, and Gastroscopy. 3rd ed. Philadelphia, W. B. Saunders Co., 1934.

Jackson, C. L., and Huber, J.: Correlated Applied Anatomy of Bronchial Tree and Lung with a System of Nomenclature. Dis. of Chest, *9*:319, 1943.

Phelps, K. A.: Foreign Bodies Lodged in Air and Food Passages. Minnesota Med., *27*:27, 1944.

Phelps, K. A.: The Diagnosis and Treatment of Non Opaque Foreign Bodies in the Air Passages, *Ibid.*, *10*:731, 1927.

Van Loon, E., and Diamond S.: Foreign Bodies in the Gastrointestinal Tract. Ann. Otol., Rhin. & Laryng., *51*:1077, 1942.

CHAPTER XXXI

TUMORS OF THE NOSE AND THROAT

Tumors of the nose and throat arise in four general locations: (1) the nasal space and sinuses; (2) the nasopharynx; (3) the tonsils and pharynx; and (4) the larynx (Fig. 164). Certain anatomical and functional characteristics of these areas determine to some extent the type of tumor, its manifestations, the course of its development, and also the method of treatment and the prognosis.

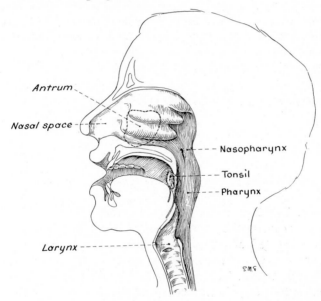

Fig. 164. Four sites of malignant disease in the nose and throat determine to some extent the type of tumor and the most effective treatment because of the type of tissue involved, its blood supply, and lymphatic drainage. These four sites are: 1. The nasal space and sinuses. 2. The nasopharynx. 3. The tonsils and pharynx. 4. The larynx.

It is important that the physician in general practice or any physician who takes the responsibility for treating nose and throat symptoms, suspect the possibility of the presence of a malignant tumor from certain symptoms and signs. Only in that way can we improve the matter of early diagnosis, granted, of course, that the patient has sought early relief of his symptoms. It is the experience of one who treats malignant disease of the nose and throat to observe that patients are often treated for "sinus trouble" who have definite evidence of a malignant lesion in the nasal space, or for simple chronic sore throat when visualization of the pharynx would reveal the ulceration of a carcinoma, or by the empirical use of prescribed sprays, gargles and so on, when a chronic hoarseness plainly warns of a laryngeal cancer.

The family doctor should know:

1. When to suspect a tumor of the nose or throat,
2. The steps necessary to a proper diagnosis, and
3. The principles underlying the modern methods of treatment.

THE NASAL SPACE AND SINUSES

Benign Tumors. These are simple nasal polyps, papilloma, fibroma, angioma, osteoma and so on. The very common nasal polyp is a myxomatous growth resulting from a hyperplastic rhinitis. It is frequently found in the presence of an allergic rhinitis and less often of an origin from purely inflammatory change in the nasal or sinus mucosa. Other benign tumors of the nasal space are relatively uncommon.

Symptoms. The prominent symptom is nasal obstruction. The presence of a tumor mass produces more or less hypersecretion so that a mucoid discharge of some degree is also noted. If infection occurs, the discharge changes in character to a purulent one. Bleeding is uncommon in cases of a benign tumor, except in some angiomas, or when an erosion of the surface of the tumor occurs. Pain is rare unless suppuration produces edema and obstruction to drainage.

Malignant Tumors. These are carcinoma, lymphosarcoma, other forms of sarcoma, endothelioma and so on.

Symptoms. The first symptom may be nasal obstruction, although discharge may concern the patient first. Unilateral fetid discharge should always be suspected of association with a malignant tumor. Pain is another symptom which may appear during the course of development of a malignant tumor. The patient with a growing carcinoma of an antrum often tells of pain in a remaining tooth or teeth in the upper jaw on the involved side. Often, these teeth are pulled by an unsuspecting dentist. An x-ray properly interpreted would focus attention on the antrum above. Swelling occurs when the tumor mass thins out the wall of the antrum or the lateral nasal margin, or it invades the orbit to cause displacement of the orbital content. Bloody discharge is not uncommon, especially from carcinoma or lymphosarcoma if either is present in the nasal fossa.

When a mass is visualized in a nasal fossa, mainpulation usually starts bleeding if the growth is malignant. A biopsy is easily made, as a rule, and confirms the diagnosis. When a mass cannot be visualized in the nasal space, x-ray studies of the sinuses may provide the suspicion that a tumor is present and indicate the need for exploration.

Treatment. Treatment of malignant tumors of the nasal space and sinuses involves *irradiation,* a combination of x-ray and the exposure of the tumor mass to radium. In the antrum, exposure for the placing of radium requires enough surgery to provide this exposure. The tumor is first removed grossly before the radium is placed and the margins co-

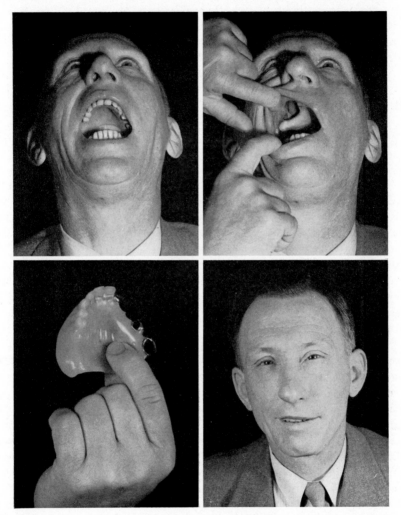

Fig. 165. Views of a healed operative cavity and dental prosthesis three years after treatment of a carcinoma of the maxillary sinus through a palate approach.

agulated with surgical diathermy. Occasionally, a lateral rhinotomy (loosening the external nose by incision on one side) is made for exposing the nasal fossa. Exposure of the contents of an antrum is through the canine fossa or through the palate (Fig. 165).

Almost one-half of the cases of primary cancer in the maxillary sinus coming into the hands of surgeons experienced in this type of surgery, are curable. With earlier diagnosis, this percentage can be greatly enlarged.

THE NASOPHARYNX

Benign Tumors. A purely benign tumor arising in the nasopharynx is rare. Occasionally nasopharyngeal polyps are encountered which originate in the nasal fossa or cysts are formed which arise in the maxillary sinus and gradually elongate through the sinus ostium and become dependent and hang into the nasopharynx.

Fibroma. A tumor which is relatively benign is one that represents a clinical entity, the fibroma of the nasopharynx. Some of the older texts refer to this as a "juvenile sarcoma." This neoplasm, though benign in the fact that it remains localized, is potentially malignant in that unchecked it may destroy by expansion and pressure necrosis, to an end in fatal complications.

Symptoms. Fibroma of the nasopharynx is usually first noted in early puberty. It is more common in males. The first symptom is one of nasal congestion, a definite obstruction which may be mostly unilateral. Subsequent symptoms may be due to the effects of the nasal obstruction, a "nasal" voice, discomfort in swallowing due to the obstructed nasopharynx, a loss of appetite and a purulent discharge due to secondary infection. Ear symptoms, such as might result from obstruction of the eustachian tube, are not uncommon. Later there may be hemorrhage. As the tumor expands, the nose and maxilla may change shape along with the result of an invasion of one or both orbits to produce the "frog face" appearance.

This tumor arises from fibrous tissue in the nasopharyngeal recess or the base of the sphenoid or any adjoining structure. The tumor substance is largely composed of fibrous tissue with an abundance of blood vessels which lack a contractile coat. The covering of the tumor is mucous membrane. In gross appearance, the tumor may appear whitish gray in color or a pinkish to a dark purple color. Depending on the texture of the tumor mass, these growths have been labeled as fibromas, fibroangiomas, or fibromyxomas. In a growth which is largely fibromatous, the tumor may feel almost "wooden" to palpation, with the consistency of soft, light wood.

Treatment. These tumors are said to regress and even disappear as growth progresses. That means that a growth noted in puberty might be safely observed through the age when physical growth is complete (at about twenty-five years) if its size is not too great to interfere with adequate physiological function. Formerly, the treatment was invariably surgical and removal by snare or avulsion was often attended by serious and even fatal hemorrhage. Today, the treatment depends on the type of tumor. Some of these growths may be suitable for destruction and removal with the use of *surgical diathermy*. Others are *irradiated* with x-ray and implantation of radon seeds and, when reduced in size and vascularity, the remaining tumor mass is removed. Some are controlled by irradiation alone.

Malignant Tumors. These lesions are the most common of the tumors which originate in the nasopharynx. Squamous celled carcinoma is the most frequently found. Lympho-epithelioma probably ranks next. Some pathologists do not recognize this tumor, believing it to be a squamous cell carcinoma of high malignancy (grade 4). Adenocarcinoma is occasionally found. Sarcomas of several types occur; the lympho-sarcoma is the one usually found.

Symptoms. The symptoms vary. Nasal obstruction, postnasal discharge which may contain blood, unilateral eustachian tube involvement with its manifestations and so on, may be relatively early symptoms. Late symptoms are pain, hemorrhage, and manifestations from an extension of the lesion to involve adjacent nerves, the intracranial cavity, or by metastasis to glands in the neck.

Treatment. The treatment is practically limited to *irradiation.* Five-year survivals are rare. However, irradiation offers considerable in the way of palliation.

THE TONSILS AND PHARYNX

Benign Tumors. Papilloma, lipoma, fibroma, angioma, mixed tumors and so on, are found in an area including the tonsils and that portion of the pharynx below the nasopharynx. The most common of these is the simple papilloma found on the tonsil. This lesion is usually of no clinical significance. Mixed tumors in this area most often originate in the soft palate. Complete enucleation usually results in a cure. Occasionally malignant change occurs.

Malignant Tumors. Malignant tumors found in this area are usually squamous cell carcinoma and less frequently lymphosarcoma. Adenocarcinoma, other forms of sarcoma (than the lymphosarcoma) and so on, are also found, but are relatively rare.

Symptoms. The first symptoms of malignant lesions in this area are common complaints, which are often overlooked. The patient usually complains of a sense of irritation in his throat, a "rawness" or "scratchiness," or a sense of something which causes him annoyance. He may think of the possibility of having a fish bone or a toothbrush bristle in his throat. The growth may produce a sense of mass or lump. The presence of the tumor usually causes hypersecretion of mucus and an increased salivation. If there is surface ulceration, the patient may spit out blood-streaked mucus. The occurrence of dysphagia, actual pain on swallowing or referred pain (usually to an ear) or of metastatic glands to the neck represent late manifestations.

Treatment. Treatment of the malignant lesions in the tonsils and pharynx is by *irradiation.* Destruction of low grade squamous cell carcinoma by surgical diathermy may be indicated, but surgery is rarely employed.

Permanent cures are not common, but can be effected when early and adequate treatment is carried out.

THE LARYNX

Benign Tumors. These include papilloma, polyp, angioma, cyst, fibroma, lipoma and chondroma.

The simple inflammatory polyp is probably the most common of the benign tumors of the larynx (Fig. 166). This is often diagnosed incorrectly as a papilloma. As its name implies, it is a polypoid type of lesion, usually localized and more or less pedunculated. The base may be broad, however. This lesion presents one symptom of importance, voice change in the form of hoarseness. Visualization of the larynx with a mirror reveals the reddish colored small tumor mass usually attached to the free margin of a vocal cord, often in the anterior one-half. Treatment consists of scalping off the tumor mass even with the surface of the vocal cord. Some laryngologists prefer to touch the site of attachment with surgical diathermy.

Simple papilloma in the adult gives the same symptom of hoarseness. Inspection with the laryngeal mirror reveals a characteristic appearance of papilloma in many cases (Fig. 167). These lesions may grow to a considerable size. There is some evidence that a papilloma is caused by a virus. The papilloma in children present a clinical entity. They are usually multiple and may become evident in early childhood. Voice change to the extent of an aphonia occurs when the tumor mass keeps the cords apart. This amount of tumor often causes obstruction to breathing, and tracheotomy may become necessary. The treatment of the tumor consists of scalping off the growth flush with the vocal cords. Recurrence is common, but as the child gets through adolescence, there is a tendency for recurrence to cease.

Claims have been made for the value of estrogenic substance in maturing the epithelium of the cord as a means of preventing recurrence of papillomas. A trial of this therapy has not proven to be convincing. X-ray and radium have also had advocates but this therapy has not proven to be a certain cure, and these agents are not without some risk, since cartilaginous reaction in the form of chondritis with subsequent stenosis has resulted.

The other benign tumors of the larynx present the one early symptom—hoarseness. Cough may occur from irritation. Lipomas and angiomas may become rather large. Lipomas are dissected out or excised; angiomas need destruction with surgical diathermy. Chondromas are rare.

Malignant Tumors. These include carcinoma, sarcoma and endothelioma. Squamous cell carcinoma is said to constitute about 93 per

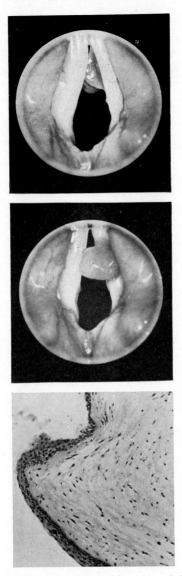

Fig. 166. Photograph of a polyp of the vocal cord, made by Dr. Paul Holinger and associates and loaned through his courtesy and the Annals of Otology, Rhinology and Laryngology.

(Upper) Pedunculated freely movable polyp of the right vocal cord, subglottic position during inspiration, showing attachment to the subglottic region of the vocal cord of a white woman, age thirty-two. Film No. 66-34 (22-f15-3/4L). History: Continuous hoarseness for past five years. No change during this time. No hemoptysis, sweats or cough. Histological Diagnosis: Myxomatous polyp of vocal cord. Microscopic Description: Polypoid structure lined by stratified squamous epithelium which overlies loose fibrous stroma. Within the latter, there are hugely dilated partly thrombosed blood vessels. (× 198). (Center) Supraglottic position during expiration. Film No. 66-35 (22-f15-3/4L). (Lower) Photomicrograph of polyp.

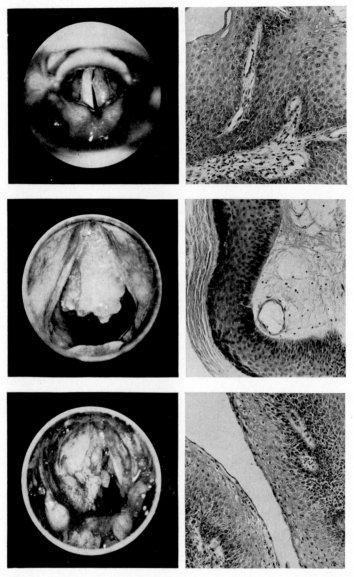

Fig. 167. Photograph of a papilloma of the vocal cord, made by Dr. Paul Holinger and associates and loaned through his courtesy and the Annals of Otology, Rhinology and Laryngology.

(Upper) Papilloma of left vocal cord, indirect view. The patient was a white female, age twenty. Film No. 56-2. History: Marked hoarseness since awakening about two weeks previously. Had some associated dyspnea. Histological Diagnosis: Papilloma of larynx. Microscopic Description: Very marked hyperplasia of squamous epithelium in a typical papilloma arrangement. These cells appear highly pyknotic but show no evidence of anaplasia. There is a hornifying layer of desquamated epithelium on all sides of the peripheral border of the tissue ($\times$ 198).

(Center) Large papilloma arising from the right vocal cord, anterior commissure, cent of all malignant growths of the larynx. Adenocarcinoma, basal cell carcinoma and sarcoma are relatively rare.

Malignant disease of the larynx is divided into two main groups: one, *intrinsic* carcinoma, in which the disease is limited to the interior of the larynx (glottis); and *extrinsic* carcinoma, in which the tumor is located on the external surface of the larynx.

The location of the lesion is of paramount importance in determining whether or not the disease is amenable to treatment by surgery, and also the extent of the surgery that is necessary. The reason for this is that growths limited to the vocal cord proper may remain localized for a considerable period of time (months), while lesions involving the ventricular bands or the posterior part of the glottis reach lymphatic channels early in the development of the disease.

INTRINSIC CARCINOMA

Symptoms and Signs. The one early symptom of intrinsic carcinoma of the larynx is a change in voice. This change occurs as a huskiness or hoarseness very early in the development of a tumor on the free margin of the true vocal cord. Other symptoms may be:

1. An easy fatigue of the voice.
2. An inability to clear the throat of phlegm.
3. A sense of rawness or dryness or of irritation as from a foreign body.

The easy fatigue occurs in the course of development of an intrinsic carcinoma; the other symptoms are more common to the extrinsic growths. Dysphagia and stridor are late symptoms. The former indicates a lesion involving the posterior wall of the larynx (postcricoid area); the latter occurs from encroachment on the glottis and suggests an intrinsic lesion. Pain from glandular involvement, especially earache (referred through the superior laryngeal branch of the vagus) is a late symptom.

The usual picture on inspection of the larynx is produced by localized edema with surface ulceration. When the lesion originates on the free

---

and anterior portion of the left vocal cord of a white female, age forty-eight. Film No. 66-21 (50-f18-3/41). History: Hoarseness for many months; increasing dyspnea for several weeks. Histological Diagnosis: Papilloma of the larynx. Microscopic Description: These tissues have the structure of a papilloma of the larynx. Stalks of edematous fibrous tissue are covered by a stratified squamous epithelium. This varies somewhat in width, but generally is wide ($\times$ 198).

(Lower) Friable, freely bleeding papilloma in a white male, age three, involving the entire larynx. Film No. 66-26 (50-f22-3/4L). History: Aphonia, dyspnea, and tracheotomy one and one-half years ago. Histological Diagnosis: Papilloma of larynx. Microscopic Description: Small fragments are of papillomatous character covered by a thick hyperplastic, stratified squamous epithelial layer permeated by polymorphonuclear cells. Papillae and base are vascular, somewhat edematous with diffuse but moderately light round cell infiltration. No evidence of malignancy ($\times$ 198).

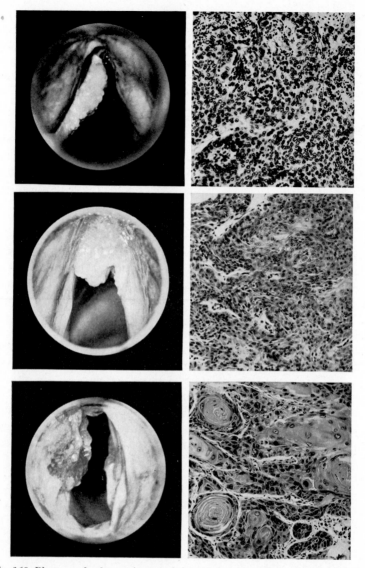

Fig. 168. Photograph of a carcinoma of the vocal cord, made by Dr. Paul Holinger. and associates and loaned through his courtesy and the Annals of Otology, Rhinology and Laryngology.

(Upper) Carcinoma involving the anterior two thirds of the vocal cord of a white male, age fifty-six. Film No. 67-1 (22-f15-5/8L). History: Hoarseness for six to eight weeks. Did not clear completely, although it improved at times. Histological Diagnosis: Stratified squamous cell carcinoma of larynx. Microscopic Description: These pieces of tissue have a fibrous stroma that is extensively ingrown by large and small irregular masses of stratified squamous epithelium. The cells repeat the middle and surface layers. There is little hornification and among the cells are some in mitosis (× 198). Therapy: Laryngofissure.

(Center) Carcinoma of the right vocal cord, anterior commissure, and anterior margin of the cord, the earliest sign may be one of thickening. This goes on to ulceration within the swelling (Fig. 168). Fixation of the true cord indicates a late stage in the disease. Persistent edema of the ventricular bands (false cords) or of an arytenoid eminence should arouse suspicion of an underlying malignancy. Lesions beginning below the level of the glottis (margins of the true cords) may be difficult to see early and are usually not detected until the true cord above has become involved.

Diagnosis. The clinical diagnosis of carcinoma of the larynx can usually be made by an inspection of the larynx with the simple laryngeal mirror. The direct view with a laryngoscope may be necessary for a clinical diagnosis in certain cases, especially when an overhanging epiglottis obscures the glottis, or the lesion is subglottic, in the ventricle, or in the postcricoid area. Direct laryngoscopy offers a satisfactory exposure for biopsy under direct vision. This provides the certain diagnosis, although it must be remembered that the surface projections of an epidermoid carcinoma sometimes show a papilloma-like projection which does not reveal malignant change.

The differential diagnosis considers two diseases which may simulate malignant lesions. These are tuberculosis and syphilis. These diseases are now less frequently encountered than was the case two decades ago.

Treatment. Opinion is almost unanimous that a *surgical removal* of the malignant lesion is necessary for a permanent cure. The cure is practically certain with lesions that originate on a vocal cord and have not extended beyond the confines of the laryngeal box.

The surgical attack may be one of three procedures:

1. Laryngofissure (thyrotomy), with a simple removal of one vocal cord (Fig. 169).

---

portion of the left cord of a white male, age seventy-three. Film No. 67-34 (50-f18-3/4L). History: Sensation of dryness in throat for two years. Hoarseness for six to eight months and cough for three months. No pain or weight loss, but stated he thinks he may have a little bronchitis. Histological Diagnosis: Stratified squamous cell carcinoma of the larynx. Microscopic Description: These tissues have only scanty fibrous stroma with inflammatory exudates. They are mainly large and small irregular masses of ingrown stratified squamous epithelium. The cells are arranged in mosaics and repeat the middle and surface layers of squamous epithelium. There is considerable hornification in the larger masses, occasionally in the form of pearls ($\times$ 198). Therapy: Laryngectomy.

(Lower) Carcinoma involving the left side of the larynx and anterior commissure. The patient was a white male, age sixty-eight. Film No. 67-27 (50-f18-5/8L). History: Hoarseness for three years. During the last month, the hoarseness had increased and he had noticed some dyspnea on exertion. Otherwise his health was excellent. Histological Diagnosis: Stratified squamous cell carcinoma of the larynx. Microscopic Description: These tissues have along one edge a surface squamous epithelium with a wide edge of hornified epidermis. Between is a fibrous stroma, rather scanty in amount, with large and small irregular masses of ingrown stratified squamous epithelium. There is considerable hornification of these masses. Many of the large and also of the small cell aggregates have centers with concentrically arranged hornified material. ($\times$ 198). Therapy: Laryngectomy.

2. Hemilaryngectomy—a wide destruction of as much of the interior of the larynx as seems necessary. This procedure is usually confined to a complete removal of one vocal cord. Occasionally the removal of a

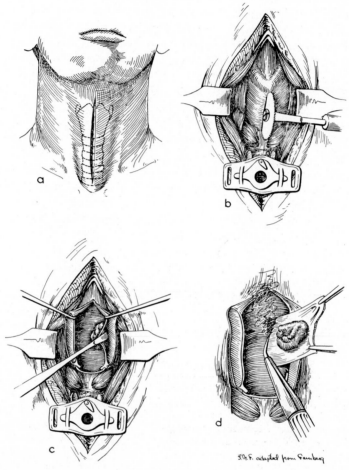

S.Ph.F. adapted from Sembery

Fig. 169. The principal maneuvers in the performance of a thyrotomy for an early cancer of the vocal cord involve (a) incision of soft tissues and exposure of the thyroid cartilage and upper end of the trachea for tracheotomy, (b) opening (fissure) of the larynx through the thyroid cartilage, (c) elevation of the involved vocal cord from the thyroid cartilage, (d) excision of a block of tissue containing the tumor and well beyond the margins of the growth. The larynx is then closed tightly.

Tracheotomy is often postponed until the procedure in (d) has been completed. In some instances it is unnecessary to perform a tracheotomy at all.

portion of the healthier vocal cord is indicated. A splitting of the larynx (laryngofissure or thyrotomy) provides the exposure.

3. Total laryngectomy. Occasionally this is supplemented with a dissection of the neck glands (Fig. 170).

A supplemental course of high voltage x-ray therapy is sometimes prescribed after hemilaryngectomy or total laryngectomy.

The choice of treatment requires an evaluation of each case. This evaluation considers:

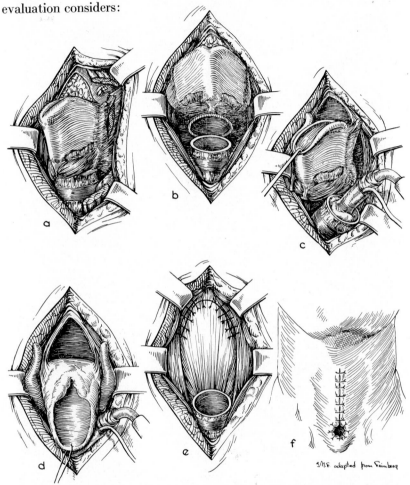

Fig. 170. The principal steps in the performance of a laryngectomy require: (a) Skeletonization of the larynx. (b) Separation of the larynx from the trachea after which the anesthesia (if intratracheal is being used) can be carried on with a short length of tubing fitted with inflatable cuff inserted into the trachea. (c-d) Removal of the larynx with due regard to preservation of as much pharyngeal mucous membrane as is feasible. (e) Careful closure of the pharyngeal stoma. (f) Anchoring the trachea to the skin to form a permanent opening there. Closure of the neck wound.

1. The location and extent of the tumor.
2. The histopathologic grading of the tumor.
3. The clinical evidence of metastasis.
4. General condition of the patient.

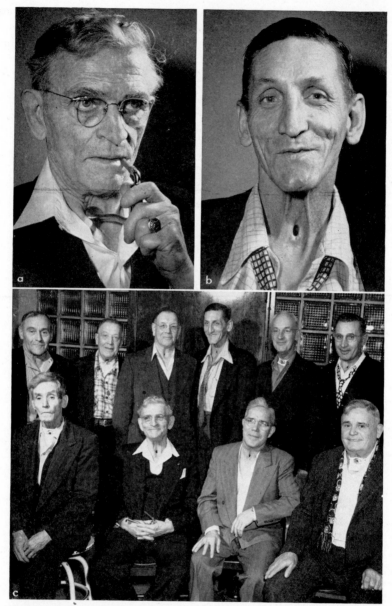

Fig. 171. *a*, The artificial larynx was largely depended upon in the past for speech production following laryngectomy. Only recently technics for teaching esophageal speech have been developed. *b*, The knack of swallowing air and expelling it past the pharyngeal opening of the esophagus to produce a sound which is then modulated with the palate, tongue and lips just as normal vocal cord sounds are modified is rather easily learned. *c*, Group instruction and practice for the development of esophageal speech is especially effective. Those wearing tracheal tubes in this group have had their surgery recently. The others have been able to discard their tubes. Most have acquired esophageal speech.

The primary consideration in the selection of treatment must be the prospect of cure of an otherwise fatal disease and, secondarily, preservation of the voice.

Laryngofissure. In general, simple laryngofissure is performed only on those lesions which involve not more than the anterior two-thirds of one vocal cord and in which there is no fixation of the cord. Occasionally, a patient is encountered in whom the lesion extends across the commissure and involves only a small portion of the anterior end of the opposite cord. This may still be suitable for a simple removal. The grade of the tumor will affect the extent of the operative procedure. New and Fletcher have shown that there is an average extension of 5.5 mm. in all grades of malignancies from the apparent margin of the growth, but in grade 4, it may be as great as 15 mm.

The study of frozen tissue sections, taken after the larynx is opened and under direct visualization, aids the surgeon in deciding on the extent of his surgical attack.

Hemilaryngectomy. The limits of hemilaryngectomy may include a destruction of one side of the larynx and occasionally a considerable portion of the opposite side. One of the factors of: (1) location and extent, (2) grade of tumor, and (3) condition of the patient, may figure prominently in the decision as to the extent of the surgical attack.

Total Laryngectomy. Total laryngectomy is usually indicated when there is fixation of a cord or extensive involvement even in slow growing tumors, subglottic extension and in most cases of rapidly growing tumors (grade 4). It is also indicated in all patients in whom an extrinsic portion of the larynx is involved and a reasonable hope of cure is present.

Cures of carcinoma of the larynx have been reported from the use of x-ray therapy and radium alone, but surgeons of large experience do not consider this single agent reliable.

Voice Production after Surgery. In laryngofissure or hemilaryngectomy, one healthy vocal cord or a major portion of one healthy vocal cord is left. When healing is complete, a shelf of scar tissue replaces the area destroyed. A useful voice ordinarily can be produced by the action of the remaining cord against the scar.

When the larynx has been completely removed, the voice production depends upon the development of esophageal speech or the use of a mechanical artificial larynx (Fig. 171a).

Esophageal speech depends upon the swallowing of air which is then "burped" out past the constriction which has formed in the lower pharynx, after the larynx has been removed. The lips and buccal cavity modulate this sound into words. Some patients develop this speech readily and talk very distinctly.

REFERENCES

Arbuckle, M. F.: Endolaryngeal Surgery Combined with Radiation in Late Laryngeal Cancer. Ann. Otol., Rhin. & Laryng., *55*:681, 1946.

Brown, J. M.: The Surgical Treatment of Nasopharyngeal Fibroma. *Ibid.*, *56*:294, 1947.

Clerf, L. H.: Sarcoma of the Larynx: Report of 8 Cases. Arch. Otol., *44*:517, 1946.

Ferguson, C., and Scott, H. W., Jr.: Papillomatosis of the Larynx in Childhood. New England J. Med., *230*:477, 1944.

Figi, F. A.: Fibromas of the Nasopharynx. J.A.M.A., *115*:665, 1940.

Holinger, P. H., Andrews, A., Jr., Anison, G., and Johnston, K.: Pathology of the Larynx. Ann. Otol., Rhin. & Laryng., *56*:583, 1947.

Lejeune, F. E.: Intralaryngeal Operation for Cancer of Vocal Cord. Ann. Otol., Rhin. & Laryng., *55*:531, 1946.

Martin, H.: Cancer of the Head and Neck. J.A.M.A., *137*:1366, 1948.

New, G. B., Figi, F. A., Havens, F. Z., and Erich, J. B.: Carcinoma of the Larynx: Methods and Results of Treatment. Surg., Gynec. & Obst., *85*:623, 1947.

Nielsen, J.: Roentgen Treatment of Malignant Tumors of the Nasopharynx. Acta Radiol., *26*:133, 1945.

Robinson, G. A.: Diagnosis, Treatment and End-Results of Malignant Tumors of the Nasal Sinuses. New York State J. Med., *44*:713, 1944.

Schall, L. A., and Ayash, J.: Cancer of the Larynx. A Statistical Study. Ann. Otol., Rhin. & Laryng., *57*:377, 1948.

Vasconcelos, E., and Barretto, P.: Total Laryngectomy. Arch. Otolaryng., *40*:275, 1944.

CHAPTER XXXII

PRESCRIPTIONS AND THERAPEUTIC PROCEDURES

The prescriptions and procedures included in this chapter have been found useful by the authors of this textbook. This does not mean, however, that any one individually favors the use of all of these medications. No attempt has been made to include all of the medication or methods which are useful. Sedatives and general analgesics have been omitted, since these preparations are usually well known by the time the average medical student is given his undergraduate instruction in otolaryngology and are, of course, well known to the physician in general practice.

The two most important medications in use today in the field of otolaryngology are: some form of an antibiotic, and a sulfonamide. Since the introduction of the sulfonamides a little more than a decade ago, and of the antibiotics about five years ago, progress has been rapid and the changes frequent. For that reason, it would seem desirable to summarize the present state of our knowledge regarding the use of these drugs.

THE SULFONAMIDES

The drugs of choice among the sulfonamides are *sulfadiazine* and *sulfamerazine* for systemic medication. These two have approximately the same antibacterial activity and toxicity. However, the use of sulfonamides has been largely replaced by penicillin because of the greater toxicity of the former. The following are the possible toxic effects:

Fever
Dermatitis
Blood dyscrasias
    anemia
    leukopenia
    granulopenia
    agranulocytosis
Renal complications
Liver dysfunction
Splenomegaly

In the field of otolaryngology, there are no infections in which a sulfonamide alone is more effective than penicillin.

In a few diseases which are not encountered in the field of otolaryngology, a sulfonamide is the drug of choice in

Nocardiosis

Meningococcic infections

Combined with penicillin for brucellosis

Combined with penicillin for pneumococcic meningitis

Combined with streptomycin for the therapy of infections caused by *Hemophilus influenzae.* (An important organism in cases of acute epiglottitis is often *Hemophilus influenzae.*)

Development of resistance to the sulfonamides is now a recognized fact. Inadequate dosage, interrupted treatment or irregular haphazard methods of treatment are factors in development of resistance. Many bacteria have become resistant to the sulfonamide drugs. These include the gonococci, Group A hemolytic streptococci, staphylococci, pneumococci and coliform bacteria.

The dosage for sulfadiazine in the adult is 4 gm. (60 grains) for the initial dose, followed by 1 gm. (15 grains) every four hours. An adequate dose (usually an equal amount) of sodium bicarbonate should be given to produce an alkaline urine.

The dosage for sulfamerazine is 3 gm. (46.3 grains) at the initial dose, then 2 gm. (30.9 grains) every eight hours and finally 1 gm. every eight hours.

ANTIBIOTICS

Penicillin and streptomycin are the most effective of the antibiotics. Tyrothrycin is effective against gram-positive bacteria, but can only be used topically because of its toxicity when used systemically.

A new antibiotic, aureomycin, has recently been reported which is especially effective against many rickettsias and certain viruses. Other new antibiotics are being evaluated, such as chloromycin and bacitracin. Probably an antibiotic will be found which is relatively nontoxic and which is absorbed well from the gastro-intestinal tract.

PENICILLIN

Because of its relatively low toxicity, this antibiotic is now the most used of our weapons against infections caused by the streptococci, pneumococci, micrococci (staphylococci) and so on. It is ineffective against all gram-negative bacillary infections, virus infections and cannot be expected to cure chronic disorders in which hyperplastic tissue changes have occurred, such as in chronic sinusitis, chronic tonsillitis and chronic otitis media.

As experience with this drug has accumulated, it seems that the only contraindication to its use would be in a person sensitive to the drug. In general, it now seems well to avoid it in an allergic person. When the toxicity of penicillin becomes apparent, it is manifest through the development of urticaria, pruritus and dermatitis, often accompanied with fever. Recently, a case of severe stomatitis following the use of penicillin has been reported.

Mode of Administration and Dosage

The dosage and mode of administration of penicillin has undergone considerable experimentation in the past year or two.

Intramuscular Administration. The most commonly used and reliable mode of administration is by the intramuscular route. The dosage has depended on the severity of the illness and the relative sensitivity of the bacteria being treated. There are apparently two schools of thought—those who believe a constant blood level is necessary, and those who believe it is unnecessary to maintain a constant level. Today, aqueous preparations of crystalline penicillin "G" is favored for injection at intervals of three to twelve hours, depending on the infection being treated. A common dosage used at the University Hospital (Minneapolis) is 100,000 to 200,000 units of aqueous penicillin every twelve hours.

In the past year, penicillin has been widely used in large doses (300,000 units) in an oil or wax medium. The chief drawback to this medium is the localized reaction which often accompanies it. Because of this, there seems to be a good argument for the use of aqueous penicillin in large doses every twelve hours.

Oral Administration. The use of penicillin by mouth, buffered so as to prevent as much destruction as possible by gastric juices, has the appeal that it can easily be self-administered. However, it is necessary to give five times the usual intramuscular dose to maintain a therapeutic level, and the ingestion of fluids and food must be limited in quantity midway between the three hourly dosage.

Aerosol Penicillin. In the past year, reports have appeared on the use of nebulized penicillin for the treatment of respiratory tract infections. Considerable interest in this has developed for the therapy of so-called "sinusitis." Since the publicity for this by lay publications has appeared, otolaryngologists have been deluged with appeals for trial of this therapy in cases of self-diagnosed sinusitis. The results have not been startling. Acute sinusitis of bacterial origin ending in suppuration usually is improved by supportive methods and certainly by parenteral administration of penicillin. However, the vasomotor states often misdiagnosed as sinusitis are, as a rule, self limiting, and any medication administered in an acute phase of these states may be credited with the improvement.

There seems no reason to the proposition that 50,000 units of penicillin in mist form blown through the nasal fossae should have any definite effect upon an empyema of the maxillary antrum or a well-established suppurative ethmoiditis. Certainly it would have no effect upon the tissue changes which develop in chronic disease. In an acute process, penicillin brought in by the blood supply combined with vasoconstriction and skillful irrigation, when needed, should insure prompt relief.

Aerosol penicillin apparently has some value in acute upper respiratory infections caused by pyogenic organisms, except in the type of sinusitis mentioned, where there is considerable soft tissue change in the form of edema of the mucosa. It seems to have value in such acute inflammations as pharyngitis, laryngitis, tracheitis, and bronchitis, and will reduce the suppuration in bronchiectasis, although the improvement is not a permanent one.

Penicillin Dust. This is the latest innovation in therapy with this antibiotic. It is being widely tried in patients complaining of "sinus trouble," many of whom do not have a suppurative sinusitis, but rather have vasomotor changes causing stuffiness and hypersecretion. On certain nasal mucous membranes, the inhalation of penicillin dust will undoubtedly cause some irritation. Again, there is no reason to believe that penicillin in powder form inhaled into the nasal fossae should produce much change in an empyema of an antrum or a suppurative ethmoiditis. More effective would be contact with the drug brought in through the blood stream and combined with adequate drainage, etc. It may prove beneficial in throat infections.

STREPTOMYCIN

Streptomycin possesses antibacterial activity for gram-positive and gram-negative organisms. Its use in otolaryngology at present is limited to disease caused by:

1. *Hemophilus influenzae*
2. *Mycobacterium tuberculosis*
3. Certain serious infections caused by micrococci (staphylococci), streptococci, pneumococci and so on, which are resistant to sulfonamides or penicillin.

The possible toxic reactions of this drug limit its use to serious infections. This reaction is not uncommon with large doses of the drug and with continued treatment. The acoustic nerve is vulnerable. Ataxia is caused by involvement of the vestibular branch and deafness is caused by involvement of the acoustic branch. If therapy is stopped at the onset of the hearing loss, the hearing is usually regained. Recovery from the vestibular damage is less likely to occur.

Contact dermatitis may occur in those handling streptomycin. Aplastic anemia, leukopenia, neutropenia and agranulocytosis are rare toxic reactions. Severe forms of stomatitis have been reported.

Bacterial resistance to streptomycin can develop with great rapidity.

Streptomycin is not absorbed from the gastrointestinal tract. The dosage is 2 gm. (30.9 grains) daily in divided doses every six to eight hours. It is not excreted as rapidly as penicillin and acts more rapidly on bacteria than does penicillin.

Topical application combined with its parenteral use is valuable in tuberculous laryngitis.

FORMULAS

The following formulas represent prescriptions used by the authors of this textbook in the practice of otolaryngology. This does not mean however, that any one individually favors the use of all of these preparations.

Ointments for Dermatitis of the External Ear:

Tincture benzoin compound	1.25
Zinc oxide	1.75
Petrolatum	8.00

Sulfathiazole or sulfadiazine cream in 5 per cent or 10 per cent strength.

Penicillin ointment with 1000 units per gram.

Solution for Wet Dressings for Dermatitis of the External Ear:

Penicillin—1000 units per cc. in sterile normal saline

Aluminum subacetate	60.0
Distilled water	120.0

Boric acid	2.0
Distilled water	90.0
Alcohol 70 per cent	90.0

Ear Drops for Use in Subacute or Chronic Diseases of the External Auditory Canal:

(Ear drops, particularly those containing alcohol, should be warmed at least to body temperature before instillation.)

Boric acid	0.6
Alcohol 70 per cent	30.0

Salicylic acid	0.6
Alcohol 70 per cent	30.0

meta-Cresylacetate (cresatin)	8.0

(This preparation is useful in acute inflammations such as diffuse dermatitis or furunculosis. It promptly relieves pain. A wick should be saturated with the medication and inserted into the canal. The patient should be supplied with about a dram of the medication and instructed to instill four or five drops of the medication against the wick every four to six hours. The wick is left in place for forty-eight hours.)

Penicillin, 1000 units per cubic centimeter of isotonic saline solution.

Ear Drops for Use in Chronic Disease of the Middle Ear:

Boric acid	0.6
Alcohol—95 per cent	30.0

Warm and instill ½ dropperful (10 drops) in ear twice daily. Allow to remain in position for ten minutes.

Urea	3.0
Sulfathiazole	2.12
Ethyl aminobenzoate (benzocaine)	0.2
Glycerol	20.0

"Glycerite of Hydrogen Peroxide"

Formula:

Hydrogen peroxide............................ 1.446%
Urea (carbamide)............................. 2.554%
8–Hydroxyquinoline........................... 0.1%
Anhydrous glycerin q.s.

Evolves active oxygen.

Antiseptic Powders for Use in Chronic Disease of the Middle Ear:

Boric acid, finely powdered..................... 15.0

Sulfanilamide, finely powdered.................. 15.0

Sulfanilamide, finely powdered.................. 10.0
Penicillin powder .... 300,000 units

Sulfanilamide, finely powdered
Zinc peroxide, finely powdered.................āā   7.5

Iodine..   0.3
Ethyl oxide (solvent ether).....................   4.0
Boric acid, finely powdered..................... 30.0

(Dissolve the iodine in the ether and mix thoroughly in a mortar with boric acid until dry again.)

Powders for use in chronically discharging ears are usually blown in by a special powder blower or dropped in by the patient. A simple,

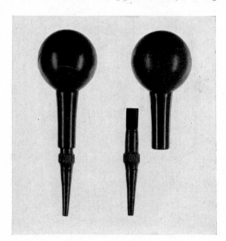

Fig. 172. A simple, inexpensive powder blower for the insufflation of powdered medication in the treatment of diseases of the external auditory canal and the middle ear. One end of a detachable tip may be dipped in the supply of powder, the blower assembled and the soft rubber end of the tip inserted in the external meatus and canal. The powder is then insufflated when the soft rubber bulb is compressed. (Manufactured by DeVilbiss.)

inexpensive powder blower is shown in Fig. 172. One end of a detachable tip may be dipped in the supply of powder, the blower assembled and the soft rubber end of the tip inserted in the external meatus and canal. The powder is then insufflated when the soft rubber bulb is compressed.

Ear Drops to Relieve the Pain of Otitis Media:

Phenol.	0.65
Glycerol.	30.0

(Warm and instill five to ten drops every two hours.)

"Auralgan". 15.0

(Warm and instill five to ten drops every two hours.)

Ointments for Dermatitis of the External Nose and Nasal Vestibule:

Ammoniated mercury ointment U.S.P. (5 per cent).

Boric acid ointment U.S.P. (10 per cent).

Sulfathiazole or sulfadiazine ointment (or cream base) 5 or 10 per cent.

Penicillin ointment 1000 units per gram.

Lanolin (hydrous).

Wet Dressings for Dermatitis of the External Nose and Nasal Vestibule:

The same solutions as are used for the external ear.

Solutions for Use as Nasal Spray or Drops by the Instillation Method:

Ephedrine sulfate 1 per cent in isotonic saline or isotonic dextrose solution.

Phenylephrine hydrochloride (neo-synephrine hydrochloride) $\frac{1}{4}$ per cent

Tuamine sulfate. . . . . .2 per cent

Naphazoline hydrochloride (privine hydrochloride). . . . . 0.05 per cent (children)
0.1 per cent (adults)

This drug represents a good vasoconstrictor but seems to produce congestion ("rhinitis medicamentosa") if used very much.

Propadrine hydrochloride. . . . . .2 per cent

"Par-Pen" (paredrine hydrochloride aqueous 10 per cent plus penicillin 500 units per cc.).

Cocaine 1 per cent sol. in mineral oil with oil of rose (.045 to the ounce) added.

A useful prescription to provide comfort in the early stage of irritation in acute rhinitis. Should not be refilled.

Solution for Irrigation of the Nasal Fossae:

(Some physicians limit the use of nasal irrigations to atrophic rhinitis; others find irrigation with isotonic saline useful in any acute or subacute purulent rhinitis, particularly in children.)

15

Sodium chloride
Sodium bicarbonate
Sodium biborate.................................āā 30

One teaspoonful to the pint of warm water.

Isotonic saline solution (may be made by dissolving one level tea-spoonful of ordinary table salt to two glasses of water which has been boiled and allowed to cool).

Stimulating Medications for Use in the Dry Nose:

Formula of Proetz:

Alcohol..   6.0
Glycerin.......................................   6.0
Normal saline...........................q.s. 120.0
Spirits of cologne.........................M   5.0

One-half dropperful in each nostril every four hours.

For use in atrophic rhinitis:

Iodine...   .065
Menthol..   .13
Camphor..   .13
Liquid petrolatum............................ 30

Estrogenic substance (Theelin, Amniotin, etc.) is dissolved in olive or corn oil and freely sprayed into the nose twice daily after the nose is cleaned. Three ampules of 10,000 units each per cubic centimeter are dissolved in 30 cc. of oil.

NASAL DOUCHING

An irrigating can or douche bag of a one-quart capacity, about two feet of rubber tubing and a nasal tip of hard rubber or glass (Fig. 173a) constitutes the necessary equipment.

The irrigating fluid should be comfortably warm when tested on the back of the hand. The can or douche bag should be about two feet above the patient's head which is held face down over a basin. The irrigating tip is inserted into one nostril and the solution allowed to flow gently into the nose and out the other nostril. This will occur if the mouth is held open and the breathing is carried on through it. After half of the fluid has been used in irrigating through one nostril, the direction of flow is reversed by changing to the opposite one. In case the patient has to cough, sneeze or gag, he closes the tube temporarily by clamping or pinching it off. At the finish of the irrigation, the patient is instructed to allow all of the fluid to run out before he attempts to blow his nose so as to avoid forcing any solution into his eustachian tubes.

A fairly efficient method of washing the nasal cavities may be carried out by snuffing a warm solution from the palm of the hand. Isotonic saline solution is commonly used.

The solution is drawn into one nostril from the palm with a strong snuff. It enters the nasopharynx from which it is hawked out and then expectorated into a basin. The snuffing is done through alternate sides until a water glass full of the solution has been used. Nose blowing is avoided until all of the fluid has run out.

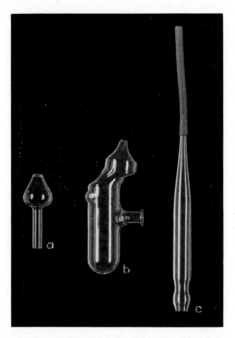

Fig. 173. (a) Glass tip for use in nasal irrigation. (b) A type of glass bulb (Bermingham) for use in nasal douching. (c) A tapered glass tube fitted with two inches of soft rubber tubing to form a tip useful for throat irrigations.

Another method of douching may be accomplished with the use of a specially constructed glass bulb, the Bermingham nasal douche (Fig. 173b). This bulb can be filled with the solution and the flow controlled by a finger held on or off the vent on the top of the bulb.

MEDICATIONS FOR RELIEF IN ALLERGIC RHINITIS

The vasoconstrictors such as ephedrine, phenylephrine hydrochloride (neo-synephrine) and naphazoline hydrochloride (privine), are not advised except for temporary relief. In the acute phase of hay fever, the following nasal spray is effective in relieving the congestion and irritation, but should not be refilled:

Cocaine hydrochloride	0.26
Phenol	0.0036
Antipyrine	.45
3 per cent ephedrine sulfate solution	14.0
Water	q.s. ad 30.0

For rest at night these capsules are helpful:

> Ephedrine with amytal or seconal..............āā $\frac{3}{8}$ grain
> One capsule every three or four hours.

Taken internally for relief of allergic symptoms:

> Diphenhydramine hydrochloride (benadryl)....... 50 mg.

> Tripelennamine hydrochloride (pyribenzamine) tablets.....50 mg.
> One capsule or tablet is taken three or four times daily (adults).

Medication to Abort an Attack of "Acute Rhinitis:"

Copavin (tablets or capsules, each contains $\frac{1}{4}$ grain of papaverine and $\frac{1}{4}$ grain of codeine). One tablet is taken after each meal and two at bedtime. Most effective when started with the earliest manifestations of an acute rhinitis.

Medication for Use in Certain Types of Headache:

Migraine:

Ergotamine tartrate (gynergen) 1 cc. ampules $\frac{1}{2}$ to 1 ampule (0.25 to 0.5 mg. of the drug) is given hypodermically (intramuscularly) and repeated once in an hour or two if symptoms are not fully abated or if they return.

Histaminic Cephalgia:

> (See "vasodilator" drugs at end of chapter.)

Medications for Use as Gargles:

> Dobell's solution (Liquor Sodii Boratis Compositus).

Formula:

Sodium borate	15.0
Sodium bicarbonate	15.0
Liquefied phenol	3.0
Glycerin	35.0
Distilled water ....q.s. ad	1000.0

One part to two or three parts of hot water.

Alkaline aromatic solution—Liquor Aromaticus Alkalinus (Seiler's formula).

Potassium bicarbonate	20.0
Sodium borate	20.0
Thymol	0.5
Eucalyptol	1.0
Methyl salicylate	0.5
Tincture cudbear	20.0
Alcohol	50.0
Glycerin	100.0
Distilled water ....q.s. ad	1000.0

This medication may be conveniently purchased in tablet form as Seiler's Tablets.

Dissolve three or four tablets to the glass of hot water for gargling.

Phenol	3.3
Tannic acid	2.6
Glycerin	60.0
Peppermint water	q.s. ad 180.0

Dilute with equal amount of hot water. Gargle every two hours.

Isotonic saline solution (1 teaspoonful of table salt to two glasses of water)

Sodium perborate powder	30.0

One teaspoonful to the glass of warm water.

(Indicated in Plaut-Vincent infections.)

The above medications may also be used for a mouth wash.

Solutions for Irrigation of the Pharynx:

Isotonic saline solution.

Sodium bicarbonate	
Sodium chloride	āā 4.0
Water (1 pint)	500.0

Liquor antisepticus N.F.	120.0
Water (1 pint)	500.0

Formula for liquor antisepticus:

Boric acid	25.0
Thymol	1 0
Chlorthymol	1.0
Menthol	1.0
Eucalyptal	2.0
Methyl salicylate	1.2
Oil of thyme	0.3
Alcohol	
Distilled water āā	q.s. ad 1000.0

HOT THROAT IRRIGATIONS

Irrigation of the inflamed area in acute tonsillitis or pharyngitis adds materially to the comfort of the patient and contributes, because of its local effects, to the cleansing and processes of repair.

The equipment required consists of a one-quart container, two or three feet of rubber tubing, a glass or rubber irrigating tip, and a pinch-cock to control the flow through the tubing (Fig. 174).

The patient is seated in bed or stands over a washbowl. The container with the irrigating fluid is held at two feet above the patient's head. The irrigating tip (Fig. 173c) is held in the patient's hand so that a stream is directed against the tonsillar area or pharyngeal wall while he breathes quietly through his nose. The flow of the solution is temporarily inter-

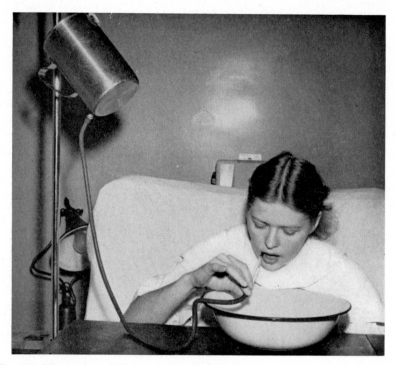

Fig. 174. The equipment for and the position of the patient taking a hot throat irrigation.

rupted in case the patient has to gag, cough or swallow. The temperature of the fluid placed in the irrigating can should be as hot as can be borne on the back of the hand. A total of two quarts of fluid should be used.

Local Applications for the Pharynx ("Throat paints"):

> Silver nitrate solution (fresh), 5 per cent. Apply thoroughly with cotton tipped applicator which has been dipped in the solution and from which the excess has been expressed. Several applications are needed.

For Use in Pharyngitis Sicca and Atrophic Pharyngitis:

Mandl's paint:

Iodine	0.3
Potassium iodide	0.3
Oil of gaultheria	0.3
Glycerin	30.0

An applicator with a rather abrupt curve, and one on which the cotton will be wound securely, is needed for applications to the nasopharynx and hypopharynx. Two types are illustrated in Fig. 175.

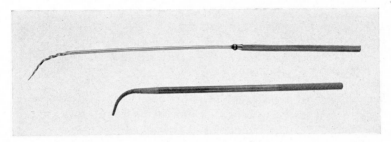

Fig. 175. Two types of metal applicators properly shaped for the application of medication to the nasopharynx and the hypopharynx.

Medicated Troches for Use in Mouth and Throat Infections:

Penicillin troches 1000 to 2500 units.
    Dissolve one between cheek and teeth every two to three hours.

Sulfathiazole gum (each piece contains $3\frac{3}{4}$ grains, 0.25 gm. of sulfathiazole).

Chew two tablets for ten to twenty minutes every three hours.

Powders for Analgesic Effect:

Ethyl aminobenzoate (benzocaine) 8.0

Orthoform 8.0

May be applied lightly to the throat with a powder blower or inhaled through a glass tube from a small saucer.

Acetylsalicylic acid 4.0
Codeine 0.26

Make 12 powders (each powder contains 5 grains of acetylsalicylic acid and $\frac{1}{3}$ grain of codeine).

Useful in relief of post-tonsillectomy sore throat. A powder is dissolved on tongue one-half hour before mealtime.

Medications for the Larynx and Trachea:

Humidity, oxygen, and controlled temperature in obstructive laryngitis. (See Figures 182, 183, 184.)

Emetic medication in croup in children:

Syrup of ipecac. 30.0

One teaspoonful in a little water every fifteen minutes until vomiting occurs.

Mono-*p*-chlorophenol, with camphor in light liquid
petrolatum. 30.0

To be dropped into the larynx in small quantity from a laryngeal syringe as the patient phonates.

Instillation of Laryngeal Medication. A specially shaped glass syringe is used for laryngeal medication. A simple inexpensive type is shown in Fig. 176. The technic for its use is as follows:

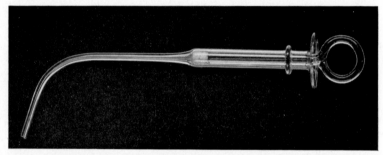

Fig. 176. A simple inexpensive glass syringe for the instillation of medication to the larynx.

The patient's tongue is grasped as for indirect laryngoscopy as the mouth is opened widely. The tip of the syringe is inserted over the back of the tongue without touching the tongue, uvula, or pharyngeal wall. As the patient phonates, several drops of the medication being used are expressed from the syringe. It drops on the vocal cords and some of it enters the subglottic space and trachea as the patient takes a deep breath.

In an average larynx in an adult, the instillation of the medication is a simple matter. In certain circumstances, such as when the epiglottis is dependent and partially covers the glottis, it is more difficult to introduce medication.

Medicated Steam Inhalation:

Menthol. 0.3
Oil of eucalyptus. 0.6
Oil of pine. 0.6
Tincture benzoin compound. . . . . .q.s. ad 30.0

Put one teaspoonful in a pint of boiling water in a bowl. Cover head with a Turkish towel and inhale the vapor deeply for five minutes. A croup kettle or electric vaporizer may also be used to provide the vaporization.

Medications for the Control of Cough:

Codeine phosphate or sulfate....................	0.25
Terpin hydrate...............................	4.0
Alcohol......................................	30.0
Syrup simplex..........................q.s. ad	120.0

One or two teaspoonfuls every two hours until cough is relieved.

Useful for an irritating laryngeal cough:

Menthol......................................	0.16
Codeine sulfate..............................	0.36
Honey.......................................	60.0
Chloroform water........................q.s. ad	240.0

Gargle with one mouthful; then swallow. Repeat as necessary.

The following formula in capsule form may be varied according to special needs:

In each capsule:

Codeine sulfate ($\frac{1}{8}$ grain).........................	0.008
Terpin hydrate (2 grains).......................	0.1

(Five grains of ammonium chloride may be substituted for the terpin hydrate when expectorant action is desired.)

One capsule every three or four hours and at bedtime.

Dilaudid......................................	0.05
Syrup of tolu................................	30.0
Water...................................q.s. ad	180.0

For allergic cough, $\frac{1}{4}$ grain of ephedrine sulfate may be added to each dose to relieve the bronchial spasm.

One teaspoonful in water every four hours for cough.

Vasodilator drugs for use in Ménière's disease, histaminic cephalgia, vasodilating head pains, and vasomotor rhinitis:

Histamine diphosphate for intravenous use. Each cc. contains 2.75 mg. (1.0 mg. of histamine base). To be dissolved in not less than 250 cc. of isotonic saline solution and used intravenously at a rate determined by patient's tolerance.

Histamine diphosphate for subcutaneous injection. Each cc. contains 0.275 mg. (0.1 mg. histamine base).

"Desensitization" is accomplished by the subcutaneous injection of small doses twice daily. The first dose consists of 0.25 cc. Each succeeding dose is increased by 0.05 cc. until 1.00 cc. is reached unless the patient experiences flushing of the face, whereupon the dose is reduced by half and then gradually increased again.

The 1.00 cc. dose is continued twice daily for two or three weeks. If this desensitization is successful, the treatment is continued one to three times weekly for an indefinite period.

Nicotinic acid may be administered by intramuscular or subcutaneous injection, or may be taken orally in tablet form.

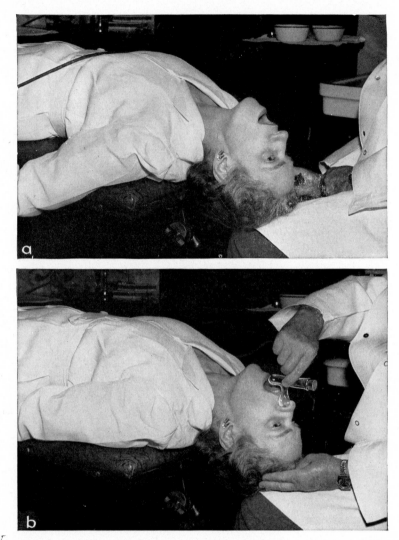

Fig. 177. (a) The position of the patient for displacement irrigation. The patient is requested to breathe entirely by mouth, the medication is instilled into the side to be treated and the tip of the suction bulb is inserted (b), and alternate action and release of negative pressure is produced by holding a finger on and off the vent in the suction bulb.

Results from injection are considered more effective than when the medication is administered by the oral route. Preparations are available in 50 mg. and 100 mg. per 2 cc.

The amide of nicotinic acid, nicotinamide, causes less reaction but the results seem to be less certain than with the nicotinic acid solution.

At the present time, there seems to be a variance of opinion among clinicians regarding the effectiveness of nicotinic acid administered orally. Since the purpose of the medication is to provide vasodilatation, there is an increasing tendency on the part of clinicians to use the medication at more frequent intervals than formerly. It seems probable that on the average, 50 mg. at two or three hourly intervals produces a more sustained vasodilation, which is the desirable effect.

DISPLACEMENT IRRIGATION

This useful therapeutic procedure is illustrated in Fig. 177. Usually $\frac{1}{4}$ per cent ephedrine in isotonic saline solution is used. The principal

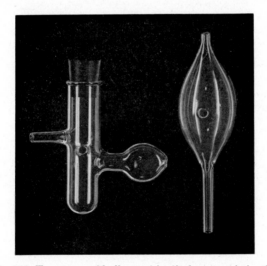

Fig. 178. Two types of bulbs used in displacement irrigation.

therapeutic action of this medication is obviously one of vasoconstriction. This shrinkage of the ostia of the sinuses combined with the actual entrance of some of the medication into the sinus and the negative pressure of the act which dislodges obstructing secretions, accounts for the value of the procedure. The introduction of medications which might have an antibacterial action has never been considered effective. An antibacterial agent in sufficient strength to be effective would be expected to have a deleterious effect on ciliary activity. Recently, however, the combination of a vasoconstrictor and penicillin has been advocated. This combination may prove to have some value. Two types of suction bulbs for this procedure are shown in Fig. 178.

Another modern method of sinus therapy is the irrigation through natural ostia by cannula for maxillary sinusitis and by way of the naso-frontal duct for frontal sinusitis. Three types of maxillary sinus cannulas

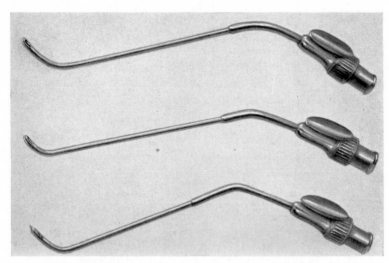

Fig. 179. Cannulas (Van Alyea) used for irrigating the maxillary sinus through the middle meatus. The pointed one is used when it is necessary to pierce the membranous portion of the middle meatus.

are shown in Fig. 179. The pointed one is used to pierce the middle meatus membrane.

PHYSICAL THERAPY

Various forms of physical therapy in the form of diathermy to produce internal heat, ultraviolet light applications, infra-red heat, etc., have been widely used in sinus disease and ear and throat infections. The advent of chemotherapy and the use of antibiotics has apparently made the use of some physical therapeutic devices less common. However, the unquestioned value of many forms of physical therapy in otolaryngological practice has never been entirely accepted. Nevertheless, simple forms of heat are of value in treating acute sinusitis with pain, acute suppurative otitis media, neck infections, laryngitis, etc. The ordinary 250 watt carbon filament bulb in a suitable reflector (Fig. 180) provides an inexpensive and easily available source of heat containing considerable infra-red radiation.

SUCTION TREATMENT FOR CLEANING TONSILS

Occasionally there is a need for ridding a tonsil of debris which clogs the tonsil crypts, particularly in adults. A tonsil suction tube (Fig. 181) fits over the tonsil and negative pressure exerted on the surface of the tonsil will withdraw debris from the crypts and may even demonstrate considerable liquid pus. Following several trials of the suction tube, a fine cotton-tipped applicator is used to apply 5 per cent silver nitrate to the

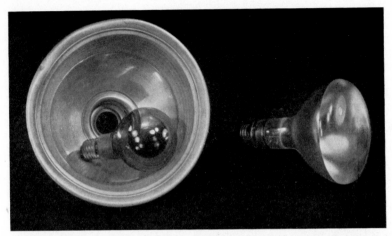

Fig. 180. Two types of inexpensive bulbs for a source of dry heat. (Left) A carbon filament bulb used with metal reflector. (Right) A newer type of specially constructed bulb which is used without reflector. Both bulbs may be used in standard sockets attached to ordinary goose neck lamp stands.

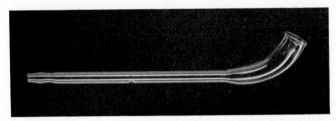

Fig. 181. A glass tube with bell-shaped tip which may be useful in cleaning tonsil crypts of debris. The large end is placed over the tonsil and negative pressure is produced by holding a finger over the vent in the side of the stem of the tube.

crypts. The benefits of this treatment are often prompt but may be only temporary.

CONTROL OF HUMIDITY, TEMPERATURE AND OXYGEN IN THE TREATMENT OF OBSTRUCTIVE LARYNGITIS

The old-fashioned croup tent provided increased humidity, but also increased the temperature of the patient's environment to an uncomfortable point. Consider the lack of comfort one experiences on a warm day in the presence of a high humidity and an inkling may be had of what one would experience in the 90 degree temperature of a croup tent with the relative humidity markedly increased over normal surroundings.

The modern therapy tent in which a humidity of 90 degrees in a

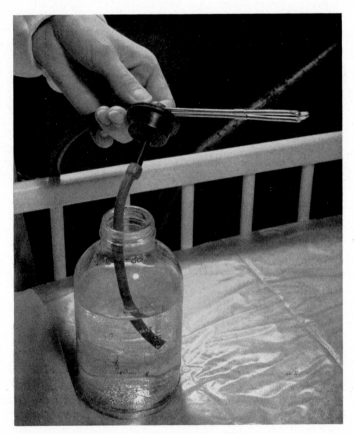

Fig. 182. An atomizer used to provide humidity in plastic tents in which children suffering from croup and acute laryngotracheitis with or without tracheotomy tubes are being treated. The atomizer is prepared using an ordinary intravenous flask and a common DeVilbiss atomizer and rubber tubing available in any hospital. Penicillin or streptomycin may be added to the solution, but there is reason to question their efficacy when administered in the large droplets used in this method. A wet and dry bulb hygrometer can be placed in the tent and the humidity will be found to be very high.

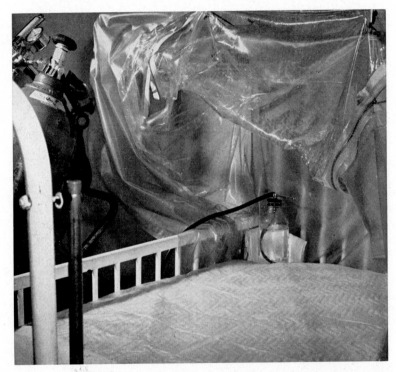

Fig. 183. This figure shows method of preparing crib for use with humidifier illustrated in Fig. 182. The humidity in tents used with this equipment is so high that it is necessary to protect the mattress with rubber or plastic sheeting and to protect the child with extra clothing.

Motive power for the humidifier is supplied by an oxygen tank connected directly to the atomizer. The rate of flow of the oxygen is sufficient to produce a good blast of atomized fluid from the nozzle of the atomizer. Usually this means that the tank runs at about 6 liters per minute.

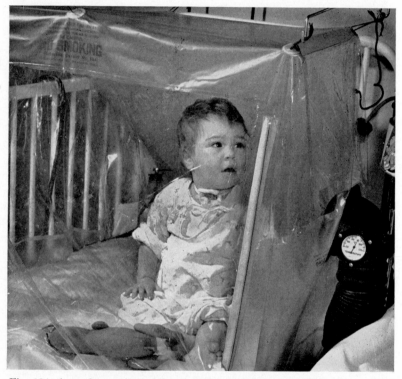

Fig. 184. A tracheotomized child in the tent with the humidifier illustrated in Figs. 182 and 183. The temperature of the tent can be changed if necessary by feeding a small amount of oxygen through the regular oxygen apparatus and using ice in the container attached thereto. Sometimes it is possible to use the atomizer in a plastic tent without regular oxygen feeding equipment. One must watch the temperature closely and be sure that it does not go too high.

temperature of approximately 72 degrees F. is maintained and in which oxygen in varying amount can be introduced, has proven to be one of the most effective measures in the treatment of obstructive laryngitis, particularly laryngotracheobronchitis (Figs. 182, 183, 184). Combined with the sulfonamides, antibiotics, and relief of the obstruction by intubation or tracheotomy, the once high mortality of acute obstructive laryngitis has been markedly reduced when the condition is recognized early and is promptly treated.

REFERENCES

Bryer, M. S., et al.: Aureomycin. J.A.M.A., *138*:117, 1948.

Chen, K. K.: Aliphatic versus Aromatic Amines as Vasoconstrictors. Ann. Otol., Rhin. & Laryng., *57*:287, 1948.

Council on Pharmacy & Chemistry: Streptomycin. J.A.M.A., *135*:839, 1947.

Dickson, J. C.: Effect of Sulfonamide Drug on Mucous Membranes. Arch. Otolaryng., *44*:474, 1946.

Dowling, H. F., et al: "Liquid" Versus "Solid" Penicillin in Oil and Wax. J.A.M.A., *135*:567, 1947.

Editorial: Acquired Resistance to Antibiotics. Ann. Int. Med., *27*:317, 1947.

Editorial: Annual Report on Streptomycin. J.A.M.A., *135*:641, 1947.

Farrington, J., et al: Stomatitis after Administration of Penicillin. J. Oral Surg., *5*:149, 1947.

Feinberg, F. M.: Histamine and Antihistaminic Agents: Their Experimental and Therapeutic Status. J.A.M.A., *132*:702, 1946.

Fowler, E. P., Jr., and Seligman, E.: Otic Complications of Streptomycin Therapy. *Ibid.*, *133*:87, 1947.

Gordon, J. S.: Studies in Oral Penicillin. Laryngoscope, *57*:202, 1947.

Greenwood, G., et al.: Effect of Zephiran Chloride, Tyrothricin, Penicillin and Streptomycin on Ciliary Action. Arch. Otolaryng., *43*:623, 1946.

Gundrum, L. K.: Paralysis of Left Vocal Cord Following Streptomycin Therapy. J.A.M.A., *138*:22, 1948.

Herrell, W. E.: Penicillin and Other Antibiotic Agents. Philadelphia, W. B. Saunders Co., 1945.

Hulse, W. F.: The Effect of Streptomycin on Eighth Nerve Function. Ohio M. J., *44*:822, 1948.

Kolmer, J. A.: Penicillin Therapy. New York, Appleton-Century-Crofts Co., 1947.

Krasno, L., et al: Inhalation of Penicillin Dust. J.A.M.A., *138*:344, 1948.

Krauss, F. H.: Penicillin Therapy in Otorhinolaryngologic Practice. Arch. Otolaryng., *44*:647, 1946.

Kully, B.: Use and Abuse of Nasal Vasoconstrictor Medications. J.A.M.A., *127*:307, 1945.

Levy, A. J.: Local Treatment of Carriers of Virulent Diphtheria with Penicillin. *Ibid.*, *136*:855, 1948.

Miller, C. P.: Development of Bacterial Resistance to Antibiotics. *Ibid.*, *135*:749, 1947.

Olsen, A. M.: Administration of Antibiotic Preparation by the Aerosol Method. M. Clin. North America, *32*:1077, 1948.

Priest, R. E.: Penicillin in Treatment of Maxillary Sinusitis. Ann. Otol., Rhin. & Laryng., *54*:786, 1945.

Pulaski, E. J., and Matthews, C. S.: Streptomycin in Surgical Infections: Otitis Externa, Otitis Media, Mastoiditis, Brain Abscess and Meningitis. Arch. Otolaryng., *45*:503, 1947.

Rabinovitch, J., and Snitkoff, N. C.: Acute Exfoliative Dermatitis and Death following Penicillin Therapy. J.A.M.A., *138*:496, 1948.

Rauchwerger, S. M., et al: Development of Sensitivity in Nursing Personnel Through Contact During Administration of the Drug to Patients. *Ibid.*, *136*:614, 1948.

Rosen, F. L.: Sensitivity to Streptomycin. *Ibid.*, *137*:1128, 1948.

Smith, H. V., Schiller, F., and Cairns, H.: Chemotherapy of Meningitis Secondary to Infections of the Ear and Nasal Sinuses. Proc. Roy. Soc. Med., *39*:613, 1946.

Spink, W. W.: Sulfanilamide and Related Compounds in General Practice. Chicago. Year Book Publishers, Inc., 1942.

Spink, W. W., and Ferris, V.: Penicillin Resistant Staphylococci Mechanisms Involved in the Development of Resistance. J. Clin. Investigation, *26*:379, 1947.

Starkey, H., and Dixon, J. H.: Oral Administration of Penicillin. Canad. M. A. J., *59*:47, 1948.

Suchett, K. A. I., and Latter, R. B.: Oral Penicillin in Young Children. Brit. M. J., p. 953, 1947.

Tucker, H. A., and Eagle, H.: Serum Concentration of Penicillin "G" in Man Following Intramuscular Injection in Aqueous Solution and in Peanut Oil and Beeswax Suspension. Am. J. Med., *4*:343, 1948.

Woodward, F., and Holt, T.: Local Use of Penicillin in Infections of Ear, Nose and Throat. J.A.M.A., *129*:589, 1945.

Wright, L. T., et al.: Aureomycin. *Ibid.*, *138*:408, 1948.

INDEX

Page numbers in *italics* refer to illustrations. Words in *italics* indicate treatment.

433